IMMUNOLOGY
A Short Course

ABOUT THE AUTHORS

Eli Benjamini is a professor emeritus of immunology in the Department of Medical Mircrobiology and Immunology at the School of Medicine of the University of California at Davis. Since 1970, Dr. Benjamini has taught immunology to undergraduate, graduate, and medical students, as well as having served for 10 years as Chairman of the Graduate Program of Immunology on the Davis campus—a program which he was instrumental in forming. His research interests include the immunobiology of protein antigens, mechanisms of immune regulation, and principles of synthetic vaccine.

Geoffrey Sunshine is a senior scientist at ImmuLogic Pharmaceutical Corporation in Waltham, Massachusetts, working on autoimmune diseases. He is also a lecturer in the Department of Pathology at Tufts University School of Medicine. For several years, he directed courses in immunology for veterinary students and for graduate dental students at Tufts University Veterinary and Dental Schools. He was also a member of the Sackler School of Graduate Biomedical Sciences at Tufts University, doing research in antigen presentation and teaching immunology to medical, graduate, and undergraduate students.

Sidney Leskowitz served as a professor in the Department of Pathology at Tufts University School of Medicine, where he taught immunology to medical and graduate students as well as veterinary and dental students. In his more than 20 years at Tufts, Dr. Leskowitz was responsible for the creation of an Immunology Training Program, organizing courses in immunology, lecturing, and writing syllabi. He also served for four years on the Microbiology Test Examination Committee for the National Board of Medical Examiners. His research activities spanned such areas as delayed hypersensitivity, cutaneous hypersensitivity, tolerance, and antigen presentation to T cells.

IMMUNOLOGY
A Short Course

THIRD EDITION

Eli Benjamini

Professor Emeritus
Department of Medical Microbiology and Immunology
University of California School of Medicine
Davis, California

Geoffrey Sunshine

Senior Scientist
ImmuLogic Pharmaceutical Corporation
Waltham, Massachusetts
and
Lecturer, Department of Pathology
Tufts University School of Medicine
Boston, Massachusetts

Sidney Leskowitz

(1922–1991)
Department of Pathology
Tufts University School of Medicine
Boston, Massachusetts

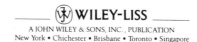

A JOHN WILEY & SONS, INC., PUBLICATION
New York • Chichester • Brisbane • Toronto • Singapore

Address all Inquiries to the Publisher
Wiley-Liss, Inc., 605 Third Avenue, New York, NY 10158-0012

Printed in the United States of America.

While the authors, editors, and publisher believe that drug selection and dosage and the specification and usage of equipment and devices, as set forth in this book, are in accord with current recommendations and practice at the time of publication, they accept no legal responsibility for any errors or omissions, and make no warranty, express or implied, with respect to material contained herein. In view of ongoing research, equipment modifications, changes in governmental regulations and the constant flow of information relating to drug therapy, drug reactions, and the use of equipment and devices, the reader is urged to review and evaluate the information provided in the package insert or instructions for each drug, piece of equipment, or device for, among other things, any changes in the instructions or indication of dosage or usage and for added warnings and precautions.

Library of Congress Cataloging-in-Publication Data

Benjamini, Eli.
    Immunology : a short course / Eli Benjamini, Geoffrey Sunshine,
Sidney Leskowitz. — 3rd ed.
       p. cm.
    Includes bibliographical references and index.
    ISBN 0-471-59791-0
    1. Immunology. I. Sunshine, Geoffrey. II. Leskowitz, Sidney.
III. Title.
    [DNLM: 1. Allergy and Immunology. 2. Immunity. QW 504 B468i
1996]
QR181.B395   1996
616.07′9—dc20
DNLM/DLC
for Library of Congress   96-1776

The text of this book is printed on acid-free paper.

CONTENTS

CHAPTER 12: CONTROL MECHANISMS IN THE IMMUNE RESPONSE

CHAPTER 13: COMPLEMENT

CHAPTER 16: HYPERSENSITIVITY REACTIONS: T-CELL-MEDIATED, TYPE IV—DELAYED-TYPE HYPERSENSITIVITY

CHAPTER 17: AUTOIMMUNITY

CHAPTER 18: IMMUNODEFICIENCY AND OTHER DISORDERS OF THE IMMUNE RESPONSE

CHAPTER 21: TUMOR IMMUNOLOGY

PREFACE AND ACKNOWLEDGMENTS TO THE THIRD EDITION

Since the last edition, the intense efforts of research scientists around the world have produced significant new findings that have reshaped our understanding of many aspects of the immune system. As a result, every chapter in the current edition has been either updated or rewritten to incorporate new findings and to delete information that no longer reflects current thinking.

As in the first and second editions, we remain committed to the motto "less is more." Our task has been to present what we consider the most relevant material in a concise, palatable, and easily digestible fashion to the introductory student. That reader will be the best judge of whether we have succeeded.

We are deeply indebted to Dr. Demosthenes Pappagianis, who contributed the chapter on immunoprophylaxis and immunotherapy, and Dr. Karen Yamaga, who contributed the chapter on control mechanisms in the immune response and on autoimmunity. We wish to thank the many co-workers and students who contributed to the first and second editions and those who were helpful in the preparation of the third edition, in particular, Dr. Robert J. Scibienski of the School of Medicine, University of California at Davis, and Dr. Donna M. Rennick, DNA

Research Institute, Palo Alto, California. Geoffrey Sunshine would like to thank the many friends who patiently answered his questions during the writing of the third edition, in particular, Peter Brodeur, Mark Exley, Paula Hochman, and Mohammad Luqman. He would also like to thank his family for their continued support: Ilene, for her encouragement and dedication to the cause, and Alex and Caroline, for their optimism. His sections are dedicated to his father Harry, who did not live to see the new edition.

PREFACE TO THE SECOND EDITION

An anxiety common to authors of textbooks in rapidly developing fields is the necessity of relatively frequent revisions to include material that, in the previous edition, was in the "twilight zone," between fact and fancy but that since has gained the status of important fact. Indeed, the rapidly developing field of immunology requires continuous revisions; hence, the present edition.

In this second edition, various concepts and findings have been updated and expanded; new information has been added on such diverse topics as the molecular biology and genes controlling antibody synthesis and isotype switch, T-cell differentiation and the T-cell receptor, antigen processing and presentation, cytokines and lymphokines, new therapeutic approaches for immunodeficiency disorders and tumors, and new aspects of prophylaxis and immunotherapy of infectious diseases. In addition, we have added a section on AIDS and several techniques such as Western blots and fluorescence-activated cell sorting. We have also expanded the glossary and added review questions as well as several clinical correlates.

Although we have deleted and shortened some sections, the expanded and added material increased somewhat the size of the book. We can, however, assure the readers that with this second edition, as with the first edition, we remain committed to the motto "less is more" and have attempted to present the principles of immunology in a concise, palatable, and easily digestible form.

Revision and change is the constant burden that authors writing about a dynamically changing field have to carry. Students, too, have to partake of that burden and must prepare themselves with the realization that science is not static and they must continually move on to new levels of understanding. Good luck to us both.

PREFACE TO THE FIRST EDITION

Why was this book written? At a time when so many excellent, extensive, and beautifully illustrated texts flood the bookstores, why offer another one? The reasons are fairly simple and rather unsophisticated. In our collective 40 some-odd years of teaching all kinds of students, we have become convinced that most texts fail their purpose because they overshoot the mark.

Anyone coming into contact with these students year after year cannot fail to appreciate the burden under which they operate. If they are to graduate, they must learn an enormous amount of material on an exceptionally diverse series of subjects, each increasing in scope yearly. As any student can tell you, every faculty lecturer considers his/her particular topic absolutely essential for future graduates, and so the pile of required "essentials" grows and grows. This is a manifestly untenable approach to curriculum.

A second cruel observation arises from long years of questioning students: many of them are not really that interested in immunology! As exciting, dynamic, and all-encompassing in its passion that we practitioners of immunology find it to be, the students have many other interests and concerns, one of which is to pass the five or six other subjects usually taken simultaneously with immunology.

This book was therefore conceived along the lines of the noted architect

Mies van der Rohe's dictum, "less is more." We have devised this text to present the bare essentials of immunology in a palatable form that will enable most students to grasp the essential principles of immunology sufficiently to pass their course. For those developing a deeper interest in the field, numerous advanced and more complete texts exist to further their interests.

The book follows the outlines of most immunology courses and is divided into chapters that mostly approximate the length of an average lecture reading assignment. A short introduction setting the stage precedes the main text of each chapter, the end of each chapter contains a summary, and a series of study questions appears at the very end. The questions are designed to enable students to evaluate their own progress and comprehension; the appended answers are meant as a further learning experience. As new terms or concepts are introduced, they are highlighted in italics and boldface and defined for easy recognition and recall.

It is our hope that students using this text will avoid that choking sensation so common in a course in immunology and even conceive a curiosity about the subject that will lead to further study.

ACKNOWLEDGMENTS TO THE FIRST AND SECOND EDITIONS

The authors are deeply indebted to a number of colleagues and students for valuable contributions to the first and/or second edition of the book.

Dr. Demosthenes Pappagianis of the University of California School of Medicine at Davis contributed the chapter on immunoprophylaxis and immunotherapy, which provides useful, practical insights into the application of immunology to the prevention and therapy of infectious diseases.

Dr. Geoffrey Sunshine of Tufts University Veterinary School was deeply involved in the revision of many chapters of the second edition. His valuable and major contributions to the second edition are gratefully acknowledged.

Drs. Linda Werner and Jacqueline Maisonnave of the University of California School of Medicine at Davis and Drs. Peter Brodeur, Arthur Rabson, and Lanny Rosenwasser of Tufts University School of Medicine were most helpful in reading and contributing valuable suggestions to portions of the first edition. Many other colleagues reviewed portions of the text, and we are grateful for their criticisms and comments. These colleagues include Drs. James R. Carlson,

Robert S. Chang, Allan C. Enders, Kent L. Erickson, Paul Luciw, Claramae H. Miller, and Robert J. Scibienski of the University of California School of Medicine, Davis; Drs. Dov Michaeli and Patricia R. Salber of the University of California School of Medicine, San Francisco; Dr. Shoshana Levy, Stanford University School of Medicine; Dr. Henry N. Claman, University of Colorado School of Medicine; Dr. Patricia Kongshavn, McGill University School of Medicine; and Dr. Karen M. Yamaga, University of Hawaii School of Medicine. Our apologies to other colleagues whose names have been unintentionally omitted.

Finally, we applaud the forbearance of our wives, Joy and Thelma, who continued to tolerate our irritability and whining during the writing of this book.

INTRODUCTION AND OVERVIEW

INTRODUCTION

The story is told about a man who visited a wise old rabbi. The man challenged the rabbi to teach him the essentials of his religion while the man stood on one foot. The rabbi, accepting the challenge, answered, "The essence of my religion is do not do unto others that which is hateful unto you; all the rest is commentary, now go and study."

The essence of immunology can be similarly stated while standing on one foot. Immunology deals with understanding how the body distinguishes between what is "self" and what is "nonself"; all the rest is technical detail.

In his penetrating essays, scientist-author Lewis Thomas, discussing parasitism and symbiosis, described the forces that would drive all living matter into one huge ball of protoplasm were it not for the recognition mechanisms of the immune response that kept "self" and "nonself" apart. The origins of these recognition mechanisms go way back in evolutionary history, and many, in fact, originated as markers for allowing cells to recognize each other to set up symbiotic households. Genetically related sponge colonies that are placed close to each other, for example, will tend to grow toward each other and fuse into one large colony. Unrelated colonies, however, will react in a different way, destroying cells that come in contact and leaving a zone of rejection between the colonies.

In the plant kingdom, similar types of recognition occur. In self-pollinating species, a pollen grain landing on the stigma of a genetically related flower will send a pollen tubule down the style to the ovary for fertilization. A pollen grain from a genetically distinct plant either will not germinate or the pollen tubule, once formed, will disintegrate in the style. The opposite occurs in cross-pollinating species: "self"-marked pollen grains disintegrate while "nonself" grains germinate and fertilize.

The nature of these primitive recognition mechanisms has not been completely worked out, but almost certainly involves cell surface molecules that are able to specifically bind and adhere to other molecules on opposing cell surfaces. This simple method of molecular recognition has evolved over time into the very complex system of the immune response, which, however, still retains as its essential feature the ability of a protein molecule to recognize and bind specifically to a particular shaped structure on another molecule. Such molecular recognition is the underlying principle involved in the discrimination between "self" and "nonself" by the immune response. It is the purpose of this book to describe how the fully mature immune response that has evolved from this simple beginning makes use of this principle of recognition in increasingly complex and sophisticated ways.

The study of immunology as a science or subspecialty of biology has gone through several periods of quiescence and active development, usually succeeding the introduction of a new technique or a changed paradigm for thinking about the subject. We are currently in a phase of feverish activity following the introduction of a whole succession of new molecular biologic techniques, so productive that every text runs a considerable risk of being outdated before it appears in print. Nevertheless the present authors take courage from the observation that new formulations generally build on and expand the old rather than replacing or negating them completely.

OVERVIEW

Innate and Acquired Immunity

The term *immunity* refers to all the mechanisms used by the body as protection against environmental agents that are foreign to the body. These agents may be microorganisms or their products, foods, chemicals, drugs, pollen, or animal hair and dander. Immunity may be innate or acquired.

INNATE IMMUNITY. Innate immunity is conferred by all those elements with which an individual is born and which are always present and available at very short notice to protect the individual from challenges by "foreign" invaders. These elements include body surfaces and internal components, such as the skin, the mucous membranes, and the cough reflex, which present effective barriers to environmental agents. Chemical influences such as pH and secreted fatty acids constitute effective barriers against invasion by many microorganisms.

Numerous internal components are also features of innate immunity: fever, interferons, and other substances released by leukocytes, as well as a variety of serum proteins such as β-lysin, the enzyme lysozyme, polyamines, and the kinins, among others. All of these elements either affect pathogenic invaders directly or enhance the effectiveness of host reactions to them. Other internal elements of innate immunity include phagocytic cells such as granulocytes, macrophages, and microglial cells of the central nervous system, which participate in the destruction and elimination of foreign material that has penetrated the physical and chemical barriers.

ACQUIRED IMMUNITY. Acquired immunity is more specialized than innate immunity, and it supplements the protection provided by innate immunity. Acquired immunity came into play relatively late, in evolutionary terms, and is present only in vertebrates.

Although an individual is born with the capacity to mount an immune response to a foreign invader, immunity is acquired by contact with the invader and is specific to that invader only, hence the term *acquired immunity*. The initial contact with the foreign agent *(immunization)* triggers a chain of events that leads to the activation of certain cells *(lymphocytes)* and the synthesis of proteins, some of which exhibit specific reactivity against the foreign agent. By this process, the individual acquires the immunity to withstand and resist a subsequent attack by, or exposure to, the same offending agent.

The discovery of acquired immunity predates many of the concepts of modern medicine. It has been recognized for centuries that people who did not die from such life-threatening diseases as bubonic plague or smallpox were subsequently more resistant to the disease than were people who had never been exposed to it. The rediscovery of acquired immunity is credited to the English physician Edward Jenner, who in the late eighteenth century experimentally induced immunity to smallpox. Jenner performed an experiment that, if done today, undoubtedly would have resulted in the revocation of his medical license and a sensational malpractice suit: he inoculated a young boy with pus from a lesion of a dairy maid who had cowpox, a relatively benign disease that is related to smallpox. He then deliberately exposed the boy to smallpox. This exposure failed to cause disease! Because of the protective effect of inoculation with cowpox (vaccinia, from the Latin word *vacca,* meaning cow), the process of inducing acquired immunity has been termed **vaccination.**

The concept of vaccination or immunization was expanded by Louis Pasteur and Paul Ehrlich almost 100 years after Jenner's experiment. By the year 1900, it had become apparent that immunity could be induced against not only microorganisms but also their products. We now know that immunity can be induced against thousands of natural and synthetic compounds, which include metals, chemicals of relatively low molecular weight, carbohydrates, proteins, and nucleotides.

The compound to which the acquired immune response is induced is termed an **antigen.**

Active, Passive, and Adoptive Immunization

Acquired immunity is induced by immunization, which can be achieved in several ways: (1) the term **active immunization** refers to immunization of an individual by administration of an antigen; (2) **passive immunization** refers to immunization through the transfer of specific antibody from an immunized individual to a nonimmunized individual; (3) **adoptive transfer** (immunization) refers to the transfer of immunity by the transfer of immune cells.

Characteristics of the Immune Response

The acquired immune response has several generalized features that characterize it and serve to distinguish it from other physiologic systems such as circulation, respiration, or reproduction. These features are:

Specificity: The ability to discriminate among different molecular entities presented to it and to respond only to those uniquely required, rather than making a random, undifferentiated response.

Adaptiveness: The ability to respond to previously unseen molecules that may in fact never have existed before on earth.

Discrimination between "self" and "nonself": A cardinal feature of the specificity of the immune response is its ability to recognize and respond to molecules that are foreign or "nonself" and avoid making a response to those molecules that are "self." This distinction and the recognition of foreign antigen is conferred by specialized cells, namely, lymphocytes, which bear on their surface receptors specific for foreign antigen. Moreover, as we shall shortly see, different lymphocytes bear different receptors specific for different antigens — each cell bears identical receptors specific for an identical antigen or a portion of the antigen.

Memory: A property shared with the nervous system is the ability to recall previous contact with a foreign molecule and respond to it in a "learned" manner, i.e., a more rapid and larger response.

By the end of this book you should understand the cellular and molecular bases of these properties of the immune response or we shall have failed in our purpose.

Cells Involved in the Acquired Immune Response

For many years immunology remained an empirical subject in which the effects of injecting various substances into hosts were studied primarily in terms of the products elicited. Most progress came in the form of more quantitative methods for detecting these products of the immune response. A major change in emphasis came in the 1950s with the recognition that *lymphocytes* were the major cellular players in the immune response, and the field of cellular immunology came to life.

It is now firmly established that there are three major cell types involved in acquired immunity and that complex interactions among these cell types are required for the expression of the full range of immune responses. Two of these cell types come from a common lymphoid precursor cell but differentiate along different developmental lines. One line matures in the thymus and is referred to as *T cell*; the other matures in the bone marrow and is referred to as *B cell*. Cells of the B- and T-lymphocyte series differ in many functional aspects but share one of the important properties of the immune response, namely, they exhibit specificity toward an antigen. Thus the major recognition and reaction functions of the immune response are contained within the lymphocytes.

Antigen-presenting cells (APC) such as macrophages, constitute the third cell type that participate in the acquired immune response. Although these cells do not have antigen-specific receptors as do the lymphocytes, their important function is to "process" the antigen and "present" the antigen to the specific receptors on T lymphocytes. The antigen-presenting cells have on their surface two types of special molecules that function in antigen presentation. These molecules, called ***MHC class I*** and ***MHC class II molecules***, are encoded by a complex set of genes that are also responsible for the rejection or acceptance of transplanted tissue. This set of genes is referred to as the ***major histocompatibility complex (MHC)*** and the class I and class II molecules are commonly referred to as MHC class I and MHC class II molecules. The processed antigen is noncovalently bound to MHC class I or class II molecules (or both) and is thus presented to the specific receptors on the T cell. Interestingly, antigen presented on MHC class I molecules is presented to and participates in the activation of one T-cell subpopulation while antigen presented on MHC class II molecules is presented to a functionally different T-cell subpopulation leading to its activation.

In addition to macrophages, other cell types such as neutrophils and mast cells participate in immune responses. In fact, they participate in both innate immunity and acquired immunity. They are involved primarily in the ***effector*** phases of the response. These cells have no specific antigen recognition properties and are activated by various substances, collectively termed ***cytokines,*** which are released by various cells including activated antigen-specific lymphocytes.

Clonal Selection Theory

A turning point in immunology came in the 1950s with the introduction of a Darwinian view of the cellular basis of specificity in the immune response. This was the now universally accepted ***clonal selection theory*** proposed and developed by Jerne and Burnet (both Nobel Prize winners) and by Talmage. The essential postulates of this theory are summarized below.

The specificity of the immune response is based on the ability of its components (namely, antigen-specific T and B lymphocytes) to recognize particular foreign molecules (antigens) and respond to them in order to eliminate them. Since, as we have already stated, the immune response is capable of recognizing literally thousands of foreign antigens, how is the response to any one accomplished? The theory proposed that

1. T and B lymphocytes of *myriad* specificities exist *before* there is any contact with the foreign antigen.

2. The lymphocytes participating in the immune response have ***antigen-specific*** receptors on their surface membranes. As a consequence of antigen binding to the lymphocyte, the cell is activated and releases various products. In the case of B lymphocytes, the receptors are molecules (antibodies) bearing the same

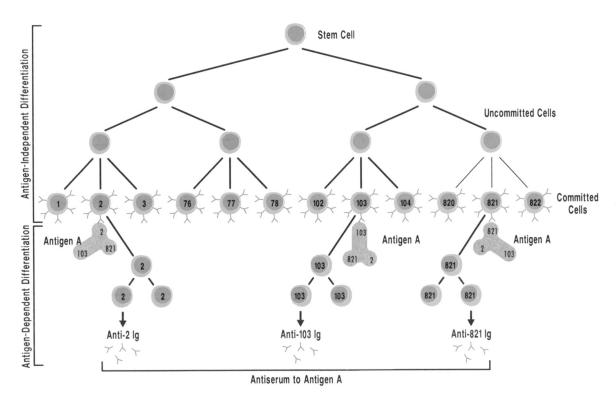

Figure 1.1.
Representation of the clonal selection theory of B cells leading to antibody production.

specificity as the antibody that the cell will subsequently produce and secrete. T cells have complex receptors denoted as ***T-cell receptors (TcRs)***. Unlike the B cell, the T-cell products are not the same as their surface receptors, but are other protein molecules that participate in elimination of the antigen.

3. Each lymphocyte carries on its surface receptor molecules of only a *single* specificity as demonstrated in Figure 1.1 for B cells, and holds true also for T cells.

These three postulates describe the existence of a large ***repertoire*** of possible specificities formed by cellular multiplication and differentiation *before* there is any contact with the foreign substance to which the response is to be made.

The introduction of the foreign antigen then selects from among all the available specificities those with specificity for the antigen enabling binding to occur (Fig. 1.1). Again, the scheme shown in Figure 1.1 for B cells also applies to T cells. However, T cells have receptors that are not antibodies and secrete molecules other than antibodies.

The remaining postulates of the clonal selection theory account for this process of selection by the antigen from among all the available cells in the repertoire.

4. Immunocompetent lymphocytes combine with the foreign antigen, or a portion of it, termed *epitope,* by virtue of their surface receptors. They are stimulated under appropriate conditions to proliferate and differentiate into clones of cells with the corresponding identical receptors to the particular portion of the antigen, termed *antigenic determinant* or *epitope*. With B-cell clones this will lead to the synthesis of monoclonal antibodies having precisely the same specificity. T cells will be similarly "selected" by appropriate antigens or portions thereof. Each selected T cell will be activated to divide and produce clones of the same specificity. Thus, the clonal response to the antigen will be amplified; the cells will release various *cytokines*, and subsequent exposure to the same antigen would now result in the activation of many cells or clones of that specificity. Instead of synthesizing and releasing antibodies as the B cells do, the T cells synthesize and release cytokines. These cytokines, which are soluble mediators, exert their effect on other cells to grow or become activated and eventually eliminate the antigen. It should be noted that several distinct regions of an antigen (epitopes) can be recognized, several different clones of cells will be stimulated, in the case of B cells, to produce antibody, the sum total of which would represent an antiserum specific for that antigen but made up of antibodies of differing specificity (Fig. 1.1), and in the case of T cells, all the T-cell clones recognizing various epitopes on the same antigen will be activated to perform their function.

A final postulate was added to account for the ability to recognize "self" antigens without making a response:

5. Circulating "self" antigens that reach the developing lymphoid system prior to some undesignated maturational step will serve to shut off those cells that recognize it specifically, and no subsequent immune response will be induced.

This formulation of the immune response had a truly revolutionary effect on the field and changed forever our way of looking at and studying immunology.

Humoral and Cellular Immunity

There are two "arms" (branches) of acquired immunity that have different sets of participants and different sets of purposes but with one common aim: to eliminate the antigen. As we shall see later, these two arms interact with each other and collaborate to achieve the final goal of eliminating the antigen. Of these two arms of the acquired immune response, one is mediated mainly by B cells and circulating antibodies, hence it is termed *humoral immunity.* The other is mediated by T cells that, as we stated before, do not synthesize antibodies but instead synthesize and release various cytokines that affect other cells. Hence, this arm of the acquired immune response is termed *cellular* or *cell-mediated immunity.*

HUMORAL IMMUNITY. Humoral immunity is mediated by serum antibodies which are the proteins secreted by the B-cell compartment of the immune response. Antibodies are a heterogeneous mixture of serum *globulins,* all of which share the ability to bind individually to specific antigens. All serum globulins with antibody activity are referred to as *immunoglobulins (Ig).*

All immunoglobulin molecules have common structural features, which enable them to do two things: (1) recognize and bind specifically to a unique structural entity on an antigen, namely, the epitope, and (2) perform a common biologic function after combining with the antigen. Basically, each immunoglobulin molecule consists of two identical *light (L) chains* and two identical *heavy (H) chains* linked by disulfide bridges. The resultant structure can be represented schematically as shown below.

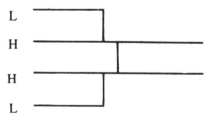

The portion of the molecule that binds antigen consists of an area composed of the amino-terminal regions of both H and L chains. Thus, each immunoglobulin molecule is symmetric and is capable of binding two identical eptitopes present on the same antigen molecule or on different molecules.

In contrast to differences in the antigen-binding portion of different immunoglobulin molecules, there are other differences, the most important of which are those in the H chains. There are five major classes of H chains (termed γ, μ, α, ϵ, and δ). On the basis of differences in their H chains, immunoglobulin molecules are divided into five major classes—IgG, IgM, IgA, IgE, and IgD—each of which has several unique biological properties. For example, IgG is the only class of immunoglobulin that crosses the placenta, conferring the mother's immunity on the fetus, and IgA is the major antibody found in secretions such as tears and saliva. It is important to remember that antibodies in all five classes may possess precisely the same specificity against an antigen (antigen combining regions), while at the same time having different functional (biological effector) properties.

The binding between antigen and antibody is not covalent but depends on many relatively weak forces, such as hydrogen bonds, van der Waals forces, and hydrophobic interactions. Since these forces are weak, successful binding between antigen and antibody depends on a very close fit over a sizable area, much like the contacts between a lock and a key.

Another important element involved in humoral immunity is the ***complement*** system. The reaction between antigen and antibody serves to activate this system, which consists of a series of serum enzymes, the end result of which is lysis of the target or enhanced phagocytosis (ingestion of the antigen) by phagocytic cells. The activation of complement (see Chapter 13) also results in the recruitment of highly phagocytic ***polymorphonuclear (PMN) cells,*** which constitute part of the innate immune system. These activities maximize the effective response made by the humoral arm of immunity against invading agents.

CELL-MEDIATED IMMUNITY. The antigen-specific arm of ***cell-mediated immunity*** consists of the ***T lymphocytes.*** Unlike B cells, which produce soluble antibody that circulates to bind its specific antigens, each T cell, bearing many identical nonsecreted complex receptors composed of several molecules, circulates directly to the site of antigen and performs its function when interacting properly with antigen.

There are several subpopulations of T cells, each of which may have the same specificity for an antigenic determinant (i.e., epitope), although each subpopulation may perform different functions. This is analogous to the different classes of immunoglobulin molecules that may have identical specificity but different biologic functions. The functions ascribed to the various subsets of T cells include:

1. *Cooperation with B cells to enhance the production of antibodies:* Such T cells are called *T helper cells* (T_H) and function by releasing cytokines that provide various activation signals for the B cells. As mentioned earlier, cytokines are soluble substances or mediators released by cells; such mediators released by lymphocytes are also termed *lymphokines*. A group of low-molecular-weight cytokines has been given the name *chemokines*. These play a role in inflammatory response as discussed below.

2. *Inflammatory effects.* On activation, a certain T-cell subpopulation releases cytokines that induce the migration and activation of monocytes and macrophages, leading to the so-called *delayed-type hypersensitivity* inflammatory reactions (Chapter 16). Some term this subpopulation of T cells T_{DTH}, for T cells participating in delayed-type hypersensitivity, and others term this subpopulation simply T_H.

3. *Cytotoxic effects.* The T cells in this subset become cytotoxic killer cells that on contact with their target, are able to deliver a lethal hit, leading to the death of the target cells. These T cells are termed *T cytotoxic cells (Tc)*.

4. *Regulatory effects.* In addition to the subsets of T helper cells, other T cells are able to suppress the immune response leading to a downward modulation or a shutoff in reactivity of other effector cells. These have been termed T suppressor (T_s) cells.

5. *Signal via cytokines.* Both T-cell subpopulations exert numerous effects on many cells, lymphoid and nonlymphoid, through many different cytokines that they release. Thus, directly or indirectly T cells communicate and collaborate with many cell types.

For many years immunologists have recognized that cells that are activated by antigen manifest a variety of effector phenomena. It is only in the last decade or so that they began to appreciate the complexity of events that take place in activation by antigen and communication with other cells. We know today that just mere contact of the T-cell receptor with antigen is not sufficient to activate the cell. In fact, antigen has to be present in the appropriate manner by antigen-presenting cells. Once this has been achieved, a series of complicated events take place and the activated cell synthesizes and releases cytokines. In turn these cytokines come in contact with appropriate receptors on different cells and exert their effect on these cells.

Although both the humoral and cellular arms of the immune response have been considered as separate and distinct components, it is important to understand that the response to any particular pathogen may involve a complex interaction between both, as well as the components of innate immunity. All this with the purpose to ensure maximal survival advantage for the host, in eliminating the antigen, and as we shall see, in protecting the host from mounting an immune response against "self".

Generation of Diversity in the Immune Response

The most recent tidal surge in immunologic research, and one that has not yet crested, represents a triumph of the marriage of molecular biology and immunology. While cellular immunology had delineated the cellular basis for the existence of a large and diverse repertoire of responses, as well as the nature of the exquisite specificity that could be achieved, arguments abounded on the exact genetic mechanisms that enabled all these specificities to become part of the repertoire in every individual of the species.

Briefly, the arguments were as follows:

1. By various calculations the number of antigenic specificities toward which an immune response can be generated could range upward of 10^6–10^7.

2. If every specific response, in the form of either antibodies or T-cell receptors, were to be encoded by a single gene, did this mean that over 10^7 genes (one for each specific antibody) would be required in every individual? How was this massive amount of DNA carried intact from individual to individual?

The pioneering studies of Tonegawa (a Nobel laureate) and Leder, using molecular biologic techniques, finally addressed these issues by describing a unique genetic mechanism by which antibodies and immunologic receptors of enormous diversity could be produced with a modest amount of DNA reserved for this purpose.

The technique evolved by nature was one of *genetic recombination* in which a protein could be encoded by a DNA molecule composed of a set of recombined minigenes that made up a complete gene. Given small sets of these minigenes, which could be randomly combined to make the complete gene, it was possible to produce an enormous repertoire of specificities from a limited number of gene fragments. (This is discussed in detail in Chapter 6.)

Although this mechanism has been first elucidated to explain the enormous diversity of antibodies that are not only released by B cells but that in fact constitute the antigen- or epitope-specific receptors on B cells, it has been subsequently established that the same mechanisms operate in generating diversity of the antigen-specific T-cell receptors. Mechanisms operating in generating diversity of B-cell receptors and antibodies are discussed in Chapter 6. Those operating in generating diversity of T-cell receptors are discussed in Chapter 9. Suffice to say at this point that various techniques of molecular biology that not only permit genes to be analyzed, but also to be moved around at will from one cell to another, have continued to provide impetus to the on-rushing tide of immunologic progress.

Benefits of Immunology

While we have thus far discussed the theoretical aspects of immunology, its practical applications are of paramount importance for survival and must be part of the education of students of medicine.

The field of immunology has been in the public limelight since the late 1960s, when successful transplantation of the human kidney was achieved. More recently, the spectacular transplantation of the human heart and other major organs, such as the liver, has been the focus of much publicity. Public interest in immunology was intensified by the potential application of the immune response to the detection and management of cancer, and in the 1980s the general public became familiar with some aspects of immunology because of the alarming spread of acquired immune deficiency syndrome (AIDS).

Less publicized, but of immense importance to the survival of the individual, is the role of acquired immunity in the prevention of and recovery from infectious diseases. Of great impact to humanity is the success of immunology in the prevention and virtual elimination of many infectious diseases. Vaccination against infectious diseases has been an effective form of prophylaxis. Immunoprophylaxis against the virus that causes poliomyelitis has reduced this dreadful disease to insignificant importance in many parts of the world and, for the first time, a previously widespread disease, smallpox, has been eliminated from the face of the earth. Recent developments in immunology hold the promise of immunoprophylaxis against malaria and several other parasitic diseases that plague many parts of the world and affect billions of people. Vaccination against diseases of domestic animals promises to increase the production of meat in developing countries, while vaccination against various substances that play roles in the reproductive processes in mammals offers the possibility of long-term contraception in humans and companion animals such as cats and dogs.

Damaging Effects of the Immune Response

The enormous survival value of the immune response is self-evident. Acquired immunity directed against a foreign material has as its ultimate goal the elimination of the invading substance. In the process some tissue damage may occur as the result of the accumulation of components with nonspecific effects. This damage is generally temporary. As soon as the invader is eliminated, the situation at that site reverts to normal.

There are instances in which the power of the immune response, although directed against innocuous foreign substances such as some medications, inhaled pollen particles, or substances deposited by insect bites, produces a response that may result in severe pathologic consequences and even death. These responses are known collectively as *hypersensitivity reactions* or *allergic reactions.* An understanding of the basic mechanisms underlying these disease processes has been fundamental in their treatment and control, but in addition has contributed much to our knowledge of the normal immune response. The latter is true since both use essentially identical mechanisms, but in hypersensitivity these mechanisms are misdirected or out of control.

Hypersensitivity reactions are divided into two major categories depending on the effectors involved. The first category is antibody-mediated and, as the term implies, may be passively transferred to another individual by the appropriate amount and type of antibody in serum. This group is, in turn, divided into three classes, depending on the specific underlying mechanisms involving either mast cells or complement and neutrophils. All these reactions have in common a rapidity of response that can range from minutes to a few hours following the injection of antigen and are therefore generally grouped as *immediate hypersensitivity reactions.*

The second major category of hypersensitivity reactions is mediated largely by T cells with consequent involvement of monocytes and is appropriately termed *cell-mediated immunity (CMI).* These responses are much more delayed in appearance, generally taking approximately 18–24 hours to reach their full expression, and have been traditionally referred to as *delayed-type hypersensitivity (DTH).* Unlike antibody-mediated hypersensitivity, which can be transferred from a sensitive individual to a nonsensitive individual via serum, DTH may be transferred not by serum but by T cells.

It should be re-emphasized that all these hypersensitivity reactions have a normal counterpart in that the same mechanisms may operate to protect the host from invading organisms. It is only when the consequences of these responses are misplaced or exaggerated that deleterious effects to the host occur and we call them hypersensitivity reactions.

Regulation of the Immune Response

Given the complexity of the immune response and its potential for inducing damage, it is self-evident that it must operate under carefully regulated conditions, as does any other physiologic system. These controls are multiple and include feedback inhibition by soluble products as well as cell–cell interactions of many types that may either heighten or reduce the response. The net result is to maintain a state of **homeostasis** such that when the system is perturbed by a foreign invader, enough response is generated to control the invader and then the system returns to equilibrium; in other words, the immune response is shut down. However, its memory of that particular invader is retained so that a more rapid and heightened response will occur should the invader return.

Disturbances in these regulatory mechanisms may be caused by conditions such as congenital defect, hormonal imbalance, or infection, any of which may have disastrous consequences. AIDS may serve as a timely example; it is associated with an infection of T lymphocytes that participate in regulating the immune response. As a result of infection with the human AIDS virus, there is a decrease in occurrence and function of one vital subpopulation of T cells that leads to immunologic deficiency, which renders the patient powerless to resist infections by microorganisms that are normally benign.

An important form of regulation concerns the prevention of immune responses against "self" antigens. For various reasons, this regulation may be defective and an immune response against "self" is mounted. This type of immune response is termed **autoimmunity,** and is the cause of diseases such as some forms of arthritis, thyroiditis, and diabetes that are very difficult to treat.

The Future of Immunology

A peek into the world of the future for the student of immunology suggests many exciting areas in which the application of molecular biologic techniques promises significant dividends. To cite just a few examples, we may take vaccine development and control of the immune response. In the former, rather than the laborious, empirical search for an attenuated virus or bacterium for use in immunization, it is now possible to obtain the nucleotide sequence of the DNA that encodes the component of the invading organism that accounts for the protective immune response. Educated guesses can be made from these sequences about the segment of the encoded protein most likely to be responsible for inducing immunity. Such segments can be readily synthesized and tested for use as a vaccine. Moreover, the identification of various genes and the proteins that they are encoding makes it possible to design vaccines against a wide spectrum of biologically important compounds. For example, there are already clinical trials to evaluate the efficacy of antifertility vaccines [anti-HCG (human chorionic gonadotropin)] and other gonadotropioc hormones.

Another area of great promise is the characterization and synthesis of various cytokines—substances that enhance and control the activation of various cells associated with the immune response as well as with other functions of the body. Again, the techniques of gene isolation, clonal reproduction, and biosynthesis have contributed to rapid progress. Powerful and important modulators have been synthesized by the methods of recombinant DNA technology and are being tested for their therapeutic efficacy in a variety of diseases, including many different cancers.

Finally, and probably one of the most exciting areas, is the technology to genetically engineer various cells and even whole animals such as mice that lack one or more specific trait ("gene knockout") or carry a specific trait (transgenic). This allows the immunologist to study the effects of these traits on the immune system and on the body as a whole with the aim of understanding the intricate regulation, expression, and function of the immune response and with the ultimate aim of controlling the trait to the benefit of the individual. Thus, our burgeoning understanding of the functioning of the immune system, combined with the recently acquired ability to alter and manipulate its components, carries enormous implications for the future of humankind.

In the following chapters of this text we attempt a more detailed account of the workings of the immune response, beginning with the cellular components of the system, followed by a description of the structure of the reactants and the general methodology for measuring their reactions. This is followed by chapters describing the formation of and the activation of the cellular and molecular components of the immune apparatus required to generate a response. A discussion of the control mechanisms that regulate the scope and intensity of the immune response completes the description of the basic nature of immunity. Next are chapters that deal with the great variety of diseases involving immunologic components. These vary from ineffective or absent immune response (immunodeficiency) to those produced by aberrant immune responses (hypersensitivity) to responses to self antigens (autoimmunity). The last chapters of the book describe the role of the immune response in transfusion, transplantation, and antitumor reactions. A final chapter deals with some practical aspects of immunization against infectious diseases.

With the enormous scope of the subject and the extraordinary richness of detail available, every effort has been made by the authors to adhere to fundamental elements and basic concepts required to achieve an integrated, if not extensive, understanding of the immune response. If the reader's interest has been aroused, many current books, articles, and reviews are available to flesh out the details on the scaffolding provided by this book.

ELEMENTS OF INNATE AND ACQUIRED IMMUNITY

INTRODUCTION

Every living organism is confronted by continual intrusions from its environment. To survive, every organism has therefore had to develop defenses that render it resistant, or immune, to such assaults. These defenses range from physical barriers, such as a cell wall, to highly sophisticated systems, such as the acquired immune response. This chapter describes the defense systems: the elements that constitute the defense, the participating cells and organs, and the action of the participants in the immune response to foreign substances that invade the body.

In vertebrates, immunity against microorganisms and their products, or against other foreign substances that may invade the body, is divided into two major categories: *innate or natural immunity* and *acquired immunity.* These two types of immunity and their origins, components, and interrelationships, are also discussed in the present chapter.

INNATE OR NATURAL IMMUNITY

Innate (natural) immunity is present from birth and consists of many factors that are relatively nonspecific; that is, they operate against almost any substance that threatens the body. Some of the important nonspecific factors that are part of innate immunity are given below.

Physiological and Chemical Barriers (Skin and Mucous Membranes)

Most organisms and foreign substances cannot penetrate intact skin, but can enter the body if the skin is damaged. Some microorganisms can enter through sebaceous glands and hair follicles. However, the *acid pH* of sweat and sebaceous secretions and the presence of various *fatty acids* and *enzymes* (e.g., lysozyme), all of which have some antimicrobial effect, minimize the importance of this route of infection.

Mucus covers the surface of many areas in the body, such as the respiratory and gastrointestinal tracts. In the respiratory tract, the mucus and microorganisms trapped in it are constantly being driven upward by ciliated cells, toward the external openings. Also, the hairs in the nostrils and the cough reflex are helpful in preventing organisms from infecting the respiratory tract. Alcohol, cigarette smoke, and narcotics suppress this entire defense system.

The elimination of microorganisms from the respiratory tract is aided by pulmonary or alveolar macrophages, which, as we shall see later, are phagocytic cells able to engulf and destroy some microorganisms. Other microorganisms that have penetrated the mucous membrane can be picked up by macrophages or otherwise transported to lymph nodes, where many are destroyed.

The environment of the gastrointestinal tract is made hostile to many microorganisms by the *hydrolytic enzymes in saliva,* by the *low pH of the stomach,* and by the *proteolytic enzymes and bile in the small intestine.* The *low pH of the vagina* serves a similar function.

Cellular Defenses

Once an invading microorganism has penetrated the various physiological and chemical barriers, the next line of defense consists of various specialized cells whose purpose is to destroy the invader. There are several cell types that fulfill this function. The interrelationship between the various cell types that will be discussed in this and subsequent chapters is shown diagramatically in Figure 2.1.

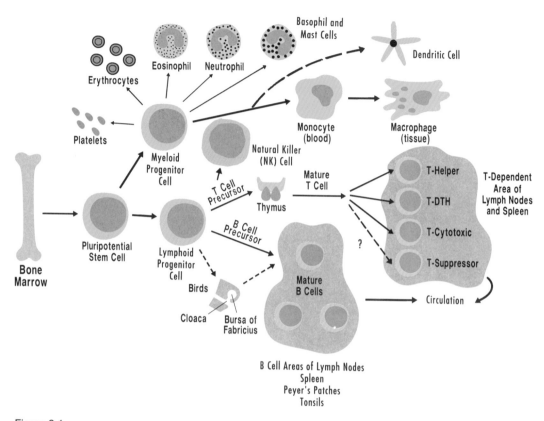

Figure 2.1.

The developmental pathway of various cell types from a pluripotential bone marrow stem cell.

Phagocytosis and Extracellular Killing

As part of its innate immunity, the body has developed defenses mediated by specialized cells that destroy the invading microorganism by first ingesting and then destroying it *(phagocytosis)*, or by killing it extracellularly (without ingesting it).

PHAGOCYTOSIS. *Phagocytosis* is the ingestion and destruction by individual cells of invading foreign particles, such as bacteria. Many microorganisms release substances that attract phagocytic cells. Phagocytosis may be enhanced by a variety of factors that make the foreign particle an easier target. These factors, collectively referred to as *opsonins* (Greek "prepare food for"), consist of antibodies and various serum components of complement (see Chapter 13). After ingestion, the foreign particle is entrapped in a ***phagocytic vacuole*** that fuses with granule-containing ***lysosomes.*** The latter release their powerful enzymes that digest the particle.

The phagocytic cells consist of certain types of polymorphonuclear leukocytes, phagocytic monocytes (i.e., macrophages), and fixed macrophages of the reticuloendothelial system. On activation, all these cells release soluble substances called ***cytokines*** that have different effects on various cells (see Chapter 11).

Polymorphonuclear (PMN) leukocytes, also referred to as ***granulocytes,*** include basophils, mast cells, eosinophils, and neutrophils. These are short-lived phagocytic cells that contain granules (lysosomes) filled with hydrolytic enzymes (Fig. 2.2). They also produce peroxide and superoxide radicals that are toxic to many microorganisms. Some granules also contain bactericidal proteins such as lactoferrin. The PMN play a major role in protection against infection. Defects in PMN function are accompanied by chronic or recurrent infection.

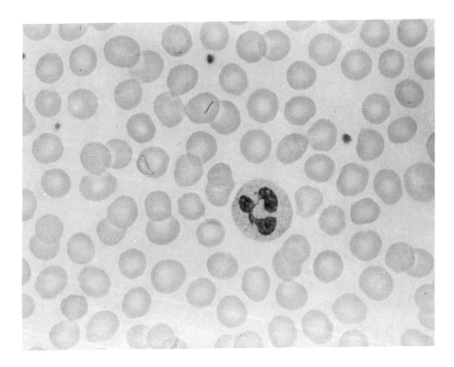

Figure 2.2.
A polymorphonuclear leukocyte (surrounded by erythrocytes in a blood smear) with a trilobed nucleus and cytoplasmic granules. ×950. (Photo courtesy of Dr. A.C. Enders, School of Medicine, University of California, Davis.)

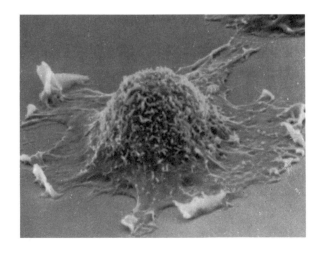

Figure 2.3.

A scanning electron micrograph of a macrophage with ruffled membranes and a surface covered with microvilli. ×5,200. (Photo courtesy of Dr. K.L. Erickson, School of Medicine, University of California, Davis; reproduced with permission of Lippincott/ Harper and Row.)

Macrophages. After entering the blood as monocytes, these cells (see Fig. 2.3) migrate to various tissues where they undergo further differentiation into a variety of histologic forms that are included in the so-called ***reticuloendothelial system (RES)***, which is widely distributed throughout the body. The major function of the RES is to trap microorganisms and foreign substances that are in the bloodstream and in various tissues and to expose them to phagocytosis. The RES also functions in the destruction of aged and imperfect cells such as erythrocytes.

The monocyte itself is a small, spherical cell with few projections, abundant cytoplasm, little endoplasmic reticulum, and many granules. Once settled in a particular tissue, the monocyte differentiates into one of a variety of forms such as

Kupffer cells in the liver; large cells with many cytoplasmic projections

Alveolar macrophages, in the lung

Splenic macrophages, in the white pulp

Peritoneal macrophages, free-floating in peritoneal fluid

Microglial cells, in the central nervous tissue

Although associated with so many diverse names and locations, many of these cells share common features, such as the ability to ***bind and engulf particulate materials and antigens.*** Their locations along capillaries make them the cells most likely to make first contact with invading pathogens and antigens, and the performance of these cells, as we shall see later, plays a large part in the success of innate as well as acquired immunity.

In general, cells of the macrophage series have two major functions. One of their functions, as their name ("large eater") implies, is to **engulf** and, with the aid of all the degradative enzymes in their lysosomal granules, **break down** trapped materials into simple amino acids, sugars, and other substances, for excretion or reutilization. Thus, these cells play a key role in the removal of bacteria and parasites from the blood. As we shall see in later chapters, the second major function of the macrophages is to take up antigens, **process** them by denaturation or by partial digestion, and **present** them, on their surfaces, to specific T cells. Thus macrophages function also as **antigen-presenting cells.**

Dendrite-shaped cells in spleen and lymph nodes **(dendritic cells), interdigitating cells** of the thymus, as well as Langerhans cells in the skin probably also belong to this lineage of cells. These cells are not very phagocytic but they are potent antigen-presenting cells.

From this outline, it can be seen that monocytes play a central role in all phases of immunity. Their role in innate immunity is phagocytosis. They also play a key role in the **afferent** or **induction** limb of the acquired immune response (by initiating T-cell responses). Finally, the macrophages play a role in the **efferent** or **effector** limb of the acquired immune response as the end cells that become activated by T-cell-released cytokines that enhance their killing of pathogens.

EXTRACELLULAR KILLING.   Unique structures on the membranes of abnormal cells, such as virus-infected or cancer cells, are recognized by cytotoxic or killer cells that destroy the target cell not by phagocytosis but by releasing biologically potent molecules that within a very short time kill the target cell. Such killer cells include the cytotoxic T lymphocytes, which constitute an arm of the acquired immune response and are dealt with in Chapters 9 and 11, and the natural-killer (NK) cells, a component of the innate immune system. NK cells probably play a role in the early stages of viral infection or tumorogenesis, before the cytotoxic T lymphocytes of the acquired immune response increase in numbers. NK cells are large granular lymphocytes. They are brought to proximity with their target cells by the help of their receptors to unique glycoproteins which appear on the target cell membrane following viral infection or oncogenic transformation. Killing is achieved by the release of various cytotoxic molecules. Some of these molecules cause the formation of pores in the membrane of the target cell leading to its lysis. Other molecules enter the target cell and cause **apoptosis** — a form of programmed cell death, of the target cell by enhanced fragmentation of its nuclear DNA. The activity of NK cells is highly increased by soluble mediators such as IL-2 (interleukin-2) and interferons. Interferons α and β are antiviral proteins synthesized and released by leukocytes, fibroblasts, and virally infected cells; IL-2 and interferon γ are released by activated T lymphocytes.

Inflammation

An important function of phagocytic cells and phagocytosis is their participation in inflammation, a major component of the body's defense mechanism. The important aspects of inflammation are summarized below.

Inflammation is a complex process, comprising many events, initiated by tissue damage caused by endogenous factors (such as tissue necrosis or bone fracture) as well as exogenous factors. These include various types of damage such as mechanical injury (e.g., cut), physical injury (e.g., burn), chemical injury (e.g., exposure to a corrosive chemical), biological injury (e.g., infection by microorganisms), and immunologic injury (e.g., hypersensitivity reactions; see Chapters 14–16). The inflammatory response constitutes an important part of both innate and acquired immunity. It has evolved as a protective response against injury and infection. Although in certain cases, such as hypersensitivity, inflammation becomes the problem rather than the solution to a problem such as infection, by and large the inflammatory response is protective; it is one of the major responses to injury and constitutes a process aimed at bringing the injured tissue back to its normal state.

The hallmark signs of inflammation, described almost 2000 years ago, are *swelling (tumor), redness (rubor), heat (calor), pain (dolor),* and *loss of function* of the inflamed area. Within minutes after injury, the inflammatory process begins with the activation and increased concentration of pharmacologically powerful substances such as a group of proteins known as *acute-phase proteins.* An important member of the acute phase proteins is the *C-reactive protein.* This protein binds to the membrane of certain microorganisms and activates the complement system (Chapter 13). This results in the lysis of the microorganism or its enhanced phagocytosis by phagocytic cells, as well as other important biologic functions, as we shall see later.

The *kinin* system also becomes activated by tissue injury, which triggers inflammation. The kinin system is initiated through activation of the clotting or coagulation system with its key player, clotting factor XII, called the *Hageman factor.* The Hageman factor is a protease zymogen that becomes activated through contact with nonmembranous high-molecular-weight surfaces such as basement membrane collagen matrices or by the action of other proteases. In addition to promoting the coagulaton cascade, the Hageman factor cleaves a zymogen called *kallikreinogen* to yield kallikrein, another protease. Kallikrein initiates the fibrinolytic system by cleaving plasmin, yet another protease, from its zymogen plasminogen. Plasmin mediates clot lysis as well as activating complement components. Moreover, kallikrein acts on kininogen to yield a series of pharmacologically active peptides called *kinins* (the prototype is the monopeptide bradykinin).

The kinins are rapidly inactivated by further cleavage but, while intact, have several important effects:

1. They act directly on local smooth muscle and cause muscle contraction.

2. They act on axons to block nervous impulses, leading to a distal muscle relaxation.

3. Most importantly, they act on vascular endothelial cells, causing them to contract, leading to increase in vascular permeability, and to express endothelial cell adhesion molecules (ECAMs), leading to leukocyte adhesion and extravasation.

4. Kinins are very potent nerve stimulators and are the molecules most responsible for pain (and itching) associated with inflammation.

In the inflammatory response the cytokines playing a most important role include IL-1 (interleukin 1), IL-6, and tumor necrosis factor α (TNF-α). These cytokines released by activated macrophages induce adhesion molecules on the walls of vascular endothelial cells to which neutrophils, monocytes, and lymphocytes adhere before moving out of the vessel through a process called *extravasation,* to the affected tissue. These cytokines also induce coagulation and increased vascular permeability. Together with IL-8 and interferon γ, they exert additional effects such as increased chemotaxis for leukocytes and increased phagocytosis. All these effects result in the accumulation of fluid (edema) and leukocytic cells in the injured areas. These, in turn, amplify the response further since additional biologically active compounds are transported in the fluid and also are released from the accumulated cells, attracting and activating still more cells.

Most of the cells involved in the inflammatory response are phagocytic cells, first consisting mainly of the *polymorphonuclear leukocytes,* which accumulate within 30–60 minutes, phagocytize the intruder or damaged tissue, and release their lysosomal enzymes in an attempt to destroy the intruder. If the cause of the inflammatory response persists beyond this point, within 5–6 hours the area will be infiltrated by *mononuclear cells,* which include macrophages and lymphocytes. The macrophages supplement the phagocytic activity of the polymorphonuclear cells, thus adding to the defense of the area. Moreover, the macrophages participate in the processing and presentation of antigen to lymphocytes, which respond to the foreign antigens of the invader by inducing the acquired immune response specific to those antigens.

If the injury or the invasion by microorganisms continues, the inflammatory response will be supplemented and augmented by elements of acquired immunity that include antibodies and cell-mediated immunity. The antibody response initiates the complement cascade in which pharmacologically active compounds are activated and released. These include substances that increase vascular permeability and capillary dilatation, as well as chemotactic substances that attract and activate additional polymorphonuclear cells and antigen-specific lymphocytes. The lymphocytes themselves are capable of destroying some foreign invaders. More importantly, they release cytokines that activate macrophages and other cells to participate in destroying and removing the invaders.

Many substances activated during the inflammatory process participate in repairing the injury. During this remarkable process many cells, including leukocytes, are being destroyed. The macrophages that are present in the area phagocytize the debris and the inflammation subsides; the tissue may be restored to its normal state, or scar tissue may be formed.

Sometimes it is difficult or impossible to remove the causes of inflammation. This results in chronic inflammation, which occurs in situations of chronic infection such as tuberculosis or chronic activation of the immune response, exemplified by rheumatoid arthritis or glomerulonephritis. In these cases the inflammatory response continues and can be only temporarily modified by the administration of anti-inflammatory agents such as aspirin, ibuprofen, or cortisone. These and other drugs act on several of the metabolic pathways involved in the elaboration and activation of some of the pharmacologic mediators of inflammation. However, they do not affect the root cause of the inflammation, and so when withdrawn, the symptoms may return.

Fever

Although fever is one of the most common manifestations of infection and inflammation, there is still limited information about the significance of fever in the course of infection in mammals. Fever is caused by many bacterial products, most notably the endotoxins of gram-negative bacteria, generally as the result of the release of endogenous *pyrogens* that derive from monocytes and macrophages and include *interleukins (IL-1)* and *interferons*.

Biologically Active Substances

Many tissues synthesize substances that are harmful to microorganisms. Examples are *degradative enzymes, toxic free radicals, acids, inhibitors of growth, acute-phase proteins*, and *interferons*. Thus, depending on their ability to synthesize these substances, certain tissues may have a heightened resistance to infection by some microorganisms.

Innate or natural immunity is related to many attributes of the individual that are determined genetically. Differences in innate immunity between various people may, in addition, be attributed to age, race, and the hormonal and metabolic conditions of the individual.

ACQUIRED IMMUNITY

In contrast to innate immunity, which is an attribute of every living organism, acquired immunity is a more specialized form of immunity. It developed late in evolution and is found only in vertebrates. The various elements that participate in innate immunity do not exhibit specificity against the foreign agents they encounter; in contrast, acquired immunity always exhibits such specificity. As its name implies, acquired immunity is a consequence of an encounter with a foreign substance. The first encounter with a foreign substance that has penetrated the body triggers a chain of events that induces an immune response with specificity against that foreign substance.

Although an individual is genetically endowed with the capacity to mount an immune response against a certain substance, acquired immunity is usually exhibited only after an initial encounter with the substance. Thus, acquired immunity develops only after exposure to, or *immunization* with, a given substance.

There are two major types of cells that participate in acquired immunity: *B lymphocytes* (so named because they originate in the bone marrow), and *T lymphocytes* (named for their differentiation in the thymus). B lymphocytes and T lymphocytes are responsible for the specificity exhibited by the acquired immune response. B lymphocytes synthesize and secrete into the bloodstream antibodies with specificity against the foreign substance. This is termed *humoral immunity*. The T lymphocytes, which also exhibit specificity against the foreign substance by virtue of their receptors, do not make antibodies, but they themselves seek out the invader to produce their effects. T lymphocytes also interact with B cells and "help" the latter make antibodies; they activate macrophages, and they have a central role in the development and regulation of acquired immunity (see Chapter 12). Acquired immunity mediated by T lymphocytes is termed *cellular immunity* or *cell-mediated immunity (CMI)*. As we have seen, macrophages are phagocytic cells; they do not exhibit specificity against a given substance, but they are involved in the processing and presentation of foreign substances to T lymphocytes and activation of T lymphocytes (see Chapters 10 and 11).

Lymphatic Organs

The *lymphatic organs* are those organs in which lymphocyte maturation, differentiation, and proliferation take place. *Lymphocytes* are derived from the pluripotential *hematopoietic bone marrow stem cells,* which give rise to all blood cells. The *erythroid* and *myeloid* cells, which differentiate into erythrocytes and granulocytes, are derived from these stem cell progenitors. Lymphoid progenitor cells differentiate into lymphocytes (see Fig. 2.1).

The lymphoid organs are generally divided into two categories. The *primary* or *central lymphoid organs* are those in which the maturation of T and B lymphocytes into antigen-recognizing lymphocytes occurs. As we shall see in subsequent chapters, developing T and B cells acquire their antigen-specific receptors in primary lymphoid organs. The *secondary lymphoid organs* are those organs in which antigen-driven proliferation and differentiation take place.

PRIMARY LYMPHOID ORGANS.   There are two major primary lymphoid organs, one in which the T cells develop and the other in which the B cells develop.

The Thymus Gland. Progenitor cells from the bone marrow migrate to the primary lymphoid organ, the *thymus gland,* where they differentiate into *T lymphocytes*. The thymus gland (Fig. 2.4A,B) is a bilobed structure, derived from the endoderm of the third and fourth pharyngeal pouches. During fetal development, the size of the thymus increases. The growth continues until puberty. Thereafter, the thymus undergoes atrophy with aging.

The thymus is a *lymphoepithelial* organ and consists of epithelial cells organized into cortical and medullary areas that are infiltrated with lymphoid cells (thymocytes). The *cortex* is densely populated with lymphocytes of various sizes, most of which are immature. T lymphocytes mature in the cortex and migrate to the *medulla,* which they then leave to enter the peripheral blood circulation, through which they are transported to the *secondary lymphoid organs* (cell development is discussed in detail in Chapter 9). It is in these secondary lymphoid organs that the T cells encounter and respond to foreign antigens.

Maturation of the T lymphocyte involves the commitment of a given T cell to recognize and respond to a given determinant or *epitope* of a foreign antigen. This

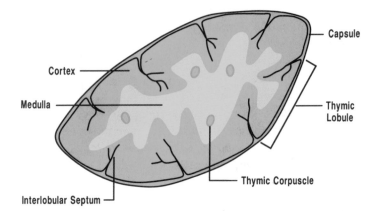

Figure 2.4A.

A diagrammatic representation of a section of the thymus gland.

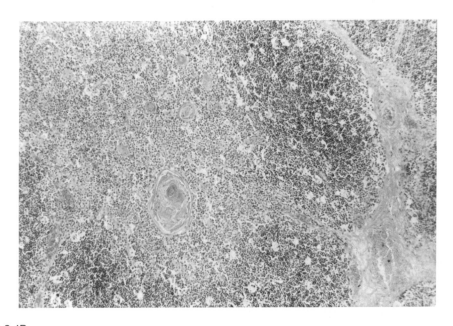

Figure 2.4B.

Section of the thymus showing interlobular septum, a thymic lobule, the cortex (darker areas), the medulla (lighter area), and a thymic corpuscle. ×140. (Photo courtesy of Dr. A.C. Enders, School of Medicine, University of California, Davis.)

recognition is achieved by a specific receptor on the T cell, which is acquired during differentiation in the thymus (see Chapter 9). Mature T lymphocytes in the medulla are capable of responding to foreign antigens in the same way that they would respond in the secondary lymphoid organs. However, the thymus is considered to be a primary lymphoid organ, where antigen-driven proliferation and differentiation (events that generally take place in secondary lymphoid organs, as described below) do not take place.

The maturation of T lymphocytes occurs mainly during fetal development and for a short time after birth. Thus, removal of the thymus gland from a neonate results in a severe reduction in the quantity and quality of T lymphocytes and produces a potentially lethal wasting disease. Removal of the thymus from an adult generally has little effect on the quantity and quality of the T lymphocytes, which have already matured and populated the secondary lymphoid organs. However, adult thymectomy could, in time, result in a deficiency of T cells if there is acute death of the T cells that originally populated the secondary lymphoid organs (such as following whole-body irradiation). Without the thymus there would be no mechanism for repopulation of the secondary organs with new T lymphocytes.

It is of interest that only 5–10% of maturing lymphocytes survive and eventually leave the thymus; 90–95% of all thymocytes die in the thymus. It is clear that the lymphocytes that die have developed specificity to "self" structures or have failed to make functional receptors and therefore, eliminated. The lymphocytes that survive develop specificity against foreign antigens. This is discussed in Chapter 9.

Bursa of Fabricius and the Bone Marrow. A primary lymphoid organ was first discovered in birds. In birds, B cells undergo maturation in the *bursa of Fabricius*. This organ, situated near the cloaca, consists of lymphoid centers that contain epithelial cells and lymphocytes. Unlike the lymphocytes in the thymus, these lymphocytes consist solely of antibody-producing *B cells* (see Chapter 8).

Mammals do not have a bursa of Fabricius. Consequently, much work has been directed toward the identification of a mammalian equivalent of the primary lymphoid organ in which B cells develop and mature. It is now clear that in embryonic life, B cells differentiate from hematopoietic stem cells in the fetal liver. After birth and for the life of the individual this function moves to the bone marrow, a structure that is considered to be a primary lymphoid organ with functions equivalent to that of the avian bursa. Each mature B lymphocyte bears antigen-specific receptors that have a structure and specificity identical to the antibody later synthesized by that B cell. The mature B cells are transported by the circulating blood to the secondary lymphoid organs, where they encounter and respond to foreign antigens.

SECONDARY LYMPHOID ORGANS. The secondary lymphoid organs consist of certain structures in which mature, antigen-committed lymphocytes are stimulated by antigen to undergo further division and differentiation. The major secondary lymphoid organs are the ***spleen*** and the ***lymph nodes***. In addition, tonsils, appendix, clusters of lymphocytes distributed in the lining of the small intestine ***(Peyer's patches),*** as well as lymphoid aggregates spread throughout mucosal tissue are considered secondary lymphoid organs. The latter comprise of various areas of the body such as the linings of the digestive tract, the respiratory and genitourinary tracts, the conjunctiva, and the salivary glands. In these secondary lymphoid organs, mature lymphocytes interact with antigen and differentiate to synthesize specific antibodies. These latter secondary lymphoid organs have been given the name ***mucosa-associated lymphoid tissue (MALT).*** Those lymphoid tissues associated with the gut are ***gut-associated lymphoid tissue (GALT);*** those associated with the bronchial tree are termed ***bronchus-associated lymphoid tissue (BALT).***

The secondary lymphoid organs have two major functions: they are highly efficient in trapping and concentrating foreign substances, and they are the main sites of production of antibodies and the generation of antigen-specific T lymphocytes.

The Spleen. The spleen (Fig. 2.5A,B) is the largest of the secondary lymphoid organs. It is highly efficient in trapping and concentrating foreign substances carried in the blood. It is the major organ in the body in which antibodies are synthesized and from which they are released into the circulation. The spleen is composed of ***white pulp,*** rich in lymphoid cells, and ***red pulp,*** which contains many sinuses as well as large quantities of erythrocytes and macrophages, some lymphocytes, and a few other cells.

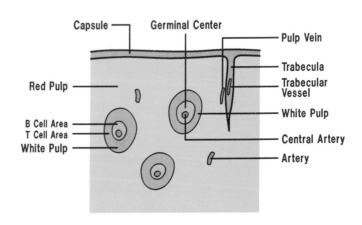

Figure 2.5A.

A diagrammatic representation of a section of the spleen.

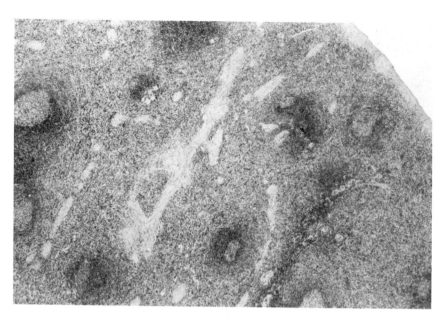

Figure 2.5B.

A section of the spleen showing the capsule (top right), trabecula (muscular area transversing from top center toward bottom left) with vein (darker region) in the trabecula, and red pulp and white pulp (darker areas) with germinal centers within the white pulp. B cells are concentrated around the germinal centers; T cells are concentrated in the interface between the white and red pulp. ×35. (Photo courtesy of Dr. A.C. Enders, School of Medicine, University of California, Davis.)

The areas of white pulp are located mainly around small arterioles, the peripheral regions of which are rich in T cells, with B cells present mainly in germinal centers. Approximately 50% of spleen cells are B lymphocytes; 30–40% are T lymphocytes. Following antigenic stimulation, the *germinal centers* contain large numbers of B cells and *plasma cells*. These cells synthesize and release antibodies.

Lymph Nodes. Lymph nodes (Fig. 2.6A,B) are small ovoid structures (normally less than one cm in diameter) found in various regions throughout the body. They are close to major junctions of the *lymphatic channels,* which are connected to the *thoracic duct*. The thoracic duct transports lymph and lymphocytes to the *vena cava,* the vessel that carries blood to the right side of the heart (see Fig. 2.7) from where it is redistributed throughout the body.

Lymph nodes are composed of a *medulla* with many sinuses and a *cortex,* which is surrounded by a capsule of connective tissue. The cortical region con-

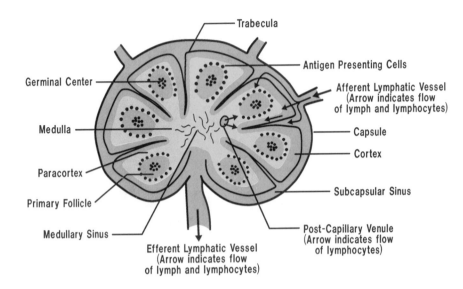

Figure 2.6A.

A diagrammatic repre-
sentation of a section of
a lymph node.

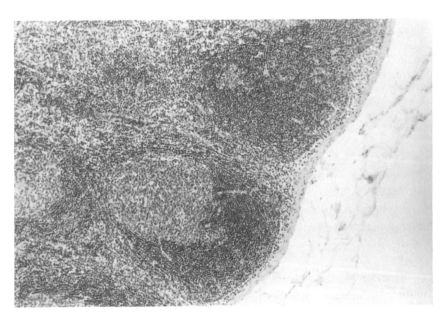

Figure 2.6B.

A section through a lymph node showing the capsule, the subcapsular sinus, the medulla (upper
left), and the cortex with primary follicles containing germinal centers. B lymphocytes are
concentrated in the paracortical areas (darker areas) around the germinal centers, and T
lymphocytes extend inward toward the medulla. Also shown (upper right) is a follicle without a
germinal center. ×140. (Photo courtesy of Dr. A.C. Enders, School of Medicine, University of
California, Davis.)

tains *primary lymphocytic follicles*. On antigenic stimulation, these structures form *germinal centers* that contain dense populations of lymphocytes—mostly B cells—that are undergoing mitosis. The deep cortical area or paracortical region contains T cells and macrophages. The macrophages trap, process, and present antigen to the T cells that have specificity against that antigen, events that result in activation of the T cells. The medullary area of the lymph node contains antibody-secreting plasma cells that have traveled from the cortex to the medulla via lymphatic vessels.

Lymph nodes are highly efficient in trapping antigen that enters through the *afferent lymphatic vessels*. In the node, the antigen interacts with macrophages, T cells, and B cells, and that interaction brings about an immune response, manifested by the generation of antibodies and antigen-specific T cells. Lymph, antibodies, and cells leave the lymph node through the *efferent lymphatic vessel,* which is just below the medullary region.

CIRCULATION OF LYMPHOCYTES

Blood lymphocytes enter the lymph nodes through *postcapillary venules* and leave the lymph nodes through efferent lymphatic vessels that eventually converge in the thoracic duct. This duct empties into the *vena cava,* the vessel that returns the blood to the heart, thus providing for the continual recirculation of lymphocytes.

The spleen functions in a similar manner. Arterial blood lymphocytes enter the spleen through the *hilus* and pass into the *trabecular artery,* which along its course becomes narrow and branched. At the farthest branches of the trabecular artery, capillaries lead to lymphoid nodules. Ultimately, the lymphocytes return to the venous circulation through the *trabecular vein*. Like lymph nodes, the spleen contains efferent lymphatic vessels through which lymph empties into the lymphatics from which the cells continue their recirculation through the body and back to the afferent vessels.

The migration of T lymphocytes between various lymphoid and nonlymphoid tissue and their "homing" to a particular site is highly regulated by means of various cell-surface adhesion molecules (CAMs) and receptors to these molecules. Thus, except in the spleen where small arterioles end in the parenchyma, allowing access to blood lymphocytes, blood lymphocytes must generally cross the endothelial vascular lining of postcapillary vascular sites termed *high endothelial venules (HEVs)*. Recirculating T lymphocytes selectively bind to specific receptors on the HEV of lymphoid tissue and appear to completely ignore other vascular endothelium. Moreover, it appears that a selective binding of finer specificity operates between the HEV and various distinct subsets of lymphocytes, further regulating the migration of lymphocytes into the various lymphoid and nonlymphoid tissue.

The traffic of lymphocytes between lymphoid and nonlymphoid tissue ensures that on exposure to an antigen, the antigen and the lymphocytes specific to that antigen are sequestered in the lymphoid tissue, where the lymphocytes undergo proliferation and differentiation. The differentiated cells (memory cells) leave the lymphoid organ and disseminate in the body to reconcentrate at the site where antigen persists and exert their protective effects.

THE FATE OF ANTIGEN AFTER PENETRATION

The reticuloendothelial system is designed to trap foreign antigens that have penetrated the body and to subject them to ingestion and degradation by the phagocytic cells of the system. Also, there is constant movement of lymphocytes throughout the body, and this movement permits deposition of lymphocytes in strategic places along the lymphatic vessels. The system not only traps antigens but also provides loci (the secondary lymphoid organs) where antigen, macrophages, T cells, and B cells can interact within a very small area to initiate an immune response.

The fate of an antigen that has penetrated the physical barriers and the cellular and antibody components of the ensuing immune response are shown in Figure 2.7.

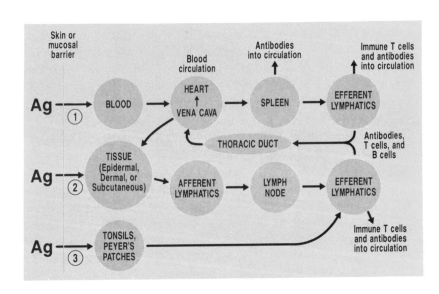

Figure 2.7.

Circulation of lymph and fate of antigen following penetration through (1) the bloodstream, (2) the skin, and (3) the gastrointestinal or respiratory tract.

As illustrated, three major routes may be followed by an antigen after it has penetrated the interior of the body:

1. The antigen may enter the body through the ***bloodstream***. In this case, it is carried to the ***spleen,*** where it interacts with antigen-presenting cells such as dentritic cells and macrophages, T cells, and B cells to generate an antigen-specific immune response. The spleen then releases the antibodies directly into the circulation. Lymphocytes also leave the spleen through the efferent lymphatics, to reenter the circulation via the thoracic duct.

2. The antigen may lodge in the ***epidermal, dermal,*** or ***subcutaneous tissue,*** where it may cause an inflammatory response. From these tissues the antigen, either free or trapped by antigen-presenting cells, is transported through the afferent lymphatic channels into the regional ***draining lymph node***. In the lymph node, the antigen, macrophages, T cells, and B cells interact to generate the immune response. Eventually, antigen-specific T cells and antibodies, which have been synthesized in the lymph node, enter the circulation and are transported to the various tissues. Antigen-specific T cells, B cells, and antibodies also enter the circulation via the thoracic duct.

3. The antigen may enter the ***gastrointestinal*** or ***respiratory tract,*** where it lodges in the mucosa-associated lymphoid tissue (MALT). There it will interact with macrophages and lymphocytes. Antibodies synthesized in these organs are deposited in the local tissue. In addition, lymphocytes entering the efferent lymphatics are carried through the ***thoracic duct*** to the circulation and are thereby redistributed to various tissue.

The induction of an acquired immune response necessitates the interaction of the foreign antigen with lymphocytes that recognize that specific antigen. It has been estimated that in a ***naive (nonimmunized)*** animal, only one in every 10^3–10^5 lymphocytes is capable of recognizing a typical antigen. Therefore, the probability that an antigen will encounter these cells is very low. The problem is compounded by the fact that, for synthesis of antibody to ensue, two different kinds of lymphocyte, the T lymphocyte and B lymphocyte, each with specificity against this particular antigen, must interact.

Statistically, the chances for the interaction of specific T lymphocytes with their particular antigen, and then with B lymphocytes specific for the same antigen, are very low. However, nature has devised an ingenious mechanism for bringing these cells into contact with antigen: the antigen is carried via the draining lymphatics to the secondary lymphoid organs. In these organs, the antigen is exposed on the surface of fixed specialized cells. Because both T and B lymphocytes circulate at a rather rapid rate, making the rounds every several days, some circulating lymphocytes with specificity for the particular antigen should pass by the fixed antigen within a relatively short time. When these lymphocytes encounter the antigen for which they are specific, the lymphocytes become activated and the acquired immune response, with specificity against this antigen, is triggered.

INTERRELATIONSHIP BETWEEN INNATE AND ACQUIRED IMMUNITY

The innate and acquired arms of the immune system have developed a beautiful interrelationship. The intricate and ingenious communication system through the various cytokines and cell adhesion molecules allows components of innate and acquired immunity to interact, send each other signals, activate each other, and work in concert toward the final goal of destroying and eliminating the invading microorganism and its products. The interrelationship between innate and acquired immunity is shown in Figure 2.8.

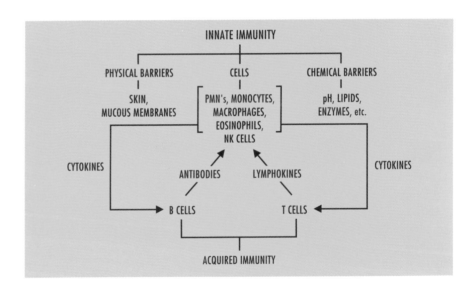

Figure 2.8.

The interrelationship between innate and acquired immunity.

   1. There are two forms of immunity: (1) innate, or natural, and (2) acquired.

2. Many elements participate in innate immunity; these include various physical barriers, chemical barriers, and cellular components.

3. Two major types of cells participate in acquired immunity: (1) B lymphocytes and (2) T lymphocytes.

4. B and T lymphocytes have receptors that are specific for particular antigens and, thus, constitute the components of acquired immunity that are responsible for antigenic specificity.

5. B and T lymphocytes develop in primary lymphoid organs. Their initial development–maturation process is independent of antigen.

6. Mature B and T lymphocytes differentiate and proliferate in response to antigenic stimulation. These events generally take place in secondary lymphoid organs.

7. B lymphocytes synthesize and secrete antibodies; T lymphocytes do not make antibodies. However, T lymphocytes participate in cell-mediated immunity; they "help" B cells make antibodies; they also participate in various regulatory aspects of the immune response by releasing soluble factors lymphokines.

8. Macrophages constitute an essential part of the reticuloendothelial system and function to trap, process, and present antigen to T lymphocytes, thus assuming an important function in innate as well as acquired immunity.

REFERENCES

Duijvestin A, Hamann A (1989): Mechanism and regulation of lymphocyte migration. Immunol Today 10:23.

Gallatin M, St John TP, Siegelman M, Reichert R, Butcher CE, Weissman I (1986): Lymphocyte homing receptors. Cell 44:673.

Mackay CR, Imhof BA (1993): Cell adhesion in the immune system. Immunol Today 14:99.

Miller JFAP (1993): The role of the thymus in immunity—thirty years of progress. The Immunologist 1:9.

Möller G (ed) (1989): Lymphocyte homing. Immunol Rev 108:5.

Picker LJ, Seigelman MH (1993): Lymphoid tissue and organs. In Paul WE (ed): Fundamental Immunology, 3rd ed. New York: Raven Press.

Shemizu Y, Newman W, Tanaka Y, Shaw S (1992): Lymphocyte interaction with endothelial cells. Immunology Today 13:106.

Strober W, James SP (1994): The mucosal immune system. In Stites DP, Terr IA, Parslow TG (eds): Basic and Clinical Immunology, 8th ed. Norwalk, CT: Appleton & Lange.

Van Furth R (1985): Mononuclear Phagocytes—Characteristics, Physiology and Function. Boston: Martinus Nijhoff.

REVIEW QUESTIONS

> For each question, choose the ONE BEST answer or completion.

1. Which of the following generally *does not* apply to *both* primary and secondary lymphoid organs:
   A) cellular proliferation
   B) differentiation of lymphocytes
   C) cellular interaction
   D) antigen-dependent response
   E) none of the above

2. Which of the following apply uniquely to secondary lymphoid organs:
   A) antigen-dependent response
   B) circulation of lymphocytes
   C) terminal differentiation
   D) cellular proliferation
   E) A and B are correct
   F) A and C are correct
   G) B and C are correct

3. Which of the following does not apply to "innate" immune mechanisms:
   A) absence of specificity
   B) activation by a stimulus
   C) involvement of multiple cell types
   D) a memory component

4. Which of the following is the major function of the lymphoid system:
   A) innate immunity
   B) inflammation
   C) phagocytosis
   D) acquired immunity

   E) none of the above
   F) all of the above

5. Removal of the bursa of Fabricius from a chicken results in
   A) a markedly decreased number of circulating T lymphocytes
   B) anemia
   C) delayed rejection of skin graft
   D) low serum levels of antibodies in serum
   E) all of the above
   F) none of the above

6. The germinal centers found in the cortical region of lymph nodes and the peripheral region of splenic periarteriolar lymphatic tissue
   A) support the development of immature B and T cells
   B) function in the removal of damaged erythrocytes from the circulation
   C) act as the major source of stem cells and thus help to maintain hematopoiesis
   D) provide an infrastructure that on antigenic stimulation contains large populations of B lymphocytes and plasma cells
   E) are the sites of NK-cell differentiation

7. Which of the following is correct:
   A) NK cells proliferate in response to antigen
   B) NK cells kill their target cells by phagocytosis and intracellular digestion
   C) NK cells are a subset of polymorphonuclear cells
   D) NK-cell killing is extracellular
   E) NK cells are particularly effective against certain bacteria
   F) all of the above

ANSWERS TO REVIEW QUESTIONS

1. **D** Cellular proliferation, differentiation of lymphocyte, and cellular interactions can take place in primary lymphoid organs (bursa of Fabricius or equivalent, thymus gland). However, antigen-dependent responses occur in the secondary lymphoid organs, such as the spleen and lymph nodes.

2. **F** Antigen-dependent responses of proliferation and differentiation (as well as terminal differentiation of B cells into plasma cells) occur only in secondary lymphoid organs, such as the spleen and lymph nodes. However, circulation of lymphocytes and cellular proliferation (but not antigen-dependent responses of terminal differentiation) also take place in the primary lymphoid organs, such as the bursa of Fabricius, or its equivalent, and the thymus.

3. **D** Innate immunity has none of the antigenic specificity exhibited by acquired immunity. It is activated by such stimuli as the invasion of foreign particles into the body. Innate immunity involves multiple cell types, such as those of the monocytic series (macrophages) and those of the granulocytic series (neutrophils, eosinophils, etc.).

4. **D** The major function of the lymphoid system is the recognition of foreign antigen by lymphocytes, which leads to the acquired immune response. Functions such as phagocytosis and inflammation do not necessarily require the lymphoid system, and they constitute part of innate immunity.

5. **D** Removal of the bursa of Fabricius from a chicken results in low levels of antibodies in serum, since this organ serves as a primary lymphoid organ in which B lymphocytes (which eventually synthesize and secrete antibodies) undergo maturation. The removal of the organ will not result in a marked decrease in the number of circulating lymphocytes, nor will it result in anemia, characterized by a marked decrease in erythrocyte count, since erythrocytes undergo maturation outside the bursa. The question has no relevance to delayed rejection of skin grafts.

6. **D** On antigenic stimulation, the germinal centers contain large populations of B lymphocytes undergoing mitosis and plasma cells secreting antibodies. Virgin immunocompetent lymphocytes are developed in the primary lymphoid organs, not in the secondary lymphoid organs, such as the spleen and lymph nodes. Germinal centers do not participate in the removal of damaged erythrocytes, nor are

they a source of stem cells, the latter found in the bone marrow.

7. **D** NK cells are large granular lymphocytes. Their number does not increase in response to antigen. Their killing is extracellular, and their target cells are virus-infected cells or tumor cells. They are not particularly effective against bacterial cells.

IMMUNOGENS AND ANTIGENS

INTRODUCTION

Acquired immune responses arise as a result of exposure to foreign stimuli. The compound that evokes the response is referred to either as "antigen" or as "immunogen." The distinction between these terms is functional. An ***immunogen*** is any agent capable of inducing an immune response. In contrast, an ***antigen*** is any agent capable of binding specifically to components of the immune response, such as lymphocytes and antibodies. The distinction between the terms is necessary because there are many compounds that are incapable of inducing an immune response, yet they are capable of binding with components of the immune system that have been induced specifically against them. Thus, all immunogens are antigens, but not all antigens need be immunogens. This difference becomes obvious in the case of low-molecular-weight compounds, a group of substances that includes many antibiotics and drugs. By themselves, these compounds are incapable of inducing an immune response, but when they are coupled with much larger entities, such as proteins, the resultant conjugate induces an immune response that is directed against various parts of the conjugate, including the low-molecular-weight compound. When manipulated in this manner, the low-molecular-weight compound is referred to as a ***hapten*** (from the Greek *hapten,* which means to grasp); the high-molecular-weight compound to which the hapten is conjugated is referred to as a ***carrier***. Thus, a hapten is a compound that, by itself, is incapable of inducing an immune response, but against which an immune response can be induced by immunization with the hapten conjugated to a carrier.

In the present chapter we deal with some attributes of compounds that render them immunogenic and antigenic.

REQUIREMENTS FOR IMMUNOGENICITY

A substance must possess the following three characteristics to be immunogenic: (1) ***foreignness,*** (2) ***high molecular weight,*** and (3) ***chemical complexity***.

Foreignness

Animals normally do not respond immunologically to *"self."* Thus, for example, if a rabbit is injected with its own serum albumin, it will not mount an immune response; it recognizes the albumin as self. In contrast, if rabbit serum albumin is injected into a guinea pig, the guinea pig recognizes the rabbit serum albumin as *"foreign"* and mounts an immune response against it. To prove that the rabbit, which did not respond to its own serum albumin, is immunologically competent, it can be injected with guinea pig albumin. The competent rabbit will mount an immune response to guinea pig serum albumin because it recognizes the substance as foreign. Thus, the first requirement for a compound to be immunogenic is foreignness. The more foreign the substance, the more immunogenic it is.

In general, compounds that are part of self are not immunogenic to the individual. However, there are exceptional cases in which an individual mounts an immune response against his or her own tissues. This condition is termed ***autoimmunity*** (see Chapter 17).

High Molecular Weight

The second requirement that determines whether a compound is immunogenic is that it must have a certain minimal molecular weight. In general, compounds that have a molecular weight of less than 1000 daltons (e.g., penicillin, progesterone, aspirin) are not immunogenic; those of molecular weight between 1000 and 6000 daltons [e.g., insulin, adrenocorticotropic hormone (ACTH)] may or may not be immunogenic; and those of molecular weight ***greater than 6000 daltons*** (e.g., albumin, tetanus toxin) ***are generally immunogenic***.

Chemical Complexity

The third characteristic necessary for a compound to be immunogenic is a certain degree of physicochemical complexity. Thus, for example, various homopolymers of amino acids, such as a polymer of lysine of molecular weight 30,000 daltons, are seldom good immunogens. Similarly, a homopolymer of poly-γ-D-glutamic acid (the capsular material of *Bacillus anthracis*) of molecular weight 50,000 daltons is not immunogenic. This absence of immunogenicity is because these compounds, although of high molecular weight, are not sufficiently chemically complex. However, if the complexity is increased by the attachment of various moieties, such as dinitrophenol or other low-molecular-weight compounds, which by themselves are not immunogenic, to the epsilon amino group of polylysine, the entire macromolecule becomes immunogenic. The resulting immune response is directed not only against the coupled low-molecular-weight compounds but also against the high-molecular-weight homopolymer. In general, an increase in the chemical complexity of a compound is accompanied by an increase in its immunogenicity. Thus, copolymers of several amino acids such as polyglutamic, alanine, and lysine (poly-GAT) are highly immunogenic.

For immunogenicity, the substance must have all three of these characteristics; it must be foreign to the individual to whom it is administered, be of a relatively high molecular weight, and possess a certain degree of chemical complexity.

Haptens

Haptens are low-molecular-weight compounds that are not immunogenic but become immunogenic if they are ***conjugated*** to high-molecular-weight ***carriers***. Thus, an immune response can be evoked to thousands of chemical compounds— those of high molecular weight and those of low molecular weight.

Immune responses have been demonstrated against all the known biochemical families of compounds—carbohydrates, lipids, proteins, and nucleic acids— as well as to drugs, antibiotics, food additives, cosmetics, and small synthetic peptides. Immunogenicity, in every case, is conferred by fulfillment of the three criteria: foreignness, high molecular weight, and chemical complexity.

Further Requirements for Immunogenicity

In addition to the above characteristics, several other factors play roles in determining whether a substance is immunogenic. These include the susceptibility of the substance to enzymatic degradation and the genetic makeup of the immunized animal. Regarding susceptibility to enzymatic degradation, on one hand the substance has to be sufficiently stable so that it can reach the site of interaction with B cells or T cells necessary for the immune response; on the other hand—and this is particularly true for proteins—the substance must be susceptible to partial enzymatic degradation that takes place during antigen "processing" by presenting cells such as macrophages. Indeed, it has been repeatedly demonstrated that peptides composed of D-amino acids, which are resistant to enzymatic degradation, are not immunogenic whereas their L-isomers are susceptible to enzymes and are immunogenic. The antigen-presenting cells have structures referred to as MHC (major histocompatibility complex) proteins to which "processed" fragments of the protein can bind noncovalently. This complex is "presented" to receptors on T cells that in turn are activated. This mechanism is discussed in detail in Chapters 10 and 11. These observations are of particular importance with respect to proteins. In contrast, carbohydrates are not processed or presented and are thus unable to activate T cells, although they can activate B cells. Finally, the genetic makeup of the immunized individual plays an important role in determining whether a given substance is immunogenic. Such genetically determined factors as the composition of the MHC molecules on antigen-presenting cells, and the B- and T-cell repertoires are crucial.

The stringent requirements given above constitute a portion of the delicate control mechanisms, expanded and elaborated in subsequent chapters, which on one hand trigger the acquired immune response and on the other hand protect the individual from responding to substances in cases where such responses are detrimental.

PRIMARY AND SECONDARY RESPONSES

The first exposure of an individual to an immunogen is referred to as the ***priming immunization.*** As we shall see in subsequent chapters, many events take place during this primary immunization—cells "process" antigen, triggering antigen-specific lymphocytes to proliferate and differentiate. T-lymphocyte subsets interact with other subsets and induce the latter to differentiate into T lymphocytes with specialized function. T lymphocytes also interact with B lymphocytes, inducing them to synthesize and secrete antibodies. The first measurable immune response is called the ***primary response.***

A second exposure to the same immunogen results in a ***secondary response.***

This second exposure may occur after the response to the first immune event has leveled off or has totally subsided (within weeks or even years). The secondary response differs from the primary response in many respects. Most notably and biologically relevant is the much *quicker onset* and the much *higher magnitude* of the response. In a sense, this secondary (and subsequent) exposure behaves as if the body "remembers" that it had been previously exposed to that same immunogen. For this reason the secondary response is also called the *memory* or *anamnestic* response and the B and T lymphocytes that participate in the memory response are termed *memory cells.* The kinetics of the antibody production following immunization is given in detail in Chapter 5 text and Figure 5.2. The cellular T-cell responses after primary and secondary immunization follow similar patterns, with a greatly hightened response following the secondary immunization.

ANTIGENICITY

An immune response induced by an antigen generates antibodies or lymphocytes that react specifically with the antigen. The antigen-binding site of an antibody or a receptor on a lymphocyte has a unique structure that allows a complementary "fit" to some structural aspect of the specific antigen. As alluded to earlier, the portion of the antigen that binds specifically with the binding site of an antibody or a receptor on a lymphocyte is termed an antigenic determinant or epitope.

Various studies indicate that the size of an epitope that combines with antibody is approximately equivalent to 5–7 amino acids, or roughly $7 \times 12 \times 35$ Å. These dimensions were calculated from experiments that involved the binding of antibodies to polysaccharides, as well as to peptide epitopes. Such dimensions would also be expected to correspond roughly to the size of the complementary antibody-combining site, termed *paratope,* and indeed this expectation has been confirmed by X-ray crystallography. Since the antigen-specific receptors on B cells are immunoglobulin molecules, the size of an epitope interacting with a B-cell receptor is roughly equivalent to 5–7 amino acid residues.

The size of an epitope that binds to a specific T cell is somewhat larger since it contains an area that binds to the MHC proteins of the antigen-presenting cell (an area referred to as *agretope*) and an area that binds to the specific receptor on the T cell, forming a trimolecular complex. Thus the size of the epitope (including the agretope) is approximately equivalent to 10–15 amino acid residues.

EPITOPES RECOGNIZED BY B CELLS AND T CELLS

It was demonstrated over 20 years ago that when the peptide glucagon (a pancreatic hormone used as a model antigen) was used to immunize an inbred strain of guinea pigs, the antibody response was directed to the N-terminal half and the T-cell response directed to the C-terminal half of the peptide, implying that B and T cells recognize different epitopes. However, when the same peptide was used to immunize guinea pigs of different inbred strains, the recognition was reversed, implying that there really were not different physicochemical attributes that distinguished the interaction with B or T cells. Other examples exist that point out that B cells and T cells can recognize the same epitope. These examples notwithstanding, there is a large body of evidence pointing out that the properties of many epitopes recognized by B cells differ from those recognized by T cells.

In general, B cells with their membrane-bound antibody, which serve as epitope receptors, recognize and bind free antigen in solution. Thus, the epitopes on the antigen must be on the "outside" of the molecule, accessible for interaction with the receptor. Terminal side chains of polysaccharides and hydrophilic portions on protein molecules generally constitute B-cell epitopes. On the other hand, the interaction of epitope with the T-cell receptor requires prior "processing" of the antigen, and the association of an area of the processed antigen with MHC molecules present on the surface of the antigen-presenting cell. Generally such "processed" epitopes are internal denatured linear hydrophobic areas of proteins. Polysaccharides do not yield such areas and indeed are not known to bind or activate T cells. In contrast, such areas are obtained following processing of proteins. Thus polysaccharides contain solely B-cell recognizable epitopes whereas proteins contain both B- and T-cell recognizable epitopes.

With respect to their epitopes, antigens may have the characteristics shown schematically in Figure 3.1. Thus, they may consist of a single epitope (hapten) or have varying numbers of the same epitope on the same molecule (polysaccharides). The most common antigens (proteins) have varying numbers of different epitopes on the same molecule.

MAJOR CLASSES OF ANTIGENS

The following major chemical families may be antigenic:

1. *Carbohydrates (polysaccharides).* Polysaccharides are potentially, but not always, immunogenic. Normally, polysaccharides, which form part of more

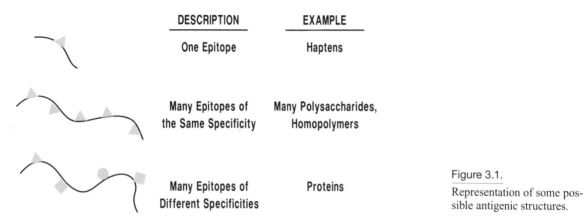

DESCRIPTION	EXAMPLE
One Epitope	Haptens
Many Epitopes of the Same Specificity	Many Polysaccharides, Homopolymers
Many Epitopes of Different Specificities	Proteins

Figure 3.1.
Representation of some possible antigenic structures.

complex molecules such as cell-surface *glycoproteins,* elicit an immune response, part of which is directed specifically against the polysaccharide moiety of the molecule. An immune response, consisting primarily of antibodies, can be induced against many kinds of polysaccharide molecules, such as components of microorganisms and of eukaryotic cells. An excellent example of antigenicity of polysaccharides is the immune response associated with the ***ABO blood groups,*** which are polysaccharides on the surface of the red blood cells (see Chapter 19).

2. *Lipids*. Lipids are rarely immunogenic, but an immune response to lipids may be induced if the lipids are conjugated to protein carriers. Thus, in a sense, lipids may be regarded as haptens. Immune responses to **sphingolipids** have been reported.

3. *Nucleic acids*. Nucleic acids are poor immunogens by themselves, but they become immunogenic when they are conjugated to protein carriers. DNA, in its native helical state, is usually nonimmunogenic in normal animals. However, immune responses to nucleic acids have been reported in many instances. One important example in clinical medicine is the appearance of anti-DNA antibodies in patients with **systemic lupus erythematosus** (discussed in detail in Chapter 17).

4. *Proteins*. Virtually all proteins are immunogenic. Thus, the most common immune responses are those to proteins. Furthermore, the greater the degree of complexity of the protein, the more vigorous will be the immune response to that protein. In general, proteins are multideterminant antigens.

The acquired immune response recognizes many structural features and physicochemical properties of compounds. For example, antibodies can recognize various structural features of a protein, such as its ***primary structure*** (the amino acid sequence), ***secondary structures*** (the structure of the backbone of the polypeptide chain, such as an α-helix or β-pleated sheet), ***tertiary structures*** (formed by the three-dimensional configuration of the protein, which is conferred by the folding of the polypeptide chain and held by disulfide bridges, hydrogen bonds, hydrophobic interactions, etc.), and ***quaternary structures*** (formed by the juxtaposition of separate parts if the molecule is composed of more than one protein subunit).

BINDING OF ANTIGEN WITH ANTIGEN-SPECIFIC ANTIBODIES OR T CELLS

The binding between antigen and antibodies is discussed in detail in Chapter 7. The interactions of antigen with both B and T cells are discussed in Chapter 10. At this point, it is important to emphasize only that the binding of antigen with antibodies or immunocompetent cells does not involve covalent bonds. The binding may involve ***electrostatic interactions, hydrophobic interactions, hydrogen bonds,*** and ***van der Waals forces.*** Since these interactive forces are relatively weak, the "fit" between antigen and its complementary site on the antigen receptor must occur over an area large enough to allow the summation of all the possible available interactions. This requirement is the basis for the exquisite specificity observed in immunologic interactions.

CROSS-REACTIVITY

Since macromolecular antigens contain several distinct epitopes, some of these macromolecules can be altered without totally changing the immunogenic and antigenic structure of the entire molecule. This concept is important in relation to immunization against highly pathogenic microorganisms or highly toxic compounds. For example, a lethal dose of tetanus toxin for mice is measured in picograms (10^{-12} g), while a dose required for immunization is measured in micrograms (10^{-6} g). Obviously, immunization with the toxin is unwise. However, it is possible to destroy the biological activity of this and a broad variety of other toxins (e.g., bacterial toxins and snake venoms) without appreciably affecting their antigenicity or immunogenicity. A toxin that has been modified to the extent that it is no longer toxic but still maintains some of its immunochemical characteristics is called a ***toxoid***. Thus we can say that a toxoid ***cross-reacts*** immunologically with the toxin. Accordingly, it is possible to immunize individuals with the toxoid and thereby induce immune responses to some of the epitopes that the toxoid still shares with the native toxin, because these epitopes have not been destroyed by the modification. Although the molecules of toxin and toxoid differ in many physicochemical and biological respects, they nevertheless cross-react immunologically: they share enough epitopes to allow the immune response to the toxoid to mount an effective defense against the toxin itself. An immunologic reaction in which the immune components, either cells or antibodies, react with two molecules that share epitopes, but are otherwise dissimilar, is called a ***cross-reaction***. When two compounds cross-react immunologically, the compounds will have one or more epitopes in common and the immune response to one of the compounds will recognize one or more of the same epitope(s) on the other compound and react with it. Another form of cross-reactivity is seen when antibodies or cells with specificity to one epitope bind, usually more weakly, to another epitope that is not quite identical, but has a structural resemblance, to the first epitope. To denote that the antigen used for immunization is different from the one with which the induced immune components are then allowed to react, the terms ***homologous*** and ***heterologous*** are used. ***Homologous*** denotes that the antigen and the immunogen are the same; ***heterologous*** denotes that the substance used to induce the immune response is different from the substance that is then used to react with the products of the induced response. In the latter case, the heterologous antigen may or may not react with the immune components. If reaction does take place, it may be concluded that the heterologous and homologous antigens exhibit ***immunologic cross-reactivity***.

Although the hallmark of immunology is specificity, immunologic cross-reactivity has been observed on many levels. This does not mean that the immunologic specificity has been diminished, but rather that the substances that cross-react share antigenic determinants. In cases of cross-reactivity, the antigenic determinants of the cross-reacting substances may have identical chemical structures, or they may be composed of similar but not identical physicochemical configurations. In the example described above, a toxin and its corresponding toxoid represent two molecules, the toxin being the ***native*** molecule and the toxoid being a ***modified*** molecule that cross-reacts with the native molecule.

There are other examples of immunologic cross-reactivity, wherein the two cross-reacting substances are unrelated to each other except that they have one or more epitopes in common, specifically, one or more areas that have similar three-dimensional characteristics. These substances are referred to as ***heterophile*** *antigens.* For example, human blood group A antigen reacts with antiserum raised against pneumococcal capsular polysaccharide (type XIV). Similarly, human blood group B antigen reacts with antibodies to certain strains of *Escherichia coli.* In these examples of cross-reactivity, the antigens of the microorganisms are referred to as the heterophile antigens (with respect to the blood group antigen).

IMMUNOLOGIC ADJUVANTS

To enhance the immune response to a given immunogen, various additives or vehicles are often used. An *adjuvant* is a substance that, when mixed with an immunogen, enhances the immune response against the immunogen. It is important to distinguish between a carrier for a hapten and an adjuvant. A hapten will become immunogenic when conjugated covalently to a carrier; it will not become immunogenic if mixed with an adjuvant. Thus, an adjuvant enhances the immune response to immunogens but does not confer immunogenicity to haptens.

There are various widely used adjuvants. One such adjuvant is *Freund's complete adjuvant (FCA),* which consists of a water-in-oil emulsion and killed *Mycobacterium tuberculosis* or *M. butyricum.* The antigen is contained in the water phase. Other microorganisms used as adjuvants are *BCG (bacille Calmette-Guérin,* an attenuated *Mycobacterium*), *Corynebacterium parvum,* and *Bordetella pertussis.* These adjuvants are presumed to release antigen slowly but continuously and to stimulate macrophages to take up, process, and present antigen to T lymphocytes as well as upregulation of expression of costimulatory molecules (discussed in detail in Chapters 10 and 11), which are essential for T-cell activation. Other adjuvants used are bacterial endotoxins and *lipopolysaccharide (LPS),* and still others contain a synthetic *muramyldipeptide* [N-acetyl-muramyl-L-alanyl-D-isoglutamine (MDP)]. In the mouse, LPS enhances the antibody response by stimulating a subpopulation of lymphocytes (B cells), while muramyldipeptide, the effective constituent of mycobacterial cell walls, stimulates macrophages and T cells.

The most widely used adjuvant in humans is *alum precipitate,* a suspension of aluminum hydroxide on which the antigen is absorbed. This adjuvant causes aggregation of a soluble antigen and allows continuous slow release of antigen. In addition, it has a slight irritant effect that enhances the ingestion and processing of antigen by macrophages which present the antigen to T cells, leading to T-cell activation.

SUMMARY

1. Immunologically, a compound may have one or both of the following two major attributes:

a) *Immunogenicity*—the capacity to induce an immune response. Immunogenicity requires that a compound (i) be foreign to the immunized individual, (ii) possesses a certain minimal molecular weight, and (iii) possesses a certain degree of chemical complexity.

b) *Antigenicity*—the ability to bind with antibodies or with cells of the immune system. This binding is highly specific; the immune components are capable of recognizing various physicochemical aspects of the compound. The binding between antigen and immune components involves several weak forces operating over short distances (van der Waals forces, electrostatic interactions, hydrophobic interactions, and hydrogen bonds); it does not involve covalent bonds.

2. The smallest unit of antigen that is capable of binding with antibodies is called an *antigenic determinant* or *epitope*. Compounds may have one or more epitopes capable of reacting with immune components. The immune response against these compounds involves the production of antibodies or the generation of cells with specificities directed against most or all of the epitopes.

3. Immunologic cross-reactivity denotes a situation in which two or more substances, which may have various degrees of dissimilarity, share epitopes and would, therefore, react with the immune components induced against any one of these substances. Thus, a toxoid, which is a modified form of toxin, may have one or more epitopes in common with the toxin. Immunization with the toxoid leads to an immune response capable of reacting not only with the toxoid but also with the native toxin.

REFERENCES

Atassi MZ (ed) (1977): Immunochemistry of Proteins, Vols 1 and 2. New York: Plenum Press.

Benjamin DC, Berzofsky JA, East IJ, Gurd FRN, Hannum C, Leach SJ, Margoliash E, Michael JG, Miller A, Prager EM, Reichlin M, Sercarz EE, Smith-Gill SJ, Todd PE, Wilson AC (1984): The antigenic structure of proteins: a reappraisal. Annu Rev Immunol 2:67.

Berzofsky JA, Berkower IJ (1993): Immunogenicity and antigen structure. In Paul WE (ed): Fundamental Immunology, 3rd ed. New York: Raven Press.

Berzofsky JA, Cease KB, Cornette JL, Spouge JL, Margalit H, Berkower IJ, Good FM, Miller LH, DeLisi C (1987): Protein antigenic structures recognized by T cells: potential applications to vaccine design. Immunol Rev 98:9.

Hopp TP, Woods KR (1981): Prediction of protein antigenic determinants from amino acid sequences. Proc Natl Acad Sci (USA) 78:3824.

Lerner RA (1983): Synthetic vaccines. Sci Am 248:66.

Novotny J, Handschumacher H, Bruccoleri RE (1987): Protein antigenicity: A static surface property. Immunol Today 8:26.

Sercarz EE, Berzofsky A (eds) (1987): Immunogenicity of Protein Anitgens: Repertoire and Regulation. Boca Raton, FL: CRC Press.

Rothbard JB, Gefter ML (1991): Interactions between immunogenic peptides and MHC proteins. Annu Rev Immunol 9:527.

REVIEW QUESTIONS

For each question, choose the ONE BEST answer or completion.

1. The following properties render a substance immunogenic:
   A) high molecular weight
   B) chemical complexity
   C) sufficient stability and persistence after injection
   D) all of the above
   E) all of the above are essential but not sufficient

2. The protection against smallpox afforded by prior infection with cowpox represents
   A) antigenic specificity
   B) antigenic cross-reactivity
   C) enhanced viral uptake by macrophages
   D) innate immunity
   E) passive protection

3. Converting a toxin to a toxoid
   A) makes the toxin more immunogenic
   B) reduces the pharmacologic activity of the toxin
   C) enhances binding with antitoxin
   D) induces only innate immunity
   E) increases phagocytosis

4. Haptens
   A) require carrier molecules in order to be immunogenic
   B) will not react with specific antibodies in vitro unless homologous carriers are employed
   C) interact with specific antibody even if the hapten is monovalent
   D) can stimulate secondary antibody responses without carriers
   E) A and B are correct
   F) A and C are correct
   G) B and C are correct
   H) B and D are correct

5. An immunologic adjuvant is a substance that
   A) reduces the toxicity of the immunogen
   B) enhances the immunogenicity of haptens
   C) enhances hematopoiesis
   D) enhances the immune response against the immunogen
   E) enchances immunologic cross-reactivity

6. An antibody made against the antigen tetanus toxoid (TT) reacts with it even when the TT is denatured by disrupting all disulfide bonds. Another antibody against TT fails to react when the TT is similarly denatured. The most likely explanation is
   A) the first antibody is not specific for TT
   B) the second antibody is specific for conformational determinants on TT
   C) the second antibody is specific for disulfide bonds
   D) the first antibody is specific for the primary amino acid sequence of TT
   E) B and D are correct
   F) A and C are correct
   G) C and D are correct

ANSWERS TO REVIEW QUESTIONS

1. **E** All of the properties are essential but not sufficient, since for immunogenicity the substance must be foreign to the immunized individual.

2. **B** The protection against smallpox provided by prior infection with cowpox is an example of antigenic cross-reactivity. Immunization with cowpox leads to the production of antibodies capable of reacting with smallpox because the two viruses share several identical, or structurally similar, determinants.

3. **B** Conversion of a toxin to a toxoid is performed in order to reduce the pharmacologic activity of the toxin, so that sufficient toxoid can be injected to induce an immune response.

4. **F** Haptens are substances, usually of low molecular weight and univalent, that by themselves cannot induce an immune response, but can do so if conjugated to high-molecular-weight carriers. The haptens can and do interact with the induced antibodies, without it being necessary that they be conjugated to the carrier. Thus **A** and **C** are correct, and the one best answer is **F**.

5. **D** An immunologic adjuvant is a substance that, when mixed with an immunogen, enhances the immune response against that immunogen. It does not enhance cross-reactivity, nor does it enhance hematopoiesis. An adjuvant does not enhance the immune response against a hapten, which requires its conjugation to an immunogenic carrier in order to induce a response against the hapten. The adjuvant has no relevance to possible toxicity of an immunogen.

6. **E** Antibodies can recognize primary sequence structures or secondary, tertiary, and quaternary conformational structures. Denaturing a protein by disrupting disulfide bonds generally destroys conformational determinants. Therefore it is likely that the first antibody reacts with a primary amino acid sequence determinant that is present on both native and denatured TT while the second antibody sees a conformational determinant only on native TT. Accordingly, **B** and **D** are correct and the one best answer is **E**.

ANTIBODY STRUCTURE

INTRODUCTION

One of the major functions of the immune system is the production of soluble proteins that circulate freely and exhibit properties that contribute specifically to immunity and protection against foreign material. These soluble proteins are the *antibodies,* which belong to the class of proteins called *globulins* because of their globular structure. Initially, owing to their migratory properties in an electrophoretic field, they were called γ-globulins (in relation to the more rapidly migrating albumin, α-globulin, and β-globulin); today they are known collectively as *immunoglobulins (Ig).*

The structure of immunoglobulins incorporates several features essential for their participation in the immune response. The two most important of these features are *specificity* and *biologic activity*. Specificity is attributed to a defined region of the antibody molecule and restricts the antibody to combine only with those substances that contain one particular antigenic structure. The existence of a vast array of potential antigenic determinants or epitopes (see Chapter 3) has necessitated the evolution of a system for producing a *repertoire* of antibody molecules, each of which is capable of combining with a particular antigenic structure. Thus, antibodies collectively exhibit great diversity, in terms of the types of molecular structure with which they are capable of reacting, but individually they exhibit a high degree of specificity, since each is able to react with only one particular antigenic structure.

Despite the large numbers of different specific individual antibodies capable of reacting with many different structural entities, the biologic effects of such reactions are rather few in number (e.g., complement fixation, crossing of the placenta, activation of mast cells). Therefore, while one part of the antibody molecule must be adaptable to allow the accommodation of a large number of epitopes, another part of the antibody molecule must be adaptable to allow the antibody molecule to participate in biologic activities common to many antibodies. This chapter and Chapter 5 deal with the ways in which the antibody molecule fulfills these two functions.

ISOLATION AND CHARACTERIZATION

Serum is the residue that is left when blood has clotted and the clot, which contains cells and clotting factors, is removed. When serum is subjected to *electrophoresis* (separation in an electrical field) at slightly alkaline pH (8.2), five major components can normally be visualized (see Fig. 4.1). The slowest, in terms of migration toward the anode, called γ-globulin, was shown by Kabat and Tiselius in 1939 to contain antibody. This demonstration entailed the simple comparison of the electrophoretic pattern of antiserum from a hyperimmune rabbit before and after the specific antibody had been removed by precipitation with the antigen. Only the size

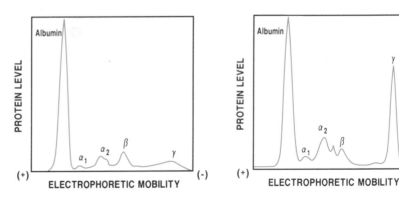

Figure 4.1.

Electrophoretic mobility of serum proteins obtained from a normal individual (left) and from a patient with IgG myeloma (right). (Courtesy of Dr. C. Miller, School of Medicine, University of California, Davis.)

of the γ-globulin fraction was diminished by this procedure. Analysis showed that when this fraction was collected separately, all measurable antibodies were contained within it. Later it was shown that antibody activity is present not only in the γ-globulin fraction but also in a slightly more anodic area. Consequently, all globular proteins with antibody activity are generically referred to as immunoglobulins (Ig), as exemplified by the γ peak (see Fig. 4.1).

From the broad electrophoretic peaks, it is clear that a ***heterogeneous*** collection of immunoglobulin molecules with slightly different charges is present. This heterogeneity was one of the early obstacles in attempts to determine the structure of antibodies, since analytical chemistry requires homogeneous, crystallizable compounds as starting material. This problem was solved, in part, by the discovery of ***myeloma proteins,*** which are homogeneous immunoglobulins produced by the progeny of a single plasma cell that has become neoplastic and reproduced itself numerous times in the malignant disease called ***multiple myeloma***. This is nicely demonstrated by the γ-globulin spike in the electrophoretic pattern of serum proteins of a patient with multiple myeloma (see Fig. 4.1). When it became clear that some myeloma proteins bound antigen, it also became apparent that they could be dealt with as typical immunoglobulin molecules.

Another aid to structural studies of antibodies was the discovery of ***Bence–Jones proteins*** in the urine. These homogeneous proteins, produced in large quantities by some patients with multiple myeloma, are ***dimers of immunoglobulin*** κ or λ ***light chains***. They were very useful in the determination of the structure of this portion of the immunoglobulin molecule. Today, the powerful technique of cell–cell hybridization (hybridomas) permits the production of large quantities of homogeneous preparations of monoclonal antibody of virtually any specificity (see Chapter 7).

STRUCTURE OF LIGHT AND HEAVY CHAINS

The analysis of the structure of antibody molecules really began in 1959 with two discoveries that, for the first time, revealed that the molecule could be separated into analyzable parts suitable for further study. In England, Porter found that proteolytic treatment with the enzyme papain split the immunoglobulin molecule (molecular weight 150,000 daltons) into three fragments of about equal size (see Fig. 4.2). Two of these fragments were found to retain the antibody's ability to bind antigen specifically, although, unlike the intact molecule, they could no longer precipitate the antigen from solution. These two fragments are referred to as ***Fab*** (fragment antigen binding) fragments and are considered to be univalent, possessing one binding site each and being in every way identical to each other.

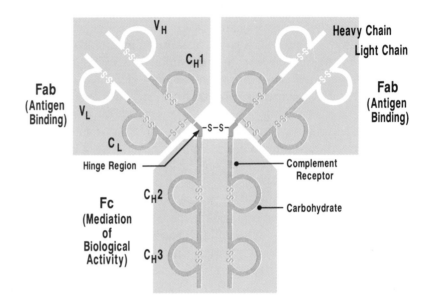

Figure 4.2.

Schematic representation of an immunoglobulin molecule. N-terminus is on top of each chain; C-terminus is at the bottom of each chain.

The third fragment could be crystallized out of solution, a property indicative of its apparent homogeneity. This fragment is called *Fc* (fragment-crystallizable). It cannot bind antigen, but, as was subsequently shown, it is responsible for the biological functions of the antibody molecule after antigen has been bound to the Fab part of the intact molecule.

At about the same time, Edelman in the United States discovered that when γ-globulin was extensively reduced by treatment with mercaptoethanol (a reagent that breaks S–S bonds), the molecule fell apart into four chains: two identical chains with a molecular weight of about 53,000 daltons each and two others of about 22,000 daltons each. The larger chains were designated *heavy (H)* and the smaller ones, *light (L).* On the basis of these results, the structure of immunoglobulin molecules, as depicted in Figure 4.2, was proposed. This model was subsequently shown to be essentially correct, and Porter and Edelman shared the Nobel Prize for the elucidation of antibody structure. Thus, all immunoglobulin molecules consist of a basic unit of four polypeptide chains, *two identical H chains* and *two identical L chains*, held together by a number of disulfide bonds. It should be noted that papain digestion of the immunoglobulin molecule results in cleavage N-terminally to the disulfide bridge between the heavy chains at the "hinge" region, yielding two monovalent Fab fragments and an Fc fragment. On the other hand, pepsin digestion results in cleavage C-terminally to the disulfide bridge, resulting in a divalent fragment referred to as F(ab')$_2$, consisting of two

Fab fragments joined by the disulfide bond and several Fc fragments. It should also be noted that the heavy chain is glycosylated as shown in Figure 4.2.

As is the case with other proteins, immunoglobulins of one species are immunogenic in another species. The use of immunoglobulins of a given species as immunogens in another species allowed the production of a variety of antisera that could distinguish between features of different immunoglobulin chains. By a combination of biochemical and *serologic* (utilizing serum antibodies) techniques, it was shown that almost all species studied have two major classes of L chains, called κ and λ. Any one individual of a species produces both types of L chain, but the ratio of κ chains to λ chains varies with the species (mouse: 95% κ; human: 60% κ). However, in any one immunoglobulin molecule, the L chains are always either both κ or both λ, never one of each.

While there are two types of L chains, the immunoglobulins of virtually all species have been shown to consist of five different *classes (isotypes)* that differ in the structure of their H chains. These H chains differ as antigens (serologically), in carbohydrate content, and in size. Most importantly, they confer different biological functions on each isotype. The H chains, derived from the various immunoglobulin isotypes, are designated with Greek letters, as follows:

Immunoglobulin class (isotype)	Heavy chain
IgM	μ
IgG	γ
IgA	α
IgD	δ
IgE	ε

Again, any individual of a species makes all H chains, in proportions characteristic of the species, but in any one antibody molecule both H chains are identical (i.e., 2γ or 2ϵ, etc.). Thus, an antibody molecule of the IgG class could have the structure $\kappa 2\gamma 2$ or $\lambda 2\gamma 2$, while an antibody of the IgE class could have the structure $\kappa 2\epsilon 2$ or $\lambda 2\epsilon 2$. In each case, it is the nature of the H chains that confers on the molecule its unique biologic properties, such as its half-life in the circulation, its ability to bind to certain receptors, and its ability to activate enzymes (see Chapter 13) on combination with antigen.

Further characterization of these isotypes by specific antisera has led to the designation of several *subclasses* (also referred to as *subisotypes*) that have more subtle differences among themselves. Thus, the major class of human IgG can be subdivided into the subclasses IgG_1, IgG_2, IgG_3, and IgG_4. IgA has been divided similarly into two subclasses, IgA_1 and IgA_2. The subclasses differ from one another in numbers and arrangement of interchain disulfide bonds, as well as by alterations in other structural features. These alterations, in turn, produce some changes in functional properties that will be discussed later.

DOMAINS

Early in the study of the structure of immunoglobulins, it became apparent that, in addition to *inter*chain disulfide bonds that hold together L and H chains, as well as H and H chains, *intra*chain disulfide bonds exist that form loops within the chain. The globular structure of immunoglobulins, and the ability of enzymes to cleave these molecules at very restricted positions into large entities instead of degrading them to oligopeptides and amino acids, is indicative of a very compact structure. Furthermore, the presence of intrachain disulfide bonds at regular, approximately equal intervals of about 100–110 amino acids each leads to the prediction that each loop in the peptide chains should form a compactly folded globular *domain*. In fact, L chains have two domains each, and H chains have four or five domains, separated by a short unfolded stretch (see Fig. 4.2). These configurations have been confirmed by direct observation and by genetic analysis (see Chapter 6).

Immunoglobulin molecules are assemblies of separate domains, each centered on a disulfide bond, and each having so much homology with the others as to suggest that they evolved from a single ancestral gene, which duplicated itself several times and then changed its amino acid sequence to enable the resultant different domains to fulfill different functions. Each domain is designated by a letter that indicates whether it is on an L chain or an H chain and a number that indicates its position. As we shall soon discuss in more detail, the first domain on L and H chains is highly *variable*, in terms of amino acid sequence, from one antibody to the next, and it is designated V_L or V_H accordingly (see Fig. 4.2). The second and subsequent domains on both chains are much more constant in amino acid sequence and are designated C_L or C_H1, C_H2, and C_H3 (Fig. 4.2). In addition to their interchain disulfide bonding, the globular domains bind to each other in homologous pairs, largely by hydrophobic interactions, as follows: V_H–V_L, C_H1–C_L, C_H2–C_H2, and C_H3–C_H3.

HINGE REGION

In the immunoglobulins (with the possible exception of IgM and IgE), a short additional segment of amino acids is found between the C_H1 and C_H2 regions of the H chains (see Fig. 4.2). This segment is made up predominantly of *cysteine and proline residues*. The cysteines are involved in formation of interchain disulfide bonds, and the proline residues prevent folding in a globular structure. This region of the H chain provides an important characteristic of immunoglobulins. It permits *flexibility* between the two Fab arms of the Y-shaped antibody molecule and is called the *hinge region*. It allows the two Fab arms to open and close to accommodate binding to two epitopes, separated by a fixed distance, as might be found on the surface of a bacterium. Additionally, since this stretch of amino acids is open and as accessible as any other nonfolded peptide, it can be cleaved by proteases, such as papain, to generate the Fab and Fc fragments described above.

VARIABLE REGION

The biological functions of the antibody molecule derive from the properties of a *constant region*, which is identical for antibodies of all specificities within a particular class. It is the variable region that contains the part of molecule which binds with an epitope. A major problem for immunologists was to determine how so many individual specificities, which are required to meet the enormous variety of antigenic challenges, are generated from the variable region. As we shall see in Chapter 6, this issue has been largely resolved.

When the amino acid sequences of proteins of sufficient homogeneity (e.g., myeloma proteins, monoclonal antibodies, Bence–Jones proteins) were determined, it was found that the greatest variability in sequence existed in the N-terminal 110 amino acids of both the L and H chains. Kabat and Wu compared the amino acid sequences of many different V_L and V_H regions. They plotted the variability in the amino acids at each position in the chain and showed that the greatest amount of variability (defined as the ratio of the number of different amino acids at a given position to the frequency of the most common amino acid at that position) occurred in three regions of the L and H chains. These regions are called *hypervariable regions*; the less variable stretches, which occur between these hypervariable regions, are called *framework regions*. It is now clear that the hypervariable regions participate in the binding with antigen and form the region complementary in structure to the antigen epitope. Consequently they are termed *complementarity-determining regions (CDRs)* of the L and H chains: CDR1, CDR2, and CDR3 (see Fig. 4.3).

The hypervariable regions, although separated in the linear, two-dimensional model of the peptide chains, are actually brought together in the folded form of the intact antibody molecule, and together they constitute the *combining site,* which is complementary to the epitope (Fig. 4.4). The variability in these CDRs provides the diversity in the shape of the combining site that is required for the

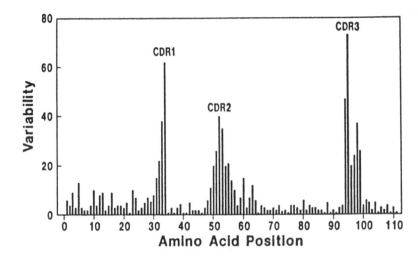

Figure 4.3.

Variability of amino acids representing the N-terminal 110 residues of an immunoglobulin chain.

function of antibodies of different specificities. All the known forces involved in antigen–antibody interactions are weak, noncovalent interactions (e.g., ionic, hydrogen-bonding, and hydrophobic interactions) (see Chapter 7). It is therefore necessary that there be a close fit between antigen and antibody over a sufficiently large region to allow a total binding force that is adequate for stable interaction. Contributions to this binding interaction by both H and L chains are involved in the overall association between epitope and antibody.

It should now be apparent that two antibody molecules with different antigenic specificities must have different amino acid sequences in their hypervariable regions and that those with similar sequences will generally have similar

Figure 4.4.

A schematic representation of the complementarity between an epitope and the antibody combining site consisting of the hypervariable areas of the L and H chains. (Numbered letters denote CDR of H and L chains; circled numbers denote the number of the amino acid residue in the CDRs.)

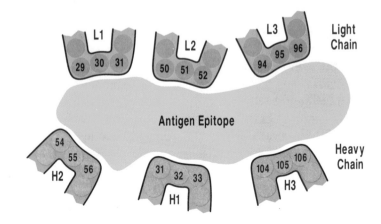

specificities. However, it is possible for two antibodies with different amino acid sequences to have specificity to the same epitope. In this case, the binding affinities of the antibodies with the epitope will probably be different because there will be differences in the number and types of binding forces available to bind identical antigens to the different binding sites of the two antibodies.

An additional source of variability involves the size of the combining site on the antibody, which is usually (but not always) considered to take the form of a depression or cleft. In some instances, especially when small, hydrophobic haptens are involved, the epitopes do not occupy the entire combining site, yet they achieve sufficient affinity of binding. It has been shown that antibodies specific for such a small hapten may, in fact, react with other antigens that have no obvious similarity to the hapten (e.g., dinitrophenol and sheep red cells). These large, dissimilar antigens bind either to a larger area or to a different area of the combining site on the antibody (see Fig. 4.5). Thus, a particular antibody combining site may have the ability to combine with two (or more) apparently diverse epitopes, a property called *redundancy*. The ability of a single antibody molecule to cross-react with an unknown number of epitopes may limit the number of different antibodies needed to defend an individual against the range of antigenic challenges.

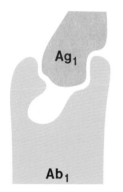
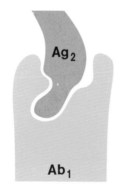

Figure 4.5.

A representation of how an antibody of a given specificity (Ab_1) can exhibit binding with two different epitopes (Ag_1 and Ag_2).

IMMUNOGLOBULIN VARIANTS

Classes of Immunoglobulins

Thus far we have described the features common to all immunoglobulin molecules, such as the four-chain unit and the structural domains. In its defense against invading foreign substances, the body has evolved a variety of mechanisms, each dependent on a somewhat different property or function of an immunoglobulin molecule. Thus, when a specific antibody molecule combines with a specific antigen or a pathogen, several different effector mechanisms come into play. These different mechanisms derive from the different classes of immunoglobulin *(isotypes),* each of which may combine with the same epitope but each of which triggers a different response. These differences result from structural variations in H chains, which have generated domains that mediate a variety of functions. ***The biological properties of each class are fully described in Chapter 5. The structural features are discussed here.*** A summary of the properties of the immunoglobulin classes is given in Tables 5.1 and 5.2.

STRUCTURAL FEATURES OF IgG. IgG is the predominant immunoglobulin in blood, lymph fluid, cerebrospinal fluid, and peritoneal fluid. The IgG molecule consists of two γ H chains of molecular weight approximately 50,000 daltons each and two L chains (either κ or λ) of molecular weight approximately 25,000 daltons each, held together by disulfide bonds (Fig. 4.2). Thus, the IgG molecule has a molecular weight of approximately 150,000 daltons and a sedimentation coefficient of 7S. Electrophoretically, the IgG molecule is the *least* anodic of all serum proteins, and it migrates to the γ range of serum globulins; hence its earlier designation as γ-*globulin* or *7S immunoglobulin*.

The IgG class of immunoglobulins in humans contains four subclasses designated IgG_1, IgG_2, IgG_3, and IgG_4. Except for their variable regions, all the immunoglobulins within a class (e.g., IgG_1 and IgG_2) have about 90% homology in their amino acid sequences, but only 60% homology exists between classes (e.g., IgG and IgA). This degree of homology means that an antiserum to IgG may be produced against a determinant that is common to, and specific for, all members of a given class (e.g., all members of the IgG class) while other antisera may be raised that are specific for determinants found in only one of the subclasses (e.g., in IgG_2). This variation was first detected antigenically by the use of antibodies against various γ chains. The IgG subclasses differ in their chemical properties and, more importantly, in their biological properties, which are discussed in Chapter 5.

STRUCTURAL FEATURES OF IgM. As we shall see in the next chapter, IgM is the first immunoglobulin produced following immunization. Its name derives from its initial description as a *macroglobulin (M)* of high molecular weight (900,000 daltons). It has a sedimentation coefficient of 19S, and it has an extra C_H domain. In comparison to the IgG molecule, which consists of one four-chain structure, the IgM molecule consists of five such units, each of which consists of

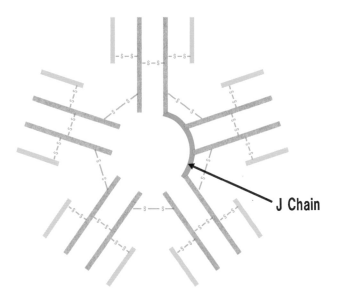

J Chain

Figure 4.6.

A schematic representation of IgM pentamer.

two L and two H chains, all joined together by additional disulfide bonds between their Fc portions and by a polypeptide chain termed the ***J chain*** (see Fig. 4.6). The J chain, which, like L and H chains, is synthesized in the B cell or plasma cell, has a molecular weight of 15,000 daltons. This pentameric ensemble of IgM, which is held together by disulfide bonds, comes apart after mild treatment with reducing agents such as mercaptoethanol.

Surprisingly, each pentameric IgM molecule appears to have a valence of 5 (i.e., five antigen combining sites), instead of the expected valence of 10 predicted by the 10 Fab segments contained in the pentamer. This apparent reduction in valence is probably the result of conformational constraints imposed by the polymerization. It is known that pentameric IgM has a planar configuration, such that each of its 10 Fab portions cannot open fully with respect to the "adjacent" Fab, when it combines with antigen, as is possible in the case of IgG. Thus, any large antigen bound to one Fab may block a neighboring site from binding with antigen, making the molecule appear pentavalent (or of even lesser valence).

STRUCTURAL FEATURES OF IgA. IgA is the major immunoglobulin in ***external secretions*** such as saliva, mucus, sweat, gastric fluid, and tears. It is, moreover, the major immunoglobulin of colostrum and milk, and it may provide the neonate with a major source of intestinal protection against pathogens. The IgA molecule consists of either two κ chains or two λ chains and two H α chains.

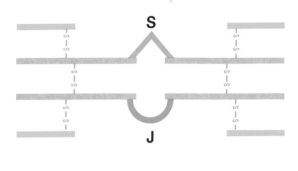

IgA

Figure 4.7.

A schematic representation
of IgA dimer.

The α chain is somewhat larger than the γ chain. The molecular weight of
monomeric IgA is approximately 165,000 daltons, and its sedimentation coefficient is 7S. Electrophoretically it migrates to the slow β or fast γ region of serum
globulins.

IgA, present in *mucous secretions,* exists as a *dimer* consisting of two four-
chain units linked by the same *joining (J) chain* found in IgM molecules (see Fig.
4.7). In addition, mucosal IgA has another attached protein, the *secretory component* (designated S in Fig. 4.7; molecular weight 70,000 daltons). Plasma cells
synthesize only the basic IgA molecules and the J chains, which form the dimers.
When these dimeric molecules are released from plasma cells, they bind to the
basal membranes of adjacent epithelial cells by a receptor on these cells, which is
the secretory component itself. This receptor transports the molecules through the
epithelial cells and releases them into extracellular fluids in fully assembled form
as dimeric IgA, with the secretory component attached.

The IgA present in *serum* is predominantly *monomeric* (one four-chain unit)
and has presumably been released before dimerization so that it fails to bind to
the secretory component. Secretory IgA is very important biologically, but little is
known of any function for serum IgA.

The IgA class of immunoglobulins contains two subclasses: IgA$_1$ (93%) and
IgA$_2$ (7%). It is interesting to note that if all production of IgA on mucosal surfaces (respiratory, gastrointestinal, and urinary tracts) is taken into account, IgA
would be the major immunoglobulin in terms of quantity.

STRUCTURAL FEATURES OF IgD. IgD is present in serum in very low
and variable amounts, probably because it is not secreted by plasma cells and be-

cause, among immunoglobulins, it is uniquely susceptible to proteolytic degradation. It is not known to have any function in serum. However, together with IgM, it has been found to be a major *surface component of many B cells.* Its presence there serves as a marker of the differentiation of B cells to a more mature form, but its exact function as a receptor for triggering or differentiation is still not completely clear.

The IgD molecule consists of either two κ or two λ L chains and two H δ-chains. IgD is present as a monomer with a molecular weight of 180,000 daltons, it has a sedimentation coefficient of 7S, and it migrates to the fast γ-region of serum globulins. No H-chain allotypes (see below) or subclasses have been reported for the IgD molecule.

STRUCTURAL FEATURES OF IgE. The IgE molecule consists of two L chains (κ or λ) and two H ε-chains. Like the IgM molecule, IgE has an extra C_H domain. IgE has a molecular weight of approximately 200,000 daltons, its sedimentation coefficient is 8S, and it migrates electrophoretically to the fast γ-region of serum globulins. To date, no H-chain allotypes or subclasses of IgE have been reported.

IgE, also called *reaginic antibody,* is present in serum in the lowest concentration of all immunoglobulins. Nevertheless, its effects are out of proportion to its concentration in the serum because of the efficiency of its behavior. The H chain of IgE contains an extra domain, by which it attaches with unusually high affinity to specific receptors on *mast cells* and *basophils,* where the IgE molecules may remain for weeks or months. When antigen reappears, it combines with and cross-links the IgE molecules on the surface of mast cells. This event leads to the discharge of the contents of the mast-cell granules and the ensuing symptoms of anaphylaxis (see Chapter 14).

The major biological role of IgE apparently involved in protection against invasion by parasites, such as helminths (worms), a protection achieved by activation of the same acute inflammatory response seen in a more pathologic form in the anaphylactic response.

Allotypes

Another form of variation in the structure of immunoglobulins is allotypy. It is based on genetic differences between individuals. It depends on the existence of allelic forms *(allotypes)* of the same protein, as a result of the presence of different forms of the same gene at a given locus. As a result of allotypy, a particular constituent of any immunoglobulin can be present in some members of a species and absent in others. This situation contrasts with that of immunoglobulin classes or subclasses, which are present in all members of a species.

Allotypic differences at known loci usually involve changes in only one or two amino acids in the constant region of a chain. With a few exceptions, the presence of allotypic differences in two identical immunoglobulin molecules does not generally affect binding with antigen, but it serves as an important marker for analysis of Mendelian inheritance.

Some known allotype markers constitute a group on the γ-chain of human IgG (called *Gm* for IgG markers), a group on the κ chain (formerly called InV, now called *Km*), and a group on the α chain (called *Am*).

Allotypic markers have been found in the immunoglobulins of several species, usually by the use of antisera generated by immunization of one member of a species with antibody from another member of the same species. As with other allelic systems, allotypes are inherited as dominant Mendelian traits. The genes encoding the markers are expressed codominantly, so that an individual may be homozygous or heterozygous for a given marker.

Idiotypes

As we have seen, the combining site of a specific antibody molecule is made up of a unique combination of amino acids in the variable regions of the L and H chains. Since this combination is not present in other antibody molecules, it should, theoretically, be immunogenic and capable of stimulating an immunologic response against itself in an animal of the same species. Such was actually found to be the case by Oudin and Kunkel, who in the early 1960s showed independently that experimental immunization with a particular antibody or myeloma protein could produce an antiserum specific only for the antibody that was used to induce the response and for no other immunoglobulin of the species. These antisera contain populations of antibodies specific for several epitopes, called ***idiotopes,*** which are present in the variable region of the antibody used for inoculation. The collection of all idiotopes on the inoculated antibody molecule is called the ***idiotype (Id)***. In some cases, anti-idiotypic sera prevent binding of the antibody with its antigen, in which event the idiotypic determinant is considered to be in or very near the combining site itself. Anti-idiotypic sera, which do not block binding of antibody with antigen, are probably directed against variable determinants of the framework area, outside the combining site (see Fig. 4.8). On theoretical grounds,

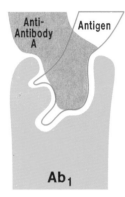 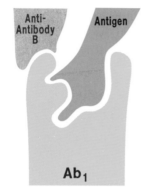

Figure 4.8.

Two anti-idiotypic antibodies to Ab_1. The anti-idiotypic antibody (A) on the left is directed to the combining site of Ab_1, preventing binding of Ab_1 with the antigen. The anti-idiotypic antibody (B) on the right binds with framework areas of Ab_1 and does not prevent its binding with antigen.

it is possible to visualize that an anti-idiotypic antibody with a combining site complementary to that of the idiotype resembles the epitope, which is also complementary to the idiotype's combining site. Thus, the anti-idiotype may represent a facsimile or an *"internal image"* of the nominal epitope. Indeed, there are examples of immunization of experimental animals using anti-idiotypic internal images as immunogens (Chapter 20). Such immunogens induce antibodies capable of reacting with the antigen that carries the epitope to which the original idiotype is directed. Such antibodies are induced without the immunized animal ever having "seen" the original antigen.

In some instances, especially with inbred animals, anti-idiotypic antibodies react with several different antibodies that are directed against the same epitope and share idiotypes. These idiotypes are called ***public*** or ***cross-reacting idiotypes,*** and this term frequently defines families of antibody molecules. By contrast, sera that react with only one particular antibody molecule define a ***private idiotype***. As we discuss in Chapter 16, the presence of idiotypic determinants on immunoglobulin molecules may have a role in the control and modulation of the immune response, as envisioned in the Jerne network theory, although this remains controversial.

SUMMARY

1. Immunoglobulins of all classes have a fundamental four-chain structure, consisting of two identical light (L) and two identical heavy (H) chains. Through disulfide bonds each light chain is linked to a heavy chain and the two heavy chains are linked to each other.

2. In the native state, the chains are coiled into domains, each of which consists of about 110 amino acids, stabilized by an intrachain disulfide bond.

3. The N-terminal domains of both H and L chains are the variable (V) regions, which together make up the combining site of the antibody and vary according to the specificity of the antibody.

4. The other domains are the constant (C) regions, and these domains are similar within each class of immunoglobulin molecule.

5. Digestion of the immunoglobulin molecule with papain yields two monovalent Fab fragments and one Fc fragment. Digestion with pepsin yields one divalent F(ab$'$)$_2$ fragment and several peptide fragments from the Fc region.

6. The classes of immunoglobulin molecules differ by virtue of the Fc regions of their H chains, which are responsible for the different biologic functions carried out by each class.

7. Certain genetic markers within the C regions of the H chains, which result from differences in one or two amino acids, are called allotypes and distinguish individuals within a species. In contrast, idiotypic markers are represented by the unique combinations of amino acids that make up the combining site of an antibody molecule and that are unique for that particular antibody.

REFERENCES

Alzari PM, Lascombe MB, Poljak RJ (1988): Three dimensional structure of antibodies. Annu Rev Immunol 6:555.

Capra D, Edmundson AB (1977): The antibody combining site. Sci Am 236:50.

Carayannopoulos L, Capra JD (1993): Immunoglobulins: structure and function. In Paul WE (ed): Fundamental Immunology, 3rd ed New York: Raven Press.

Davies DR, Metzger H (1983): Structural basis of antibody function. Annu Rev Immunol 1:87.

Jefferis R (1993): What is an idiotype. Immunol Today 14:19.

Koshland ME (1985): The coming of age of the immunoglobulin J chain. Annu Rev Immunol 3:425.

Nisonoff A (1984): Introduction to Molecular Immunology. Sunderland, MA: Sinauer.

Stanfield RL, Fisher TM, Lerner R, Wilson IA (1990): Crystal structure of an antibody to a peptide and its complex with peptide antigen at 2.8 Å. Science 248:712.

Williams AF, Barclay AN (1988): The immunoglobulin superfamily. Annu Rev Immunol 6:381.

REVIEW QUESTIONS

For each question choose the ONE BEST answer or completion.

1. The hinge region of an IgG heavy chain is located
   A) within the C_H1 intrachain loops
   B) between C_H1 and C_H2
   C) between C_H2 and C_H3
   D) between C_H3 and C_H4
   E) between V_H and C_H1

2. The class-specific antigenic determinants (epitopes) of immunoglobulins are associated with
   A) L chains
   B) J chains
   C) disulfide bonds
   D) H chains
   E) variable regions

3. The idiotype of an antibody molecule is determined by the amino acid sequence of the
   A) constant region of the L chain
   B) variable region of the L chain
   C) constant region of the H chain
   D) constant regions of the H and L chains
   E) variable regions of the H and L chains

4. An immunoglobulin molecule contains
   A) two identical light chains
   B) variable and constant regions on each chain present
   C) two identical heavy chains
   D) polypeptide chains, divided into domains

   E) A and B are correct
   F) C and D are correct
   G) all are correct

5. Injection into rabbits of a preparation of pooled human IgG could stimulate production of
   A) anti-γ heavy-chain antibody
   B) anti-κ chain antibody
   C) anti-λ chain antibody
   D) anti-Fc antibody
   E) A and B are correct
   F) B and D are correct
   G) all are correct

6. Antibodies to human IgA will react with
   A) human IgM
   B) κ light chains
   C) human IgG
   D) J chain
   E) A and B are correct
   F) C and D are correct
   G) A and C are correct
   H) all are correct

7. The statements about the domains of immunoglobulin H chain are correct *except*
   A) define separate units with different functions
   B) probably arose from the same primordial gene
   C) may carry allotypic markers
   D) lack disulfide bonds

8. The antigen binding site of an Ig molecule

A) is in the first domain of the N-terminal end of L and H chains

B) is destroyed by removal of sugar residues

C) has a specificity determined predominantly by variations in the hypervariable regions

D) has a size that cannot be determined from studies on the binding of antigen fragments

E) A and C are correct

F) B and D are correct

G) all are correct

9. An individual was found to be heterologous for IgG_1 allotypes 3 and 12. The different possible IgG_1 antibodies produced by this individual will never have

A) two H chains of allotype 12

B) two L chains of either κ or λ

C) two H chains of allotype 3

D) two H chains, one of allotype 3 and one of allotype 12

10. The pepsin digest of an IgG preparation of antibody specific for the antigen hen egg albumin (HEA) will

A) consist of four polypeptide chains

B) lose all its heavy (H) chains

C) precipitate with HEA

D) lose all interchain disulfide bonds

E) A and C are correct

F) B and D are correct

ANSWERS TO REVIEW QUESTIONS

---

1. **B** Correct location of hinge region is between C_H1 and C_H2, where the Fc portion begins.

2. **D** The five classes of Ig molecules are defined by the H chains (γ, μ, α, λ, ε).

3. **E** The idiotype is the antigenic determinant of an Ig molecule, which involves its antigen combining site, which in turn consists of contributions from the variable regions of both L and H chains.

4. **G** All are correct statements.

5. **G** All are correct statements. Since a pool of IgG is injected, it can be assumed that both κ and λ chains will be present and that antibodies will be made against them, as well as against the other determinants (H chain and Fc region) present in all IgG molecules.

6. **H** All are correct statements. Antibody to IgA will have antibody specific for κ and λ light chains, which, of course, will react with IgG and IgM, both of which have κ- and λ-chains. Antibody will also be present against J chain if the IgA used for immunization was dimeric.

7. **D** *A, B,* and *C* are correct. All domains are formed around an intrachain disulfide bond; thus, statement *D* is wrong.

8. **E** The antigen-binding site is made up of the contribution of the hypervariable regions on the H and L chains, which are at the N-terminal ends of the chains. The size of the site can be estimated by binding studies with various fragments of antigen. Loss of sugar residues does not affect this site. Thus statements **A** and **C** are correct, and the appropriate one best answer is **E**.

9. **D** In any immunoglobulin produced by a single cell, the two H chains and the two L chains are identical. Therefore, any antibody molecule in this individual would have either allotype 3 H chains or allotype 12 H chains, not a mixture. Similarly, the antibody would have either two κ or two λ chains.

10. **E** Pepsin digestion cleaves the Fc portion of the IgG molecule into smaller fragments, leaving intact one divalent F(ab')$_2$ molecules. This molecule consists of two L chains and two partial H chains held together by an interchain disulfide bridge. Since the divalence of the original IgG is retained, it will precipitate the HEA. Thus statements **A** and **C** are true, and the correct answer is **E**.

BIOLOGICAL PROPERTIES OF IMMUNOGLOBULINS

INTRODUCTION

Many important biological functions are attributed to antibodies. These include *neutralization* of toxins, *immobilization* of microorganisms, neutralization of viral activity, *agglutination* (clumping together) of microorganisms or of antigenic particles (see Chapter 7), binding with soluble antigen leading to the formation of *precipitates* (which are readily phagocytized and destroyed by phagocytic cells; see Chapter 7), and activating serum complement to facilitate the *lysis* of microorganisms (see Chapter 13) or their phagocytosis and destruction either by phagocytic cells or by killer lymphocytes. Still another important biological function of antibodies is their ability to *cross the placenta* from the mother to the fetus. Not all antibody isotypes are equal in the performance of all of these biological tasks. Indeed, prior to 1960, before the elucidation of the structure of the various isotypes, it was already recognized that antibody populations, even if directed against the same epitope, differ in their capacity to fulfill these biological functions. Consequently, those antibodies that exhibited the capacity to agglutinate particulate antigens or microorganisms were called *agglutinating antibodies* or *agglutinins;* other antibodies that activated or "fixed" complement in the presence of antigen were termed *complement-fixing* antibodies, and so on. Today, it is well established that the differences in the various biological activities of the antibodies are attributed to their isotypic (class) structure.

The determination of the structure of antibody, the establishment of the relationship between this structure and function, and the elucidation of the genetic organization of the Ig molecule have led to an understanding of the evolution of a sophisticated, highly specialized system in which diverse structures (immunoglobulins) all recognize the same antigen, but in which combination of immunoglobulin with antigen leads to an array of diverse biological effects. In the sections that follow, the structural characteristics of the Ig isotypes are related to their biological properties. The structural features of the immunoglobulin isotypes are described in Chapter 4; their metabolism, distribution, and biological properties are dealt with here. *The important features of the various immunoglobulin isotypes are presented in Tables 5.1 and 5.2*.

BIOLOGICAL PROPERTIES OF IgG

IgG present in the serum of human adults represents about 15% of the total protein (other proteins include albumins, globulins, and enzymes). *IgG is distributed approximately equally between the intravascular and extravascular spaces*.

Except for the IgG_3 subclass, which has a rapid turnover, with a *half-life* of 7 days, the half-life of IgG (i.e., IgG_1, IgG_2, and IgG_4) is approximately *23 days,* which is the longest half-life of all Ig isotypes. This persistence in the serum makes IgG the most suitable for passive immunization by transfer of antibodies. Interestingly, as the concentration of IgG in the serum increases (as in cases of multiple myeloma or after the transfer of very high concentrations of IgG), the rate of catabolism of IgG increases, and the half-life of IgG decreases to 15–20 days or even less.

IgG molecules may be made to *aggregate* by a variety of procedures. For example, precipitation with alcohol, a method employed in the purification of IgG for passive immunization (see Chapter 22), or heating at 63°C for 10 minutes, a method used to inactivate complement (see Chapter 13), cause aggregation. Aggregated IgG can still combine with antigen.

Many of the properties that are attributed to antigen–antibody complexes are exhibited by aggregated IgG (without antigen)—for example, attachment to phagocytic cells, as well as the activation of complement and other biologically active substances that may be harmful to the body. Such activation is attributable

TABLE 5.1 The Most Important Features of Immunoglobulin Isotypes

	Isotype				
	IgG	IgA	IgM	IgD	IgE
Molecular weight	150,000	160,000 for monomer	900,000	180,000	200,000
Additional protein subunits	–	J and S	J	–	–
Approximate concentration in serum (mg/ml)	12	1.8	1	0–0.04	0.00002
Percent of total Ig	80	13	6	0.2	0.002
Distribution	~Equal: intravascular and extravascular	Intravascular and secretions	Mostly intravascular	Present on lymphocyte surface	On basophils and mast cells present in saliva and nasal secretions
Half-life (days)	23	5.5	5	2.8	2.0
Placental passage	++	–	–	–	–
Presence in secretion	–	++	–	–	–
Presence in milk	+	+	0 to trace	–	–
Activation of complement	+	–	+++	–	–
Binding to Fc receptors on macrophages, polymorphonuclear cells, and NK[a] cells	++	–	–	–	–
Relative agglutinating capacity	+	++	+++	–	–
Antiviral activity	+++	+++	+	–	–
Antibacterial activity (gram-negative)	+++	++ (with lysozyme)	+++ (with complement)	–	–
Antitoxin activity	+++	–	–	–	–
"Allergic activity"	–	–	–	–	++

[a]Natural killer.

TABLE 5.2   Important Differences Between Human IgG Subclasses

	IgG_1	IgG_2	IgG_3	IgG_4
Occurrence (% of total IgG)	70	20	7	3
Half-life	23	23	7	23
Complement binding	+	+	+++	–
Placental passage	++	±	++	++
Binding of monocytes	+++	+	+++	±

to the juxtaposition of Fc domains by the aggregation process in a way analogous to that produced by antigen-induced complex formation. It is therefore imperative that no aggregated IgG be present in passively administered IgG.

Agglutination and Formation of Precipitate

IgG molecules can cause the **agglutination** or clumping of particulate (insoluble) antigens such as microorganisms. The reaction of IgG with soluble, multivalent antigens can generate **precipitates** (see Chapter 7). This property of IgG is undoubtedly of considerable survival value since insoluble antigen–antibody complexes are easily phagocytized and destroyed by phagocytic cells.

Passage Through the Placenta

The IgG isotype (except for subclass IgG_2) is the only class of immunoglobulin that can pass through the placenta, enabling the mother to transfer her immunity to the fetus. Analysis of fetal immunoglobulins (see Fig. 22.2) shows that, at the third or fourth month of pregnancy, there is a rapid increase in the concentration of IgG. This IgG must be of maternal origin, since the fetus is unable to synthesize immunoglobulins at this age. Then, during the fifth month of pregnancy, the fetus begins to synthesize IgM and trace amounts of IgA. It is not until 3 or 4 months after birth, when the level of inherited maternal IgG drops as a result of catabolism (the half-life of IgG is 23 days), that the infant begins to synthesize its own IgG antibodies. Thus, the resistance of the fetus and the neonate to infection is conferred almost entirely by the mother's IgG, which passes across the placenta. It has been established that passage across the placenta is mediated by the Fc portion of the IgG molecule; $F(ab')_2$ or Fab fragments of IgG do not pass through the placenta.

While passage of IgG molecules across the placenta confers immunity to infection on the fetus, it may also be responsible for ***hemolytic disease of the newborn (erythroblastosis fetalis)*** (see Chapter 19). This is caused by maternal antibodies to fetal red blood cells. The maternal IgG antibodies, produced by an Rh^- mother, to Rh antigen pass across the placenta and attack the fetal red blood cells that carry Rh antigens (Rh^+).

Opsonization

IgG is an ***opsonizing*** antibody (from the Greek *opsonin*, which means to prepare for eating). It reacts with epitopes on microorganisms via its Fab portions; but it is the Fc portion that confers the opsonizing property, since many phagocytic cells, including macrophages and polymorphonuclear phagocytes, bear receptors for the Fc portion of the IgG molecule. These cells adhere to the antibody-coated bacteria by virtue of their receptors for Fc. The net effect is a zipper-like closure of the surface membrane of the phagocytic cell around the organism, as receptors for Fc and the Fc regions on the antibodies continue to combine, leading to the final engulfing and destruction of the microorganism (see Fig. 5.1).

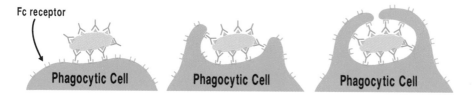

Figure 5.1.

A diagrammatic representation of phagocytosis of a particle coated with antibodies.

Antibody-Dependent, Cell-Mediated Cytotoxicity

The IgG molecule plays an important role in antibody-dependent, cell-mediated cytotoxicity (ADCC). In this form of cytotoxicity, the Fab portion binds with the target cell, whether it is a microorganism or a tumor cell, and the Fc portion binds with specific receptors for Fc that are found on certain large granular lymphocytic cells called ***natural killer (*or *NK) cells*** (see Chapter 2). By this mechanism, the IgG molecule "focuses" the killer cells on their target, and the killer cells destroy the target, not by phagocytosis but with the various substances that they release.

Activation of Complement

The IgG molecule can activate the **complement** system (see Chapter 13). Activation of complement results in the release of several important biologically active molecules and leads to lysis if the antibody is bound to antigen on the surface of a cell. Some of the complement components are also **opsonins**; they bind to the target antigen and thereby direct phagocytes, which carry receptors specific for these opsonins, to focus their phagocytic activity on the target antigen. Other components from the activation of complement are **chemotactic;** specifically, they attract phagocytic cells. All in all, the activation of complement by IgG has profound biological effects on the host and on the target antigen, whether it is a live cell, a microorganism, or a tumor cell.

Neutralization of Toxin

The IgG molecule is an excellent antibody for the neutralization of such toxins as tetanus and botulinus, or for the inactivation of, for example, snake and scorpion venoms. Because of its ability to neutralize such poisons (mostly by blocking their active sites) and because of its long half-life, compared to that of other isotypes, the IgG molecule is the isotype of choice for **passive immunization** (i.e., the transfer of antibodies) against toxins and venoms (see Chapter 22).

Immobilization of Bacteria

IgG molecules are efficient in immobilizing various motile bacteria. Reaction of antibodies specific for the **flagella** and **cilia** of certain microorganisms causes them to clump, thereby arresting their movement and preventing their ability to spread or invade tissue.

Neutralization of Viruses

The IgG antibody is an efficient virus neutralizing antibody. One mechanism of neutralization is that in which the antibody binds with antigenic determinants present on various portions of the virus coat, among which is the region used by the virus for attachment to the target cell. ***Inhibition of viral attachment*** effectively arrests infection. Other antibodies are thought to inhibit viral penetration or shedding of the viral coat required for release of the viral DNA or RNA needed to induce infection.

Summary

To reiterate, the versatility in function of the IgG molecule makes it a very important molecule in the immune response. Its importance is underscored in those immune deficiency disorders in which an individual is unable to synthesize IgG molecules (see Chapter 18). Such individuals are prone to infections that may result in toxemias and death.

BIOLOGICAL PROPERTIES OF IgA

Serum IgA, which has no known biological function, has a ***half-life of 5.5 days. Most IgA is present not in the serum, but in secretions such as tears, saliva, colostrum, sweat, and mucus,*** where it serves an important biological function such as being part of the mucosa-associated lymphoid tissue (MALT) as alluded to in Chapter 2.

It has already been mentioned (see Chapter 4) that during the synthesis of IgA by plasma cells situated in various epithelia of the body (e.g., in the parotid gland, along the gastrointestinal tract in the intestinal villi, in tear glands, in the lactating breast, or beneath bronchial mucosa), two monomeric IgA molecules become joined by a J chain. The J chain, synthesized by the same cell that makes the IgA, is attached to the IgA molecules by disulfide bonds. The IgA dimer is released into the lamina propria and transported across the epithelial cells of the mucosa into the lumen. This transport is mediated by another protein called the ***secretory component,*** which is a receptor on epithelial cells that becomes attached to the dimer of IgA. The secretory component (***S*** in Fig. 4.7) is synthesized by epithelial cells situated near the mucous membrane, and it binds to the IgA dimer by strong, noncovalent bonds. (Secretory component also binds and transports pentameric IgM to mucosal surfaces in small amounts.)

The IgA found in secretions (i.e., ***secretory IgA***) is always present in ***dimeric*** form (see Fig. 4.7) and has a molecular weight of 400,000 daltons. As noted before, if all secretion of IgA from various sources is taken into account, it is the major immunoglobulin synthesized in the body. Its protective effect is thought to be due to its ability to prevent the invading organism from attaching to and penetrating the epithelial surface.

Role in Mucosal Infections

Because of its presence in secretions, such as saliva, urine, and gastric fluid, secretory IgA is of importance in the primary immunologic defense against local infections in such areas as the respiratory or gastrointestinal tract. For example, in the case of cholera, the pathogenic *Vibrio* organism attaches to, but never penetrates beyond, the cells that line the gastrointestinal tract, where it secretes an exotoxin responsible for all symptoms. IgA antibody, which can prevent attachment of the organism to the cells, provides protection from the pathogen. Thus, for protection against local infections, routes of immunization that result in local production of IgA are much more effective than routes that primarily produce antibodies in serum.

Bactericidal Activity

The IgA molecule does not contain receptors for complement and, thus, it is not a complement-activating or complement-fixing immunoglobulin. Consequently, IgA does not induce complement-mediated bacterial lysis. However, IgA has been shown to possess bactericidal activity against *gram-negative organisms,* but only in the presence of *lysozyme,* which, interestingly, is also present in the same secretions that contain secretory IgA.

Antiviral Activity

Secretory IgA is an efficient antiviral antibody, preventing the viruses from entering host cells. In addition, secretory IgA is an efficient agglutinating antibody.

BIOLOGICAL PROPERTIES OF IgM

IgM present in adult human serum is found predominantly in the *intravascular* spaces. The *half-life* of the IgM molecule is approximately *5 days*. IgM is also found on the surface of mature B cells, where it serves as the specific receptor for antigen. IgM antibodies do not pass through the placenta; however, since this is the only class of immunoglobulins that is synthesized by the fetus beginning at approximately 5 months of gestation, *elevated levels of IgM in the fetus are indicative of congenital or perinatal infection.*

IgM is the isotype synthesized by children and adults in appreciable amounts after immunization or exposure to T-independent antigens, and it is the first isotype that is synthesized after immunization with T-dependent antigens (see Fig. 5.2). Thus, elevated levels of IgM usually indicate either recent infection or recent exposure to antigen.

Agglutination

IgM molecules are efficient agglutinating antibodies. Because of their pentameric form, IgM antibodies can form macromolecular bridges between epitopes on molecules that may be too distant from each other to be bridged by the smaller IgG antibodies. Furthermore, because of their pentameric form and multiple valence, the IgM antibodies are particularly well suited to combine with antigens that contain repeated patterns of the same antigenic determinant, as in the case of polysaccharide antigens or cellular antigens, which are multiply expressed on cell surfaces.

Isohemagglutinins

The IgM antibodies include the so-called *natural isohemagglutinins*—the naturally occurring antibodies against the red blood cell antigens of the ABO blood groups (see Chapter 19). These antibodies are presumed to arise as a result of immunization by bacteria in the gastrointestinal and respiratory tracts, which bear determinants similar to the oligosaccharides of the ABO blood groups. Thus, without known prior immunization, people with the type O blood group have isohemagglutinins to the A and B antigens; those with the type A blood group have antibodies to the B antigens; and those with the B antigen have antibodies to the A antigen. An individual of the AB group has neither anti-A nor anti-B antibodies. Fortunately, the IgM isohemagglutinins do not pass through the placenta, so incompatibility of the ABO groups between mother and fetus poses no danger to the fetus. However, *transfusion* reactions, which arise as a result of *ABO incompatibility,* and in which the recipient's isohemagglutinins react with the donor's red blood cells, may have disastrous consequences (see Chapter 19).

Activation of Complement

Because of its pentameric form, IgM is an excellent complement-fixing or complement-activating antibody. Unlike other classes of immunoglobulins, a single molecule of IgM, on binding to antigen with at least two of its Fab arms, can initiate the complement sequence, making it the most efficient immunoglobulin as an initiator of the complement-mediated lysis of microorganisms and other cells. This ability, taken together with the appearance of IgM as the first class of antibodies generated after immunization or infection, makes IgM antibodies very important as providers of an early line of immunological defense against bacterial infections.

In contrast to IgG, the IgM antibodies are not very versatile; they are poor toxin-neutralizing antibodies, and they are not efficient in the neutralization of viruses.

BIOLOGICAL PROPERTIES OF IgD

IgD is present on the surface of B lymphocytes during certain stages of maturation. It has been suggested to be involved in the maturation of these cells (see Chapter 9). IgD is present in the serum in very small amounts. It is thought that serum IgD represents molecules that came off the B lymphocyte surface (rather than having been secreted). Serum IgD has a half-life of 2.8 days; its rate of turnover is unknown.

Although there are isolated reports of serum IgD with specificity against certain antigens, generally, the antibodies in serum that belong to this class of immunoglobulins have not been demonstrated to serve a protective function.

BIOLOGICAL PROPERTIES OF IgE

IgE, also termed *reaginic antibody,* has a *half-life* in serum of *2 days,* the shortest half-life of all classes of immunoglobulins. Another distinction of IgE antibodies is that they are present in serum at the lowest concentrations of all immunoglobulins. These low levels are due in part to a low rate of synthesis and, in part, to the unique ability of the Fc portion of IgE to bind with very high affinity to mast cells and basophils. Both mast cells and basophils have specific receptors for this region, and thus they effectively remove the IgE from the circulation.

Importance of IgE in Parasitic Infections and Hypersensitivity Reactions

IgE is not an agglutinating or complement-activating antibody; nevertheless, it has a role in protection against microorganisms that is becoming better appreciated. Elevated levels of IgE in serum have been shown to occur during infections with certain *parasites*. For example, induction of IgE production has been demonstrated in cases of infection with *ascaris* (a roundworm). In fact, immunization with ascaris antigen induces the formation of IgE.

The IgE class of antibodies is of great importance in some immune responses that have a pathologic outcome (*hypersensitivity* or *allergy*; see Chapter 14). The surfaces of the highly granulated basophils or mast cells contain receptors for the Fc portion of the IgE molecule, and IgE molecules are found predominantly attached to these cells. When antigen binds with the Fab portion of the IgE attached to these cells, the cells become activated and release the contents of their granules: histamine, heparin, leukotrienes, and other pharmacologically active compounds that trigger the hypersensitivity reactions. These reactions may be mild, as in the case of a mosquito bite, or severe, as in the case of bronchial asthma; they may even result in systemic anaphylaxis, which can cause death within minutes.

KINETICS OF THE ANTIBODY RESPONSE FOLLOWING IMMUNIZATION

Primary Response

As mentioned in Chapter 3, the first exposure of an individual to a particular immunogen is referred to as the *priming immunization* and the measurable response that ensues is called the *primary response.* As shown in Figure 5.2, the primary antibody response may be divided into several phases, as follows:

1. *Latent or lag phase:* After initial injection of antigen, a significant amount of time elapses before antibody is detectable in the serum. The length of this period is generally 1–2 weeks, depending on the species immunized, the antigen, and other factors that will become apparent in subsequent chapters. The length of the latent period is also greatly dependent on the sensitivity of the assay used to measure the product of the response. As we shall see in more detail in subsequent chapters, the latent period includes the time taken for T and B cells to

make contact with the antigen, to proliferate, and to differentiate. B cells must also secrete antibody in sufficient quantity so that it can be detected in the serum. The less sensitive the assay used for detection of antibody, the more antibody will be required for detection and the longer the apparent latent period will be.

2. *Exponential production phase:* During this phase, the concentration of antibody in the serum increases exponentially.

3. *Steady state:* During this period, production and degradation of antibody are balanced.

4. *Declining phase:* Finally, the immune response begins to shut down, and the concentration of antibody in serum declines rapidly.

In the primary response, the first class of antibody detected is generally *IgM,* which in some instances may be the only class of immunoglobulin that is made. If production of IgG antibody ensues, its appearance is generally accompanied by a rapid cessation of production of IgM (see Fig. 5.2).

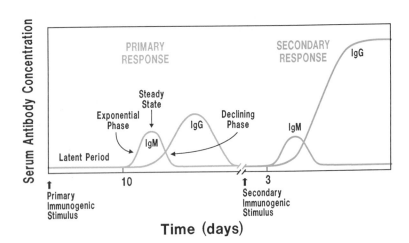

Figure 5.2.

The kinetics of an antibody response.

Secondary Response

Although production of antibody after a priming contact with antigen may cease entirely within a few weeks (see Fig. 5.2), the immunized individual is left with a cellular memory (i.e., long-lasting *memory cells*) of this contact. This memory becomes apparent when a response is triggered by a *second injection* of the same antigen. After the second injection, the lag phase is considerably shorter and antibody may appear in less than half the time required for the primary response. The production of antibody is much greater, and higher concentrations of antibody are detectable in the serum. The production of antibody may also continue for a longer period, with persistent levels remaining in serum months, or even years, later.

There is a marked change in the type and quality of antibody produced in the secondary response. There is a *shift in class response,* with IgG antibodies appearing at higher concentrations, and with greater persistence, than IgM, which may be greatly reduced or disappear altogether. This may be also accompanied by the appearance of IgA and IgE. In addition, a *maturation* of the response occurs, such that the average affinity (binding constant) of the antibodies for the antigen increases as the secondary response develops. The driving force for this increase in affinity may be a selection process during which B cells compete with free antibody to capture a decreasing amount of antigen. Thus, only those B-cell clones with high-affinity Ig receptors on their surfaces will bind enough antigen to ensure that the B cells are triggered to differentiate into plasma cells. These plasma cells, which arise from preferentially selected B cells, synthesize this antibody with high affinity for antigen.

The capacity to make secondary or *anamnestic* (memory) response may persist for a long time (months in mice; years in humans), and it provides an obvious selective advantage for an individual that survives the first contact with an invading pathogen. Establishment of this memory for generating a specific response is, of course, the purpose of public health immunization programs.

SUMMARY

1. There are many biological functions that antibodies carry out in addition to binding with antigen.

2. These properties are conferred on the antibody by the heavy chain, and the biological functions (excluding binding with antigen) are mediated by the Fc portion of the antibody and by the hinge region.

3. IgG is the most versatile class of antibody, capable of carrying out numerous biological functions that range from neutralization of toxin to activation of complement and opsonization. IgG is the only class of immunoglobulin that passes through the placenta and confers maternal immunity on the fetus. The half-life of IgG (23 days) is the longest of all immunoglobulin classes.

4. IgA antibody is present in monomeric as well as dimeric form. The dimeric IgA found in secretions and referred to as secretory IgA is an important antiviral immunoglobulin.

5. IgM antibody is present in pentameric form; of all classes of immunoglobulin it is the best agglutinating and complement-activating antibody.

6. IgD antibodies are present on the surface of B lymphocytes at certain developmental stages of these cells and appear to be involved in their differentiation.

7. IgE, also called reaginic antibody, is of paramount importance in hypersensitivity reactions. It also appears to be of importance in protection against parasitic infections. The Fc portion of IgE binds with high affinity to receptors on mast cells and, on contact with antigen, it triggers the degranulation of mast cells, resulting in the release of pharmacologically active substances that mediate the hypersensitivity reactions.

8. Following first immunization, the primary response consists mainly of the production of IgM antibodies. The second exposure to the same antigen results in a secondary or anamnestic (memory) response, which is much quicker than the primary response and in which the response shifts from IgM production to the synthesis of IgG and other isotypes. The secondary response lasts much longer than the primary response.

REFERENCES

Carayanopoulos L, Capra JD (1993): Immunoglobulins: structure and function. In Paul WE (ed): Fundamental Immunology, 3rd ed. New York: Raven Press.

Davies DR, Metzger H (1983): Structural basis of antibody function. Annu Rev Immunol 1:87.

Koshland ME (1985): The coming of age of the immunoglobulin J chain. Annu Rev Immunol 3:425.

Mestecky J, McGhee JR (1987): Immunoglobulin A (IgA): Molecular and cellular interactions involved in IgA biosynthesis and immune response. Adv Immunol 40:153.

Möller G (ed) (1977): Immunoglobulin D: Structure, synthesis, membrane representation and function. Immunol Rev 37.

Möller G (ed) (1978): Immunoglobulin E. Immunol Rev 41.

Nisonoff A, Hopper JR, Spring SB (1975): The Antibody Molecule. New York: Academic Press.

Tomasi TB (1992): The discovery of secretory IgA and the mucosal immune system. Immunol Today 13:416.

Walker WA, Isselbacher KJ (1977): Intestinal antibodies. New Engl J Med 297:767.

REVIEW QUESTIONS

For each question, choose the ONE BEST answer or completion.

1. Agglutinins are useful in detection of infection caused by *Mycoplasma pneumoniae*. They are mainly IgM molecules. Assuming that successful treatment of infection caused abrupt cessation of synthesis of agglutinins, how long would it take for a fourfold drop in the concentration of IgM molecules in serum to take place?
   A) approximately 2 days
   B) approximately 10 days
   C) approximately 2 months
   D) approximately 2 years
   E) approximately 2 hours

2. The first immunoglobulin synthesized by the fetus is
   A) IgA
   B) IgE
   C) Ig G
   D) IgM
   E) none; the fetus does not synthesize immunoglobulins

3. The antibody isotype that acts in concert with lysozyme against gram-negative organisms is
   A) IgA
   B) IgG
   C) Ig D
   D) IgM
   E) IgE

4. The following properties of human IgG are true *except*
   A) it can pass the placenta
   B) it can be cleaved by pepsin and yet remain divalent
   C) its half-life is approximately 23 days
   D) it induces the formation of leukocytes
   E) it participates in the activation of complement
   F) it has the longest half-life of all Ig isotopes

5. The relative level of specific IgM antibodies can be of diagnostic significance because
   A) IgM is easier to detect than the other isotypes
   B) viral infection often results in very high IgM responses
   C) IgM antibodies are more often protective against reinfections than are the other isotypes
   D) relative high levels of IgM often correlate with a first recent exposure to the inducing agent
   E) A and B are correct
   F) C and D are correct

6. The primary and secondary responses differ in
   A) the predominant isotype generated
   B) the number of lymphocytes responding to antigen
   C) the speed at which antibodies appear in the serum.
   D) the phenomenon of isotype switch
   E) all of the above

ANSWERS TO REVIEW QUESTIONS

1. **B** The half-life of serum IgM is approximately 5 days. Therefore a fourfold drop will occur after two half-lives, i.e., after approximately 10 days.

2. **D** The first (and only) immunoglobulin synthesized by the fetus is IgM. The IgG present in the fetus is maternal IgG which has passed through the placenta. No other immunoglobulins are found in the fetus.

3. **A** Secretory IgA works in concert with lysozyme, which is found in many secretions.

4. **D** Human IgG is the only Ig that passes across the placenta. It has a half-life of 23 days, the longest of all Ig isotypes. It can be cleaved by pepsin to yield a divalent antibody portion $F(ab')_2$, and it participates in the activation of complement. It does not induce the formation of leukocytes. Thus all the statements are true except **D**.

5. **D** Only the last statement is correct. Relatively high levels of IgM often correlate with first recent exposure to an inducing agent since IgM is the first isotype synthesized in response to an immunogen. All other statements are not true.

6. **E** All are correct. The statements are self-explanatory.

THE GENETIC BASIS OF ANTIBODY STRUCTURE

INTRODUCTION

One characteristic of the immune response is its enormous diversity. Estimates of the number of B and T cells with different antigenic specificities in a given individual range from 10^6 to 10^8. If every immunoglobulin (Ig) or T-cell receptor (TcR) were coded for by one gene, then an individual would have to have this same number of genes (10^6–10^8) devoted exclusively to coding for these structures. Since such a large number of genes would occupy a significant percentage of the individual's genome (inherited DNA), it seemed hard to understand how all these genes could be fitted in. As a result of the work of several investigators over the last twenty years, however, we now know that genes coding for Ig and TcR use a unique strategy to achieve the degree of diversity required. This strategy uses a much more limited set of genes, numbering in the thousands rather than millions, which we shall discuss below.

The first key finding was that the variable and constant regions of an immunoglobulin molecule were coded for by different genes. In fact, many different variable region (V) genes can be linked up to a single constant region (C) gene. The combining of V and C region genes (rather than having a single gene coding for every individual antibody molecule) considerably reduces the amount of genetic information required to encode different antibody molecules.

A subsequent crucial finding by Susumu Tonegawa (who won the Nobel Prize) was that antibody genes could move and *rearrange* themselves within the genome of a differentiating cell. A V region gene can be located in one position in the DNA of an inherited chromosome (the *germ line*), and can then move to another position on the chromosome during lymphocyte differentiation. This process of rearrangement during differentiation brings together an appropriate set of genes for the V and C regions. The set of genes is then transcribed and translated into a complete H or L chain.

Subsequent studies of Mark Davis and others have shown that the organization of genes that code for the TcR and the mechanisms used to generate TcR diversity obey many of the same principles (this is discussed in more detail in Chapter 8). Thus, the generation of diversity of antigen-specific receptors on both B and T lymphocytes has many common features.

We stress again that the mechanisms used to generate antigen-specific receptors on T and B cells seem to be unique in the entire body: to date, no other genes behave in the same way, because they do not use these rearrangement strategies. In the paragraphs that follow we will describe the steps involved in synthesizing a complete Ig molecule.

A BRIEF REVIEW OF NONIMMUNOGLOBULIN GENE STRUCTURE AND GENE EXPRESSION

Before discussing the molecular arrangement and rearrangement of the genes involved in immunoglobulin synthesis, we will first review the organization and expression of nonimmunoglobulin genes. We will focus on the components of genes that code for a typical protein expressed at the cell surface. This is illustrated diagrammatically in Figure 6.1.

1. The *genome* (total inherited DNA) of an individual consists of linear arrays of genes in the DNA strands of the various chromosomes. Genes are transcribed into RNA, and RNA is translated into protein.

2. Every diploid cell in an individual's body contains the same set of genes as every other cell. (The only exceptions are lymphocytes, which, as we shall discuss shortly, differ from other cells and each other in the actual content of genes

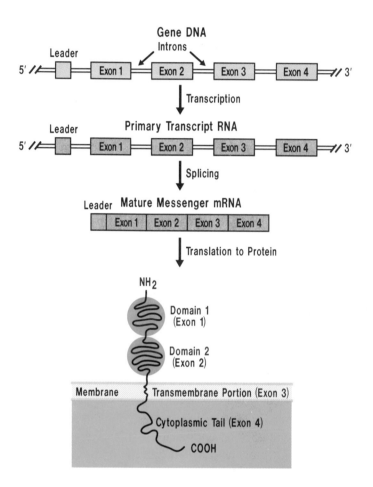

Figure 6.1.

A prototypical gene coding for a membrane protein.

coding for their antigen-specific receptor.) Cells in an individual differ from each other because they transcribe and translate different genes. We say that these genes *express* different patterns of genes.

3. The expression of a specific pattern of genes determines the cell's function. Thus, for example, while every cell contains an insulin gene, only pancreatic β cells express that gene, enabling them to make insulin. Similarly, all cells contain immunoglobulin genes; however, only B lymphocytes (and their differentiated form, plasma cells) express immunoglobulin genes and therefore synthesize immunoglobulin molecules. Like all other cells except B cells, T cells contain immunoglobulin genes but do not express them.

Control of gene expression exists at multiple levels. These levels of control include the rate of transcription, the activity of transcription factors, transport of RNA to the cytoplasm, and the rate of translation of mRNA into protein on ribosomes. Understanding the molecular mechanisms that regulate gene expression and in particular how genes are turned on and off in different cell types is an area of intense research interest. Aberrant gene expression can lead to disease, so studying how genes are turned on or off in lymphocytes and other cells will help to design therapies for treating diseases at the molecular level.

4. Most genes coding for a protein have a characteristic structure comprising *exons* and *introns*. Exons are sequences of base pairs that are later transcribed into mature messenger RNA. Exons are separated from each other by introns, noncoding regions of base pairs.

5. When a gene is transcribed into RNA, the entire stretch of DNA (exons plus introns) is transcribed into a primary RNA transcript. Enzymes modify this primary RNA transcript to *splice* out the noncoding introns, bringing together all the coding exons needed to encode the final protein. This gives a processed mature messenger RNA (mRNA) segment that is much shorter than the original transcript by virtue of having lost all its noncoding introns. This mRNA is translated into protein on ribosomes. Notice (Fig. 6.1) that exons generally code for a discrete region of the protein which is a structural entity, such as a domain or a transmembrane piece or a cytoplasmic tail. Thus, proteins are assembled by putting together functional regions, each coded by multiple gene segments.

6. Preceding each gene that codes for a protein expressed at the cell surface is a *leader sequence* (L exon) at the 5′ end coding for a signal peptide that is about 20 amino acids in length. This provides a hydrophobic amino-terminus that is used to transport the nascent polypeptide chain through the membrane of the endoplasmic reticulum and into the Golgi apparatus, where the signal peptide is cleaved off and the protein is inserted into the cell membrane.

There are many ways in which membrane immunoglobulin structure differs from the structure of the surface molecule depicted in Figure 6.1. Most obviously, an immunoglobulin molecule is a multichain glycoprotein. To make a complete immunoglobulin, the newly synthesized individual heavy and light chains must be assembled and glycosylated inside the cell before the four-chain multimer reaches the cell surface. Another important difference is that each Ig chain has a very short cytoplasmic tail.

The surface molecule depicted in Figure 6.1 is shown with its amino terminus outside the cell, a single transmembrane region, and the carboxy terminus inside the cell. For the surface molecule in the figure, its large cytoplasmic tail would also allow it to interact with other molecules inside the cell. It is worth noting, however, that other molecules involved in the immune response are expressed at the cell surface with different configurations, for example, with their C terminus extracellular and their N terminus intracellular. Other membrane molecules, such as LFA-3 (CD58)—an adhesion molecule—are completely extracellular but are linked to the surface of the cell via a covalent bond to an oligosaccharide, which in turn is bound to a phospholipid in the membrane, phosphatidylinositol. These molecules are thus referred to as glycosyl phosphatidylinositol (GPI)-linked membrane molecules. Some molecules, such as the high-affinity Fc receptor (CD16), may be expressed at the surface in both GPI-linked as well as classic transmembrane versions.

GENETIC EVENTS IN THE SYNTHESIS OF IMMUNOGLOBULIN CHAINS

Organization and Rearrangement of Light-Chain Genes

As we have seen in Chapter 4, the light-chain polypeptides κ and λ each consists of two major domains, a variable region and a constant region (V_L and C_L). A crucial point is that the variable region of the light chain, V_L, the amino-terminal portion of approximately 108 residues (see Chapter 4), is coded for by *two separate gene segments:* a *V (variable) segment* that codes for the amino-terminal 95 residues and a small *J (joining) segment* coding for about 13 residues (96–108) at the carboxy-terminal end of the variable region. To generate an immunoglobulin light chain, one V and one J gene are brought together in the genome and joined with a C-region gene to create a gene unit that codes for an entire immunoglobulin light chain. This unique mechanism, known as *gene rearrangement,* is used only by genes coding for immunoglobulin light and heavy chains and, as we shall see in Chapter 9, by genes coding for T-cell receptors.

The molecular events involved in rearrangement are only just beginning to be understood. It is known, however, that many of the steps in rearrangement appear to be common to both B cells and T cells. Thus, rearrangement of receptor genes in B and T cells is mediated by a family of enzymes, known as *recombinases,* which catalyze the joining. Furthermore, two genes whose products are required to activate the recombinase are active in both B- and T-cell precursors;

mice lacking either of these two genes RAG-1 or RAG-2 (so called "RAG knockout mice") are deficient in both B and T cells.

κ-CHAIN SYNTHESIS. We will first examine the synthesis of κ light chains. κ-chain genes are found on chromosome 2 in humans. Genetic analysis has shown that there are approximately 100–200 different V_κ genes, each of which can code for the N-terminal 95 aminoacids of a κ variable region. These V_κ genes are arranged linearly, each with its own L (leader) sequence, all separated by introns, as shown in Figure 6.2 (for simplicity the leader sequences have been omitted in Fig. 6.2). Downstream (3') of this region, a series of about 5 J_κ gene segments is found, each of which can encode the remaining 13 amino acid residues (96–108) of the κ variable region. Separated by another long intron is the single gene segment coding for the single constant region of the κ-chain (C_κ). This then is the arrangement of κ genes in the **germ line,** that is, in *any* cell in the body.

To make a κ chain, an early cell in the B-lymphocyte lineage selects one of the Vκ genes from its DNA and physically joins it to one of the Jκ segments (Fig. 6.2). (How this selection of V and J genes is made is not known but is probably a random process.) Joining involves the linking of conserved recognition sequences that are found at the 5' and 3' ends of the V and J regions. (By "conserved," we mean that these same sequences are found at the 5' and 3' ends of all genes that

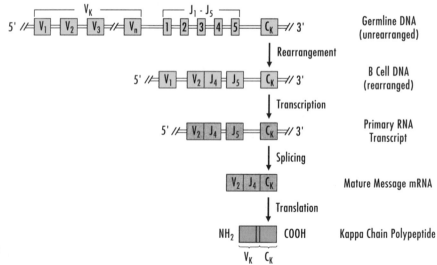

Figure 6.2.

The genetic events leading to the synthesis of light chain.

use rearranging gene segments to generate polypeptides.) In most cases, when joining occurs during rearrangement, the intervening DNA is looped, cut out, and ultimately broken down, as shown in Figure 6.3.

As a consequence of these DNA rearrangement events, a cell that has committed to using one V and one J segment brings the selected V- and J-gene segments adjacent to each other in the genome. From this rearranged DNA, a primary RNA transcript is made, which is then spliced to remove all intervening noncoding sequences to bring the Vκ, Jκ, and Cκ exons together, yielding a mature mRNA. This mRNA is then translated into the κ polypeptide chain on the cell's rough endoplasmic reticulum, and, after transport, the leader sequence is cleaved off and the κ chain is free to join with an H chain to form an immunoglobulin molecule.

λ-CHAIN SYNTHESIS. λ genes are found on chromosome 22 in humans; that is, on a chromosome distinct from both κ and heavy chain genes. The synthesis of λ chains is similar in principle to the synthesis of κ chains, in that it involves rearrangement of DNA that joins a Vλ gene, coding for the N-terminal region of a λ variable region, with a Jλ segment, coding for the remaining 13 aminoacids of the λ variable region. The human λ locus contains about 100 Vλ genes that can be joined to at least six different Jλ segments. The genetic organization of λ is slightly different from the organization of the κ-gene locus, which contains only one Cκ gene; in contrast, each Jλ is associated with a different Cλ gene. Thus, there are six different types of Cλ polypeptides in humans.

It should be stressed that the immunoglobulin gene rearrangement events de-

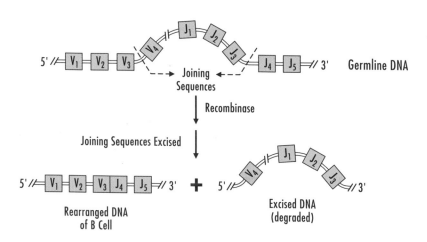

Figure 6.3.

Rearrangement of DNA coding for an immunoglobulin light chain.

scribed above for both κ and λ chains that occur in early cells of the B-lymphocyte lineage take place in the apparent *absence of antigen*. Nonetheless, the result
of the process of rearrangement (common to all B and T lymphocytes) is that the
antigenic specificity of a single lymphocyte becomes fixed; that is, once the
genes coding for a specific variable region have been rearranged and start to
make a particular receptor molecule, the specificity remains the same throughout
the lifetime of the cell. This fixing of receptor specificity in the absence of antigen also holds for immunoglobulin heavy chains and T-cell receptors.

Organization and Rearrangement of Heavy-Chain Genes

Heavy-chain genes are found on a chromosome distinct from either light chain
(chromosome 14 in humans). The organization of genes encoding the heavy chain
is different from those encoding light chains (see Fig. 6.4). In contrast to the variable region of a light chain, which is constructed from two gene segments, the
variable region of a heavy chain is constructed from three gene segments (V_H,
D_H, and J_H). Thus, in addition to V and J segments, genes coding for the variable
region of a heavy chain also use a *D (D* for *diversity) segment*. The D and J segments code for amino acid sequences in the third hypervariable region of the

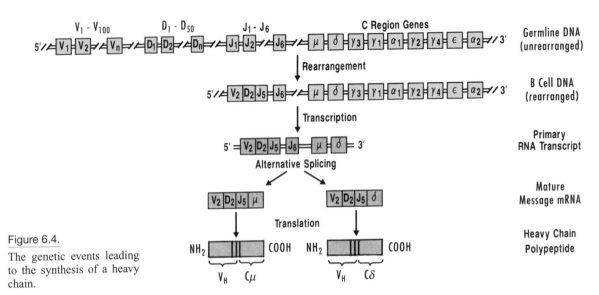

Figure 6.4.
The genetic events leading
to the synthesis of a heavy
chain.

heavy chain (see Chapter 4). A cluster of about 12 D_H gene segments is found between about 200 V_H genes and 6 J_H genes (see Fig. 6.4). There are approximately 50 D_H gene segments in the human and about 12 in the mouse.

The second key feature of the H-chain genes is the presence in the germ line of multiple genes coding for the C region of the immunoglobulin. The C region determines the class and hence biological function of the particular antibody (see Chapter 5 on the function of antibody molecules). The C genes, each flanked by introns, are separated from the V_H genes by a large intron. The order of C genes in the human is shown in Figure 6.4. The C genes closest to the V region genes are μ and δ, which are transcribed first during B-cell development.

The assembly of the H chain follows the same principles of rearrangement described for light chains, namely, the use of recombinase enzymes to mediate the joining of different segments. In the early stages of the life of a particular B cell, two rearrangements of germ line DNA must occur. The first brings one D segment alongside one J segment. The second brings one V segment next to the DJ unit ($V_2 D_2 J_5$ in Fig. 6.4), fixing the antigen specificity of the heavy chain. The rearranged DNA is then transcribed along with the closest C region genes, μ and δ. This primary transcript can be spliced in two different ways *("alternate splicing")* to yield a VDJ-μ or a VDJ-δ mRNA (see Fig. 6.4). These two messages may then be translated in rough endoplasmic reticulum to yield either a μ- or δ-expressing polypeptide. In this way an individual resting B cell may express both μ and δ with identical antigenic specificity.

Regulation of Immunoglobulin Gene Expression

Theoretically, any one B cell has many genes to choose from to synthesize an immunoglobulin molecule: multiple V, D, and J genes to form the variable regions, and different genes for the light chains, κ and λ. Interestingly, a single B cell uses only one set of VDJ genes and one type of light chain, so the result is that a *single B cell produces an immunoglobulin of only one antigenic specificity.*

Furthermore, a given B cell has two sets of chromosomes, one set from each parent. As stated earlier, H and L chains are coded for by genes found on three different chromosomes. Since each parental chromosome contains genes coding for H and L chains, theoretically six possible chromosomes could participate in synthesizing one Ig molecule. This does not occur. In contrast to all other gene products, which are derived from genes from both parental chromosomes, Ig (and T-cell receptor) molecules are coded for by only maternal or paternal genes; for example, the H chain may be coded for by genes on the paternal chromosome and the L chain by genes on the maternal chromosome. This phenomenon of using genes of only one parental chromosome is known as ***allelic exclusion***.

We now know that the steps in rearrangement, allelic exclusion, and hence the synthesis of a complete immunoglobulin (and, as we shall see later, T-cell receptor) molecule are very tightly controlled, although all the controlling mechanisms are not yet completely clear. It seems that in the differentiating cell the clusters of H chain genes on both chromosomes begin to rearrange. If a successful rearrangement of V-, D-, and J-gene DNA occurs on one of the parental chromosomes, and an H chain polypeptide is produced, then the other parental H chain DNA stops rearranging as a result of some kind of suppressive mechanism. If the first attempt to rearrange the V, D, and J genes is unsuccessful (i.e., if it fails to produce a polypeptide chain), then the second parental chromosome continues to rearrange. Thus, even though there are two chromosomal copies of the H chain in each cell, only one is functionally expressed. The same process then occurs with the light chain, first with the κ- and then with the λ-chain genes. Successful rearrangement by V-to-J fusion of any one of these genes causes the others to remain in germ line form. In this way, the cell progresses through some or all of its chromosomal copies until it has successfully completed the productive rearrangement of genes for one H and one L chain. These chains then become the basis of the antibody specificity of that particular cell. (A cell that fails to make functional H- and L-chain rearrangements makes no immunoglobulin receptors; it is incapable of responding to further stimulation and it dies.) This mechanism of gene exclusion ensures that every B cell and the antibody that it synthesizes is monospecific, that is, specific for only one epitope. In this way B cells are prevented from forming immunoglobulin molecules with different antigenic specificities on the same cell surface.

CLASS OR ISOTYPE SWITCHING

As we have described, one B cell forms antibody of just one single specificity that is fixed by the nature of VJ and VDJ rearrangements. However, during the lifetime of this cell ***it can switch to make a different class of antibody, such as IgG or IgE, while retaining the same antigenic specificity.*** This phenomenon is known as ***class*** or ***isotype switch*** (see Chapter 5 for more on the function of antibody isotypes). It involves further DNA rearrangement, juxtaposing the rearranged VDJ genes with a different heavy-chain C region gene (Fig. 6.5). In contrast to the previously described VJ and VDJ rearrangements, which occur prior to

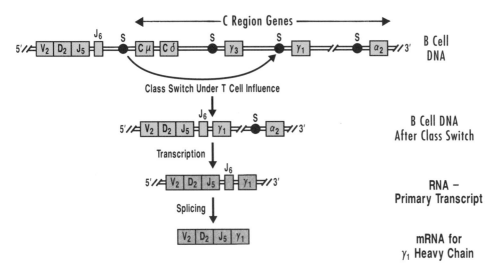

Figure 6.5.

Mechanism of class switching in immunoglobulin synthesis. S = switch region, upstream of each heavy-chain constant region gene except δ.

antigen exposure in the differentiating early B cell, class switching occurs in mature B cells and is dependent on antigenic stimulation of the cell and the presence of factors released by T cells. These factors are known as cytokines (see below and further discussion in Chapter 11). In the absence of such T-cell-derived cytokines there is little or no class switching by B cells.

The cytokines that affect class switch induce further rearrangement of B cell DNA and produce switching to other immunoglobulin classes in a downstream progression (e.g., to IgG_4 or IgE). Thus, a single B cell with a unique specificity is capable of making an antibody of all possible classes depending on the switches occurring in the DNA coding for its heavy chain.

The mechanism by which mature B cells undergo class switch is as follows: each C region gene of the H chain (C_H) has at its 5′ end a stretch of repeating base sequences called a ***switch (S) region*** (Fig. 6.5). This S region permits any of the C_H regions to associate with the VDJ unit. (The only exception is the δ gene, which has no switch region.) Under the stimulating influence of antigen and T-cell-derived cytokines, a B cell with a VDJ unit linked to Cμ and Cδ further rearranges its DNA to link the VDJ to an S region in front of another C region gene (γ_1 in Fig. 6.5). In so doing, the intervening C region DNA is removed. Thus, at this stage the cell loses its ability to revert to making a class of antibody whose C-region gene has been deleted (e.g., IgM, IgD, or IgG_3). Again, a primary RNA transcript is made from this rearranged DNA. The transcript has all the introns spliced out to give a mRNA coding for the IgG_1 heavy chain.

It is important to note that this phenomenon of class switching is unique to immunoglobulin H chains. Whereas gene rearrangement mechanisms are used for synthesizing individual H and L Ig and TcR chains, only genes coding for Ig H chains undergo DNA rearrangement using switch regions $5'$ of their C_H genes. Class switching is a unique mechanism that allows an antibody with a single antigenic specificity to associate with a variety of different effector functions.

It is also noteworthy that the C_H gene selected in isotype switching is critically dependent on the nature of the cytokine present at the time of antigen activation of the B cell. Thus, in the mouse, if the cytokine interferon γ is present, the B cell can rearrange its VDJ to the $C\gamma_2$ heavy chain and the cell will switch to IgG_2 synthesis. In contrast, if the cytokine IL-4 is present, a human or mouse B cell can rearrange its VDJ to $C\gamma_4$ or $C\epsilon$ and the cell will switch to IgG_4 or IgE synthesis. The cytokines that affect class switch are believed to induce the loosening of the structure of the DNA double helix at only certain points along the immunoglobulin gene, allowing the recombinase access only to specific C regions.

GENERATION OF ANTIBODY DIVERSITY

Thus far we have described the unique genetic mechanisms involved in generating an enormously varied set of antibodies to cope with the universe of antigens without using a great deal of DNA. Still more mechanisms for generating diversity exist, each of which is discussed briefly below.

Presence of Multiple V Genes in the Germ Line

The number of different genes for the V region in the germ line constitutes the baseline from which antibody is derived and represents the minimum number of different antibodies that could be produced.

DJ–VDJ Combinatorial Association

As we have already seen, the association of any V-gene segment with any J-gene segment can occur to form a light-chain variable region, and similarly, any V can associate with any J- or D-gene segments in heavy-chain gene rearrangement. All these distinct segments contribute to the structure of the variable region. As there are about 200 Vκ and 5 Jκ genes coding for the κ-chain variable region, assuming random association, then 200 × 5 or 1000 κ chains can be formed; with 100 V_λ and 6 J_λ genes, 600 λ chains can be formed. Similarly, if there are about 200 V genes, 12 D genes, and 6 J genes that can code for an H-chain variable region, and these may also associate in any combination, then 200 × 12 × 6 or 14,400 different heavy chains can be formed.

Random Assortment of H and L Chains

In addition to DJ–VDJ combinatorial association, any H chain may associate with any L chain. Thus, if any H chain can associate with any κ or λ chain, a total of 14.4×10^6 different κ-containing immunoglobulin molecules (1000 × 14,400), and 8.6×10^6 (600 × 14,400) λ-containing molecules can be generated from just 529 different genes by adding up all the H, κ, and λ segments! This illustrates very effectively how a limited set of genes can generate a large number of different antibodies.

Junctional and Insertional Diversity

The precise positions at which the genes for the V and J, or the V, D, and J, segments are joined are not constant, and imprecise DNA recombination can lead to changes in the amino acids at these junction sites. The absence of precision in joining during DNA rearrangement leads to deletions or changes of amino acids *(junctional diversity)* that affect the antigen-binding site, since they occur in parts of the hypervariable region, where complementarity to antigen is determined. In addition, small sets of nucleotides may be inserted *(insertional diversity)* at the V–D and D–J junctions by the enzyme terminal deoxynucleotidyl transferase without the need for a template. The additional diversity provided is termed *N region diversity.*

Somatic Cell Mutation

Mutations that occur in V genes during the lifetime of an individual B cell can increase the variety of antibodies produced by the B cell. Such mutations may provide a mechanism for fine-tuning an immune response. It has been shown by sequencing of DNA and polypeptides that an antibody formed in a primary response follows very closely the sequence of the protein that would be encoded by germ line DNA. As the response matures, especially after secondary stimulation by the antigen, an increase in affinity of the antibody for the antigen occurs, and a divergence is found from the amino acid sequence that is encoded in germ line DNA. This divergence occurs predominantly as a result of point mutations, which affect individual amino acids in the hypervariable regions, although other mechanism such as gene conversion may also be involved. Recent evidence suggests that there is a narrow window for somatic mutation to occur, that is, after antigenic stimulation in the germinal centers of spleen and lymph node, as we shall see in Chapter 8.

Thus, it is believed that an immune response commences with the formation of low-affinity antibodies, built according to information provided by germ line genes. As the immune response continues, somatic mutations may occur that are then positively selected for, since they lead to the production of antibody with greater affinity for antigen.

All these mechanisms—the presence of multiple VDJ genes, combinatorial association, junctional diversity, and somatic mutation—contribute to the formation of a huge *library* or *repertoire* of B lymphocytes that contain all the specificities required to deal with the universe of diverse epitopes.

SUMMARY

1. Every individual synthesizes an enormous number of different immunoglobulin (Ig) molecules, each of which can act as a receptor on the B-cell surface, specific for a particular epitope.

2. The variable region of a heavy-chain Ig molecule is coded for by three separate genes, referred to as V_H (variable), D_H (diversity), and J_H (joining) gene segments. A distinct gene segment codes for the constant region of the heavy chain, C_H. The variable region of a light-chain Ig molecule is coded for by two gene segments, V_L and J_L, distinct from the gene segments used for heavy-chain synthesis. Every cell in the body (the germ line) contains multiple V, D, and J gene segments for immunoglobulin H- and L-chain synthesis.

3. In the course of differentiation, a B cell *rearranges* its heavy-chain DNA so as to join one V_H gene segment to one D_H gene segment and one J_H gene segment. The joined VDJ unit codes for the entire variable region of the heavy chain. These gene rearrangements put the VDJ unit next to the heavy-chain constant region genes, C_μ and C_δ.

4. The same type of rearrangement occurs to produce a gene unit coding for the entire V region of an Ig L chain; one V_L gene segment is joined to one J_L segment. This VJ unit is put next to a light-chain constant region gene. In a B cell committed to making a κ chain, the $V_κ J_κ$ unit is put next to the $C_κ$ gene. In a B cell committed to making a λ chain, $V_λ J_λ$ is juxtaposed to a $C_λ$ gene.

5. When DNA rearrangement has occurred, the antigenic specificity of that particular cell is fixed. Primary RNA transcripts are made from the re-arranged DNA. Unnecessary RNA is spliced out of the primary transcripts, resulting in mRNA for light and heavy chains, which are then translated into the L and H chains of IgM and IgD.

6. After antigenic stimulation, a B cell can further rearrange its DNA. The VDJ unit, which has joined to the Cμ and Cγ genes, can rearrange to join another C region gene, such as Cγ, Cα, or Cε. This phenomenon is known as *class switching*. As a result, the B cell that was synthesizing IgM and IgD can now synthesize antibody of a different isotype (IgG, IgA, or IgE) but with the same antigenic specificity.

7. Diversity in antibody specificity is achieved by (a) multiple inherited genes for the V regions of both L and H chains; (b) rearrangement of V, J, and D segments in different combinations and random assortment of H and L chains; (c) junctional and insertional diversity when V, D, and J genes are joined; and (d) somatic mutation, which primarily occurs after stimulation by antigen, leading to selection for mutations that endow the antibody with higher affinity for the antigen. Thus, these mechanisms allow a small number of genes to generate a vast number of antibody molecules with different antigenic specificites.

REFERENCES

Chen J, Alt FW (1992): Gene rearrangement and B-cell development. Current Opinion Immunol 5:194.

Mombaerts J, Iacomini J, Johnson RS, Herrup K, Tonegawa S, Papaioannou VE (1992): RAG-1 deficient mice have no mature B and T lymphocytes. Cell 68:869.

Oettinger MA, Schatz DG, Gorka C, Baltimore D (1990): RAG-1 and RAG-2, adjacent genes that synergistically activate V(D)J recombination. Science 248:1517.

Schatz DG, Oettinger MA, Schissel MS (1992): V(D)J recombination: molecular biology and regulation. Annu Rev Immunol 10:359.

REVIEW QUESTIONS

For each question, choose the ONE BEST answer or completion.

1. The DNA for an H chain in a B cell making IgG2 antibody for diphtheria toxoid has the following structure:

   $5'-V_{17}D_5J_2C\gamma2-C\gamma4-C\epsilon-C\alpha2-3'$

   How many individual rearrangements were required to go from the embryonic DNA to this B-cell DNA?
   A) 1
   B) 2
   C) 3
   D) 4
   E) none

2. If you had 200 V and 5 J region genes able to code for a light chain and 300 V, 10 D, and 5 J regions able to code for a heavy chain, you could have
   A) exactly 520 antibody specificities
   B) exactly 1000 antibody specificities
   C) exactly 15,000 antibody specificities
   D) exactly 15,000,000 specificities
   E) more than 15,000,000 specificities

3. The antigen specificity of a particular B cell
   A) is induced by interaction with antigen
   B) is determined only by the L-chain sequence
   C) is determined by H + L-chain variable region sequences
   D) changes after isotype switching
   E) is determined by the heavy-chain constant region

4. If you could analyze, at the molecular level, a plasma cell making IgA antibody, you would find all of the following except
   A) a DNA sequence for V, D, and J genes translocated near the αDNA exon
   B) mRNA specific for either κ or λ light chains
   C) mRNA specific for J chains
   D) mRNA specific for μ chains
   E) a DNA sequence coding for the T-cell receptor for antigen

5. The ability of a single B cell to express both IgM and IgD receptor molecules on its surface at the same time is made possible by
   A) allelic exclusion
   B) isotype switching
   C) simultaneous recognition of two distinct antigens
   D) selective RNA splicing
   E) use of genes from both parental chromosomes

6. Which of the following statements concerning the organization of immunoglobulin genes is correct?
   A) V and J regions of embryonic DNA have already undergone a rearrangement
   B) Light-chain genes undergo further rearrangement after surface IgM is expressed.
   C) V_H gene segments can rearrange with Jκ or Jλ gene segments
   D) The VDJ segments coding for an im-

munoglobulin V_H region may associate with different heavy-chain constant region genes

E) After VDJ joining has occurred, a further rearrangement is required to bring the VDJ unit next to the $C\mu$ gene.

7. Which of the following *does not* contribute

to the generation of diversity of B-cell antigen receptors?

A) multiple V genes in the germ line
B) random assortment of L and H chains
C) imprecise recombination of V and J or V, D, and J segments
D) inheritance of multiple C-region genes
E) somatic mutation

Case study: As a member of an investigatory team studying a primitive tribe found in a remote region of New Guinea, you make the astonishing discovery that these people have only two V genes for the L chain and three V genes for the H chain of immunoglobulins. Nevertheless, they seem healthy and able to resist the diversity of pathogenic organisms endemic to the area. Suggest how this might be accomplished.

ANSWERS TO REVIEW QUESTIONS

---

1. *C* Three DNA rearrangements are required. First, $D_5 \rightarrow J_2$ rearrangement occurs, followed by the $V_{17} \rightarrow D_5J_2$. This permits synthesis of IgM and IgD molecules using $V_{17}D_5J_2$. The third rearrangement is the class switch of $V_{17}D_5J_2C\mu C\delta$ to $V_{17}D_5J_2C\gamma2$, leading to the synthesis of IgG_2 molecules.

2. *E* While 15,000,000 would be the product of all possible combinations of genes, there would still be many other possibilities due to imprecise recombinations of VJ or VDJ segments as well as somatic mutation.

3. *C* The antigenic specificity is determined by the sequences and hence the structure formed by the combination of heavy- and light-chain variable regions.

4. *D* As a consequence of the rearrangement of the VDJ to $C\alpha$ in the IgA producing cell, the $C\mu$ gene will have been deleted. The other DNA sequences and mRNA species will be found in the cell.

5. *D* The simultaneous synthesis of IgM and IgD is made possible by the alternate splicing of the primary RNA transcript $5'$–VDJ–$C\mu$–$C\delta$–$3'$ to give either VDJ $C\mu$ or VDJ $C\delta$ messages.

6. *D* This is the basis of isotype or class switching.

7. *D* The presence of multiple C_H region genes, although the basis for functional diversity, does not contribute to the diversity of antigen-specific receptors.

Case study: Despite the paucity of V-region genes, these people presumably still have other mechanisms for generating diversity. These include the presence of multiple J and D gene segments in the germ line, junctional diversity due to deletion or insertion of bases at joining sites, random assortment of H and L chains, and finally, somatic mutation. It is therefore conceivable that even with the limited V-gene repertoire available to them, they can generate sufficient diversity of antibody specificity to survive.

ANTIGEN–ANTIBODY INTERACTIONS

INTRODUCTION

Antibodies constitute the humoral arm of acquired immunity that provides protection against infectious organisms and their toxic products. Therefore, the interaction between antigen and antibody is of paramount importance. In addition, because of the exquisite specificity of the immune response, the interaction between antigen and antibody in vitro is widely used for diagnostic purposes, for the detection and identification of either antigen or antibody. The utilization of the in vitro reaction between antigen and serum antibodies is termed *serology*. An example of the use of serology for the identification and classification of antigens is the *serotyping* of various microorganisms by the use of specific antisera.

The interaction of antigen with antibodies may result in a variety of consequences, including *precipitation* (if the antigen is soluble), *agglutination* (if the antigen is particulate), and *activation of complement*. All of these outcomes are caused by the interactions between multivalent antigens and antibodies that have at least two combining sites per molecule. The consequences of antigen–antibody interaction listed above do not represent the primary interaction between antibodies and a given epitope but, rather, depend on secondary phenomena, which result from the interactions between multivalent antigens and antibodies. Such phenomena as the formation of precipitate, agglutination, and complement activation would not occur if the antibody with two or more combining sites reacted with a hapten (i.e., a unideterminant, univalent antigen), nor would they occur as a result of the interaction between a univalent fragment of antibody, such as Fab, and an antigen, even if the antigen is multivalent. The reasons for these differences are depicted in Figure 7.1A–E. ***Cross-linking*** of various antigen molecules by antibody is required for precipitation, agglutination, or complement activation, and it is possible only if the antigen is multivalent and the antibody is divalent [either intact, or F(ab′)₂] (see Fig. 7.1B, D, E). In contrast, no cross-linking is possible if the antigen or the antibody is univalent (Fig. 7.1A, C).

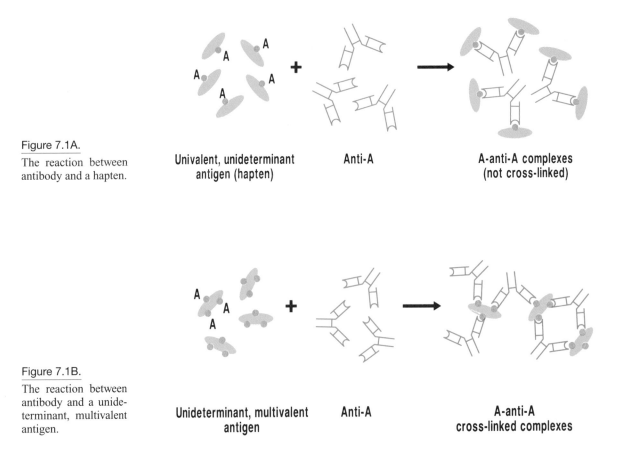

Figure 7.1A.

The reaction between antibody and a hapten.

Univalent, unideterminant antigen (hapten)   **Anti-A**   **A-anti-A complexes (not cross-linked)**

Figure 7.1B.

The reaction between antibody and a unideterminant, multivalent antigen.

Unideterminant, multivalent antigen   **Anti-A**   **A-anti-A cross-linked complexes**

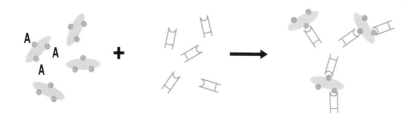

Unideterminant multivalent antigen   **Anti-A Fab**   **A-anti-A Fab complexes (not cross-linked)**

Figure 7.1C.

The reaction between Fab and a unideterminant, multivalent antigen.

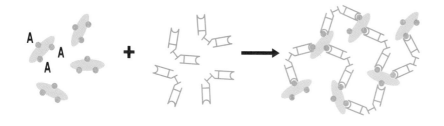

Unideterminant, multivalent antigen   **F(ab′)₂ anti-A**   **A-anti-A cross-linked complexes**

Figure 7.1D.

The reaction between F(ab′)₂ and a unideterminant, multivalent antigen.

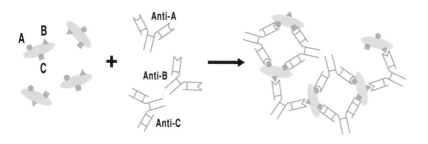

Multideterminant, multivalent antigen   **A-anti-A, B-anti-B, C-anti-C cross-linked complexes**

Figure 7.1E.

The reaction between antibodies to determinants A, B, and C, and a multivalent, multideterminant antigen with determinants A, B, and C.

There are many serologic reactions that demonstrate the binding between antigen and antibodies. This chapter describes selected reactions that are used in diagnosis; many others, not included here, are mostly variations of the reactions described here.

PRIMARY INTERACTIONS BETWEEN ANTIBODY AND ANTIGEN

No covalent bonds are involved in the interaction between antibody and an epitope. Consequently, the binding forces are relatively weak. They consist mainly of *van der Waals forces, electrostatic forces,* and *hydrophobic forces,* all of which require a very close proximity between the interacting moieties. Thus the interaction requires a very close fit between an epitope and the antibody, a fit that is often compared to that between a lock and a key. Because of the low levels of energy involved in the interaction between antigen and antibody, antigen–antibody complexes can be readily *dissociated* by *low or high pH,* by *high salt concentrations,* or by *chaotropic ions,* such as cyanates, which efficiently interfere with the hydrogen bonding of water molecules.

Association Constant

The reaction between an antibody and an epitope of an antigen is exemplified by the reaction between antibody and a univalent hapten. Because an antibody molecule is symmetric, with two identical Fab antigen combining sites, one antibody molecule binds with two identical hapten molecules, each Fab binding in an independent fashion with one hapten molecule. The binding of a hapten (H) with each site can be represented by the equation

$$Ab + H \rightleftharpoons AbH$$

and the association constant between the reactants is expressed as

$$K = \frac{[Ab\,H]}{[Ab][H]}$$

When all the antibody molecules that bind a given hapten or epitope are identical (as in the case of monoclonal antibodies), then K represents the *intrinsic associa-*

tion constant. However, because serum antibodies—even those binding to a single epitope—are heterogeneous, an *average association constant* of all the antibodies to the epitope is referred to as K_0. The interaction between antibodies and each epitope of a multivalent antigen follows the same kinetics and energetics as those involved in the interaction between antibodies and haptens, because each epitope of the antigen reacts with its corresponding antibody in the same manner as that described above.

Affinity and Avidity

The intrinsic association constant that characterizes the binding of an antibody with an epitope or a hapten is termed *affinity*. When the antigen consists of many repeating identical epitopes or when antigens are multivalent, the association between the entire antigen molecule and antibodies depends not only on the affinity between each epitope and its corresponding antibody but also on the sum of the affinities of all the epitopes involved. For example, the affinity of binding of anti-A with multivalent A (shown in Fig. 7.1B) may be four or five orders of magnitude higher than between the same antibody (i.e., anti-A) and univalent A (Fig. 7.1A). This is because the pairing of anti-A with A (where A is multivalent) is influenced by the increased number of sites on A with which anti-A can react.

While the term *affinity* denotes the intrinsic association constant between antibody and a univalent ligand such as a hapten, the term *avidity* is used to denote the overall binding energy between antibodies and a multivalent antigen. Thus, in general, IgM antibodies are of higher avidity than IgG antibodies, although the binding of each Fab in the IgM antibody with ligand may be of the same affinity as that of the Fab from IgG.

SECONDARY INTERACTIONS BETWEEN ANTIBODY AND ANTIGEN

Agglutination Reactions

Referring again to the representations given in Figure 7.1, the reactions of antibody with a multivalent antigen that is *particulate* (i.e., an insoluble particle) results in the cross-linking of the various antigen particles by the antibodies. This cross-linking eventually results in the clumping or agglutination of the antigen particles by the antibodies.

TITER. The agglutination of an antigen as a result of cross-linking by antibodies is dependent on the correct proportion of antigen to antibody. Figure 7.2 depicts an example of an agglutination test for antibodies to the bacterium *Brucella abortus* present in the serum of an infected individual. The figure shows 10 tubes containing twofold serial dilution of the serum, ranging from 1:4 to 1:2048, to which equal amounts of a suspension of *B. abortus* (a particulate antigen) are added. The plus and minus signs denote the presence or absence of agglutination. The results of the test (shown below each tube) indicate that agglutination occurs at dilutions of serum of 1:16 to 1:1024. There is no agglutination at higher dilutions because at such dilutions there are not enough antibodies to cause appreciable, visible agglutination. The highest dilution of serum that still causes agglutination, but beyond which no agglutination occurs, is termed the *titer*. In the example depicted in Figure 7.2, the titer is 1:1024.

PROZONE. The left-hand side of Figure 7.2 shows tubes with no agglutination, although they contain a suspension of antigen and concentrated serum (diluted only 1:4 or 1:8). It is a common observation that agglutination may not occur at high concentrations of antibody, even though it does take place at higher dilutions of serum. The tubes with high concentrations of serum, where agglutination does not occur, represent a ***prozone***. In the prozone, antibodies are present in excess. Agglutination may not occur at high ratio of antibody to antigen because

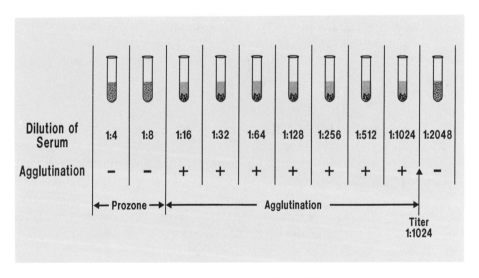

Figure 7.2.
A representation of the agglutination test.

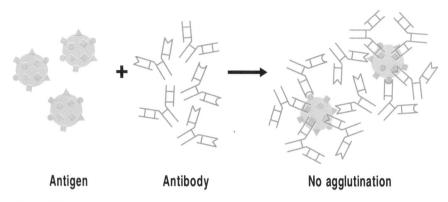

Antigen   **Antibody**   **No agglutination**

Figure 7.3.

A representation of a prozone (when antibody is present in excess) in the agglutination reaction.

every epitope on one particle may bind only to a single antibody molecule, preventing cross-linking between different particles (see Fig. 7.3).

Because of the prozone phenomenon, in testing for the presence of agglutinating antibodies to a certain antigen, it is imperative that the antiserum be tested at several dilutions. Testing serum at only one concentration may give misleading conclusions if no agglutination occurs, because the absence of agglutination might reflect either a prozone or a lack of antibody.

The agglutinating titer of a certain serum is only a *semiquantitative* expression of the antibodies present in the serum; it is not a quantitative measure of the concentration of antibody (weight/volume). Rather, the titer represents the ability of a certain dilution (i.e., volume) of the serum containing the antibodies to cause agglutination. As such, the titer of a given antiserum may be used for comparison with the agglutinating titer to another antiserum to the same antigen. For example, a change in titer of anti-*B. abortus* antibodies, in an individual, from 1:4 to 1:1024 would indicate an acute infection, while on the other hand a drop in titer might suggest that antimicrobial therapy was working. Thus, agglutination titers are useful for comparisons of the relative concentrations of agglutinating antibodies in various sera specific for the same antigen. Since the titer in any agglutination assay depends on a variety of factors, such as size, charge, and density of epitopes on an antigen, it is of little use to compare titers of antisera to different antigens.

ZETA POTENTIAL. The surfaces of certain particulate antigens may possess an electrical charge, as, for example, the net negative charge on the surface of red blood cells caused by the presence of sialic acid. When such charged particles are suspended in saline solution, an electrical potential termed the *zeta potential* is created between particles, preventing them from getting very close to each other. This introduces a difficulty in agglutinating charged particles by antibodies, in particular red blood cells by IgG antibodies. The distance between the Fab arms of the IgG molecule, even in its most extended form, is too short to allow effective bridging between two red blood cells across the zeta potential. Thus, although IgG antibodies may be directed against antigens on the charged erythrocyte, agglutination may not occur because of the repulsion by the zeta potential. On the other hand, some of the Fab areas of *IgM pentamers* are far enough apart and can bridge red blood cells separated by the zeta potential. This property of IgM antibodies, together with their pentavalence, is a major reason for their effectiveness as agglutinating antibodies.

Through the years attempts were made to improve agglutination reactions by decreasing the zeta potential in various ways, none of which was universally applicable or effective. However, an ingenious method was devised in the 1950s by Coombs to overcome this problem. This method, described below, facilitates the agglutination of erythrocytes by IgG antibodies specific for erythrocyte antigens. It is also useful for the detection of antibodies that are present on the surface of erythrocytes but that are unable to agglutinate them.

THE COOMBS TEST. The Coombs test employs antibodies to immunoglobulins (hence, it is also called the *anti-immunoglobulin test*). It is based on two important facts: (1) that immunoglobulins of one species (e.g, human) are immunogenic when injected into another species (e.g., rabbit) and lead to the production of antibodies against the immunoglobulins, and (2) that many of the anti-immunoglobulins (e.g., rabbit antihuman Ig) bind with antigenic determinants present on the Fc portion of the antibody, and leave the Fab portions free to react with antigen. Thus, for example, if human IgG antibodies are attached to their respective epitopes on erythrocyte, then the addition of rabbit antibodies to human IgG will result in their binding with the Fc portions of the human antibodies bound to the erythrocytes by their Fab portion (see Fig. 7.4). These rabbit antibodies not only bind with the human antibodies that are bound to the erythrocyte but also, by so doing, they cross-link (form bridges) between human IgG on relatively distant erythrocytes, across the separation caused by the zeta potential, and cause agglutination. The addition of anti-immunoglobulin brings about agglutination, even if the antibodies directed against the erythrocytes are present at sufficiently high concentrations to cause the prozone phenomenon.

There are two versions of the Coombs test: the *direct Coombs test* and the *indirect Coombs test*. The two versions differ somewhat in the mechanics of the test

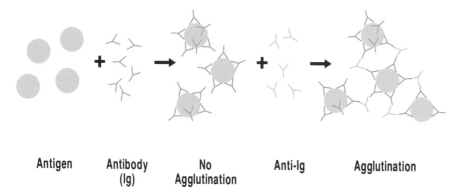

| Antigen | Antibody (Ig) | No Agglutination | Anti-Ig | Agglutination |

Figure 7.4.

A representation of the anti-immunoglobulin (Coombs) test.

but both are based on the same principle: using heterologous anti-immunoglobu-lins to detect a reaction between immunoglobulins and antigen. In the ***direct Coombs test***, anti-immunoglobulins are added to the particles (e.g., red blood cells) that are suspected of having antibodies bound to antigens on their surfaces. For example, a newborn baby is suspected of having hemolytic disease of the newborn caused by maternal anti-Rh IgG antibodies that are bound to the baby's erythrocytes. If that suspicion proved to be correct, the direct Coombs test would have the following results: the addition of anti-immunoglobulin to a suspension of the baby's erythrocytes would result in the binding of the anti-immunoglobulin to the maternal IgG on the surface of the erythrocytes and would cause agglutination (Fig. 7.5A). The ***indirect Coombs test*** is used to detect the presence, ***in the serum,*** of antibodies specific to antigens on the particle. The serum antibodies, when added to the particles, may fail to cause agglutination because of the zeta poten-tial. The subsequent addition of anti-Ig will cause agglutination. A common appli-cation of the indirect Coombs test is in the detection of anti-Rh IgG antibodies in the blood of an Rh-negative woman (see Chapter 19). This consists, first, of the reaction of the woman's serum with Rh^+ erythrocytes, and then the addition of the anti-immunoglobulin reagents (as in the direct Coombs test) (Fig. 7.5B). Thus, the direct Coombs test measures bound antibody while the indirect test measures serum antibody.

Originally, the Coombs test was used for the detection of human antibodies on the surface of erythrocytes. Today the term is applied to the detection, by the use of anti-immunoglobulin, of any Ig that is bound to antigen.

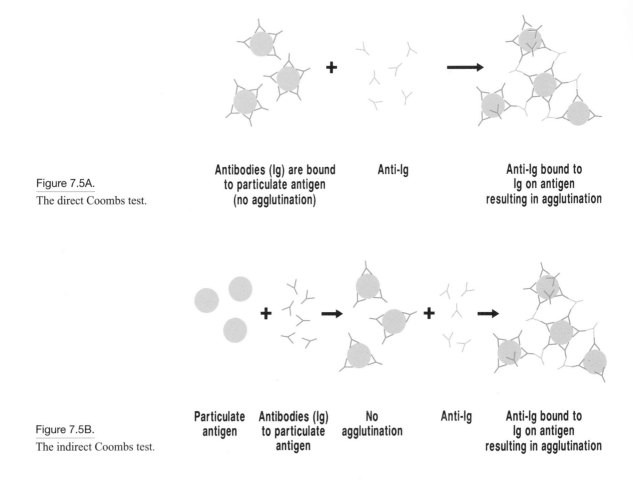

Figure 7.5A.
The direct Coombs test.

Figure 7.5B.
The indirect Coombs test.

PASSIVE AGGLUTINATION. The agglutination reaction can be used with particulate antigens (e.g., erythrocytes or bacteria) and also with soluble antigens, provided that the soluble antigen can be firmly attached to insoluble particles. For example, the soluble antigen thyroglobulin can be attached to latex particles, so that the addition of antibodies to the thyroglobulin antigen will cause agglutination of the latex particles coated with thyroglobulin. Of course, the addition of soluble antigen to the antibodies prior to the introduction of the thyroglobulin cortex latex particles will inhibit the agglutination because the antibodies will first combine with the soluble antigen, and if the soluble antigen is present in excess, the antibodies will not be able to bind with the particulate antigen. This latter example is referred to as ***agglutination inhibition.*** It should be distinguished from agglutination inhibition in which antibodies to certain viruses inhibit the agglutination of red blood cells by the virus. In these cases, the antibodies are directed to the area or areas on the virus that bind with the appropriate virus receptors on the red blood cells.

When the antigen is a natural constituent of a particle, the agglutination reaction is referred to as ***direct agglutination.*** When the agglutination reaction takes place between antibodies and soluble antigen that had been attached to an insoluble particle, the reaction is referred to as ***passive agglutination.***

The agglutination reaction (direct or passive, either employing or not employing the Coombs test) is widely used clinically. In addition to the examples already given, major applications include erythrocyte typing in blood banks, diagnosis of various immunologically mediated hemolytic diseases, such as drug-induced autohemolytic anemia, tests for rheumatoid factor (human IgM anti-human IgG), confirmatory test for syphilis, and the latex test for pregnancy, which involves the detection of human chorionic gonadotropin (HCG) in the urine of pregnant women.

Precipitation Reaction

REACTION IN SOLUTIONS. In contrast to the agglutination reaction, which takes place between antibodies and particulate antigen, the ***precipitation reaction*** takes place when antibodies and ***soluble antigen*** are mixed. As in the case of agglutination, precipitation of antigen–antibody complexes occurs because the divalent antibody molecules cross-link multivalent antigen molecules to form a ***lattice***. When it reaches a certain size, this antigen-antibody complex loses its solubility and precipitates out of solution. The phenomenon of precipitation is termed the ***precipitin reaction***.

Figure 7.6 depicts a qualitative precipitin reaction. When increasing concentrations of antigen are added to a series of tubes that contain a constant concentration of antibodies, variable amounts of precipitate form. The weight of the precipitate in each tube may be determined by a variety of methods. If the amount of the precipitate is plotted against the amount of antigen added, a precipitin curve like the one shown in Figure 7.6 is obtained.

There are three important areas under the curve shown in Figure 7.6: (1) the ***zone of antibody excess,*** (2) the ***equivalence zone,*** and (3) the ***zone of antigen excess***. In the equivalence zone, the proportion of antigen to antibody is optimal for maximal precipitation; in the zones of antibody excess or antigen excess, the proportions of the reactants do not lead to efficient cross-linking and formation of precipitate.

It should be emphasized that the zones of the precipitin curve are based on

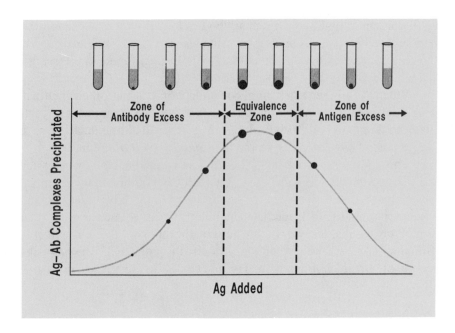

Figure 7.6.

A representation of the precipitin reaction.

the amount of antigen–antibody complexes precipitated. However, the zones of antigen or antibody excess may contain soluble antigen–antibody complexes, particularly the zone of antigen excess where a minimal amount of precipitate is formed, but large amounts of *antigen–antibody complexes* are present in the supernatant. Thus, the amount of precipitate formed is dependent on the proportions of the reactant antigens and antibodies: the correct proportion of the reactions result in maximal formation of precipitate; excess of antigen (or antibody) results in soluble complexes.

PRECIPITATION REACTIONS IN GELS. Precipitation reactions between soluble antigens and antibodies can take place not only in solution but also in semisolid media such as agar gels. When soluble antigen and antibodies are placed in wells cut in the gel (Fig. 7.7A), the reactants diffuse in the gel and form gradients of concentration, with the highest concentrations closest to the wells. Somewhere between the two wells, the reacting antigen and antibodies will be present at proportions that are optimal for formation of a precipitate.

If the antibody well contains antibodies 1, 2, and 3 specific for antigens 1, 2, and 3, respectively, and if antigens 1, 2, and 3, placed in the antigen well, diffuse at different rates (with diffusion rates of $1 \gg 2 \gg 3$), then three distinct precipitin lines will form. These three precipitin lines form because anti-1, anti-2, and anti-

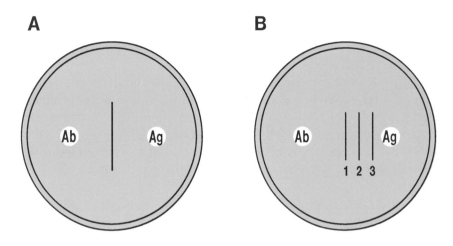

Figure 7.7.
Gel diffusion by antibodies and a single antigen (A) and antibodies to antigens 1, 2, and 3 and their respective antigents (B).

3, which diffuse at the same rate, react independently with antigens 1, 2, and 3, respectively, to form three equivalence zones and thus three separate lines of precipitate (Fig. 7.7B). Different rates of diffusion of both antibody and antibody and antigen result from differences in concentration, molecular size, or shape.

This ***double-diffusion*** method, developed by Ouchterlony, where antigen and antibody diffuse toward each other, is very useful for establishing the antigenic relationship between various substances, as shown in Figure 7.8. Three reaction patterns are seen in gel diffusion, each of which is illustrated in Figure 7.8: patterns of identity, patterns of nonidentity, and patterns of partial identity.

Patterns of Identity. In the example given on the left in Figure 7.8, the central well contains antibodies and the peripheral wells contain identical antigens. The antibodies diffuse from the central well toward the antigens that, since they are identical, form one ***continuous, coalescing*** precipitin line. This pattern, formed when the two antigens are identical, is termed a ***pattern of identity***.

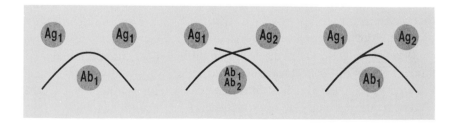

Figure 7.8.
Double gel-diffusion patterns showing pattern of identity (left), pattern of nonidentity (center), and pattern of partial identity (right).

Patterns of Nonidentity. In the example in the center of Figure 7.8, the central well contains antibodies to antigen 1 and antibodies to antigen 2, two nonrelated antigens, and the peripheral wells contain the two nonrelated antigens, antigen 1 and antigen 2. The two antibody (immunoglobulin) populations diffuse toward the peripheral wells. Antigen 1 and antigen 2 diffuse from the two peripheral wells toward the antibodies. Each antigen forms an independent precipitin line with its corresponding antibody at an equivalent point. The precipitin lines cross each other since each antigen diffuses across the band formed by the other antigen until it meets its specific antibody diffusing toward it. A pattern where the precipitin lines *cross each other* denotes *nonidentity* of the two antigens.

Patterns of Partial Identity. The pattern of partial identity is shown in the right-hand portion of Figure 7.8, where the center well contains antibodies to various epitopes of antigen 1. The reaction of these antibodies with antigen 1 results in a precipitin line. Antigen 2, however, contains some (but not all) of the epitopes present on antigen 1. Thus, some of the antibodies to antigen 1 will also combine with antigen 2. This *partial identity* between the two antigens is responsible for the coalescence of the two lines to give a line of identity. However, antibodies that do not bind with antigen 2 will pass through this line of precipitate, combine with antigen 1 on the other side, and form a *spur*. This pattern, with the formation of a spur, denotes partial identity, signifying that antigen 1 and antigen 2 share epitopes, with antigen 1 having more epitopes (and being able to react with more antibody populations) than antigen 2.

RADIAL IMMUNODIFFUSION. The radial immunodiffusion test, depicted in Figure 7.9, represents a variation of the diffusion test. The wells contain antigen at different concentrations, while the antibodies are distributed uniformly in the agar gel. Thus, the precipitin line is replaced by a precipitin ring around the well. The distance the precipitin ring migrates from the center of the antigen well is directly proportional to the concentration of antigen in the well. The relationship between concentration of antigen in a well and the diameter of the precipitin ring can be plotted as shown in Figure 7.9. If wells, such as F and G, contain unknown amounts of the same antigen, the concentration of that antigen in these wells can be determined by comparing the diameter of the precipitin ring with the *diameter* of the ring formed by a known concentration of the antigen.

An important application of radial immunodiffusion is its use clinically to measure concentrations of serum proteins. To do so, antiserum to various serum proteins is incorporated in the gel; concentration of a particular protein in a serum sample is determined by comparing the diameter of the resulting precipitin ring with the diameter obtained by known concentrations of the protein in question.

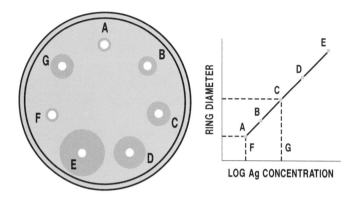

Figure 7.9.

Radial diffusion, A, B, C, D, and E represent known concentrations of antigen; F and G represent unknown concentrations that can be determined from the graph.

IMMUNOELECTROPHORESIS.   Immunoelectrophoresis involves separating a mixture of proteins in an electrical field (electrophoresis) followed by their detection with antibodies diffusing into the gel. It is very useful for the analysis of a mixture of antigens by antiserum that contains antibodies to the antigens in the mixture. For example, in the clinical characterization of human serum proteins, a small drop of human serum is placed in a well cut in the center of a slide that is coated with agar gel. The serum is then subjected to electrophoresis, which separates the various components according to their mobilities in the electrical field. After electrophoresis, a trough is cut along the side of the slides, and antibodies to human serum proteins are placed in the trough. The antibodies diffuse in the agar, as do the separated serum proteins. At an optimal antigen:antibody ratio for each antigen and its corresponding antibodies, they form precipitin lines. The result is a pattern similar to that depicted in Figure 7.10. Comparison of the pattern and intensity of lines of normal human serum with the patterns and intensity of lines obtained with sera of patients may reveal an absence, overabundance, or other abnormality of one or more serum proteins.

WESTERN BLOTS (IMMUNOBLOTS). In the Western blot (immunoblot) technique, antigen (or a mixture of antigens) is first separated in gel. The separat-

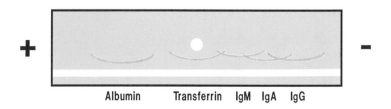

Albumin   Transferrin   IgM IgA   IgG

Figure 7.10.

Patterns of immunoelectrophoresis of serum proteins.

ed material is then "blotted" onto nitrocellulose sheets to which the antigen binds strongly. Antibody, which is then applied to the nitrocellulose sheet, binds with its specific antigen. The antibody may be labeled (e.g., with radioactivity), or a labeled anti-immunoglobulin may be used to localize the antibody and the antigen to which the first antibody is bound. These so-called "Western blots" are gaining wide application in research and clinical laboratories for the characterization of antigen. A particularly useful example is the confirmatory diagnosis of AIDS (see Chapter 18, Fig. 18.1) by the application of a patient's serum to the nitrocellulose sheets on which human immunodeficiency virus (HIV) antigens are bound. The finding of specific antibody is strong evidence of infection by the virus.

IMMUNOASSAYS

Direct Binding Immunoassays

Radioimmunoassay (RIA) employs isotopically labeled molecules and permits measurements of extremely small amounts of antigen, antibody, or antigen–antibody complexes. The concentration of such labeled molecules is determined by measuring their radioactivity, rather than by chemical analysis. The sensitivity of detection is thus increased by several orders of magnitude. For the development of this highly sensitive analytical method that has tremendous applications in hormone assays as well as assays of other substances of biological importance, RosalynYalow received the Nobel Prize.

The principle of radioimmunoassay is illustrated in Figure 7.11A,B. A known amount of radioactively labeled antigen is reacted with a limited amount of antibody. The solution now contains antibody-bound labeled antigen, as well as some unbound labeled antigen. After separating the antigen bound to antibody from free antigen, the amount of radioactivity bound to antibody is determined (Fig. 7.11A). The test continues with performance of a similar procedure in which the same amount of labeled antigen is premixed with unlabeled antigen (Fig. 7.11B). The mixture is reacted with the same amount of antibody as before, and the antibody-bound antigen is separated from the unbound antigen. The unlabeled antigen *competes* with the labeled antigen for the antibody and, as a result, less label is bound to antibody than in the absence of unlabeled antigen. The more unlabeled antigen present in the reaction mixture, the smaller the ratio of antibody-bound, radiolabeled antigen to free, radiolabeled antigen. This ratio can be plotted as a function of the concentration of the unlabeled antigen used for competition. A typical plot is shown in Figure 7.12.

To determine an unknown concentration of antigen in a solution, a sample of

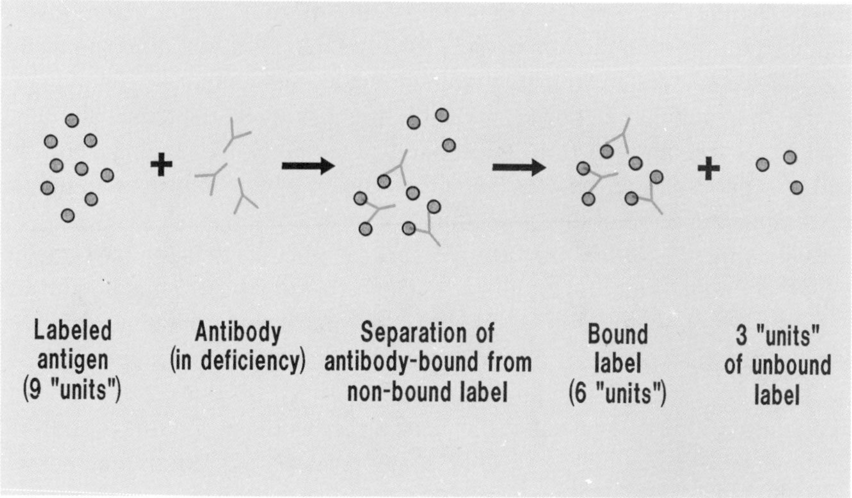

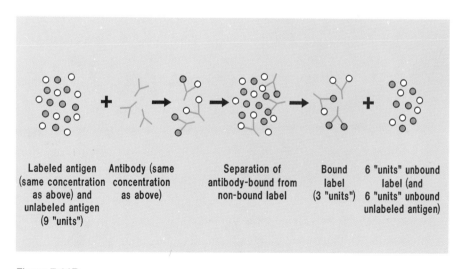

Figure 7.11A.

Amount of label bound to antibody after incubation of constant amounts of antibody and labeled antigen.

Figure 7.11B.

Radioimmunoassay, based on the competition of nonlabeled and labeled antigens for antibody.

the solution is mixed with predetermined amounts of labeled antigen and antibody. The ratio of ***bound/free radioactivity*** is compared with that obtained in the absence of unlabeled antigen (the latter value is set at 100%).

An important step in performing a radioimmunoassay, as described above, is the separation of free antigen from that bound to antibody. Depending upon the antigen, this separation can be achieved in a variety of ways, principal among which is the anti-immunoglobulin procedure.

The ***anti-immunoglobulin procedure*** is based on the fact that antigen (labeled or unlabeled) bound to immunoglobulin will also be precipitated, following the addition of anti-immunoglobulin antibodies, so that only unbound antigen remains in the supernatant. Radioimmunoassays commonly employ rabbit antibodies to the desired antigens. These rabbit antibody–antigen complexes may be precipitated by the addition of goat antibodies raised against rabbit immunoglobulins.

Since the amounts of antigen and antibody required for radioimmunoassay are extremely small, the antigen–antibody complexes reacted with anti-immunoglobulin would form only tiny precipitates. It is difficult, if not impossible, to recover these precipitates quantitatively by conventional means, in order to determine their radioactivity. To overcome this problem, it is customary to add nonspecific immunoglobulins to the reaction mixture, thereby increasing the amount of total immunoglobulins to an amount that can easily be precipitated by anti-immunoglobulins and recovered quantitatively. Such precipitates consist mainly of

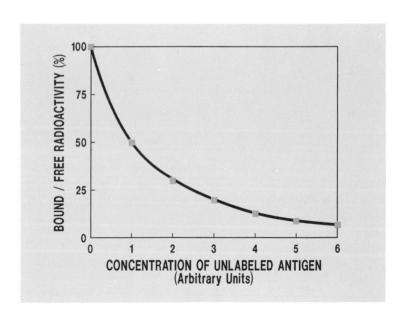

Figure 7.12.

A standard curve showing the inhibition of binding of labeled antigens to antibodies by nonlabeled antigens.

nonspecific immunoglobulins to which radioactive antigen does not bind. However, they also contain the extremely small amount of antigen-specific immunoglobulin and any radioactive antigen bound to it.

An alternative method of separating complexes of antigen bound to antibody from free antigen is based on the fact that immunoglobulins become insoluble and precipitate in a solution containing 33% saturated ammonium sulfate. If the antigen does not precipitate in 33% ammonium sulfate, the addition of ammonium sulfate to 33% will cause the antibody complexed to antigen to precipitate, leaving the free antigen in solution. Here again, the amounts of antibodies reacting with antigen (or free antibodies) is so small, unable to form precipitates. As described for the radioimmunoassay where anti-immunoglobulins are used for the separation of antibody-bound antigen from free antigen, a sufficient amount of nonspecific immunoglobulins is added to the mixture so that an appreciable precipitate will form at 33% saturation ammonium sulfate to enable the separation of free antigen from antigen bound to antibody.

Solid-Phase Immunoassays

Solid-phase immunoassay is one of the most widely used immunologic techniques. It is now automated and is widely used in clinical medicine for the detection of antigen or antibody. A good example is the use of solid-phase immunoassay for the detection of antibodies to the AIDS virus (see Chapter 18).

Solid-phase immunoassays employ the property of various plastics (e.g., polyvinyl or polystyrene) to adsorb monomolecular layers of proteins onto their surface. Although the adsorbed molecules may lose some of their antigenic determinants, enough remain unaltered and can still react with their corresponding antibodies. The presence of these antibodies, bound to antigen adsorbed onto the plastic, may be detected by the use of anti-immunoglobulins (Fig. 7.13) labeled with a radioactive tracer or with an enzyme. A solid-phase assay that uses radioactive anti-immunoglobulins is termed a solid-phase radioimmunoassay (SPRIA). If the test uses anti-immunoglobulins that are labeled with an enzyme that can be detected by the appearance of a color on addition of proper substrate, the test is called an *enzyme-linked immunosorbent assay (ELISA).* Because of problems associated with disposal or radioactive waste and the cost of radiation measuring instruments, the ELISA is rapidly replacing SPRIA.

It should be emphasized that after coating the plastic surface with antigen, it is imperative to "block" any uncoated plastic surface to prevent it from absorbing the other reagents, most importantly the labeled reagent. Such "blocking" is

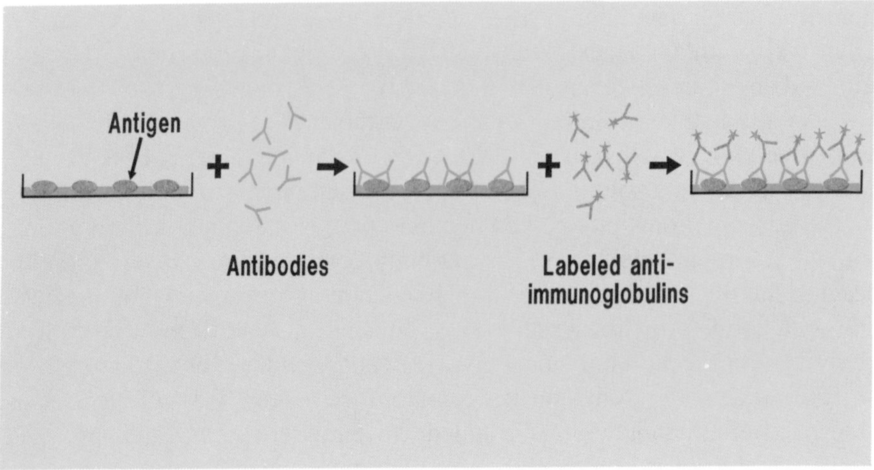

Figure 7.13.

A schematic representation of a solid-phase immunoassay.

achieved by coating the plastic surface with a high concentration of an unrelated protein, such as gelatin, after the application of the antigen.

Solid-phase immunoassay may be used to detect the presence of antibodies to the antigen that coats the plastic. Since the plastic wells are usually coated with relatively large amounts of antigen, the higher the concentration of antibodies bound with the antigen, the higher the amount of labeled anti-immunoglobulin that can bind to the antibodies. Thus, it is important always to use an excess of labeled anti-immunoglobulin to assure saturation.

Solid-phase immunoassay may be used for the qualitative or quantitative determinations of antigen. Such determinations are performed by mixing the antiserum with varying known amounts of antigen before adding the antiserum to the antigen-coated plastic wells. This preliminary procedure results in the binding of the antibodies with the soluble antigen, decreasing the availability of free antibodies for binding with the antigen that is coating the plastic. The higher the concentration of the soluble antigen that reacts with antibodies prior to addition of the antibody to the wells, the lower the number of antibodies that can bind with the antigen on the plate, and the lower the number of labeled anti-immunoglobulin that can bind to these antibodies. The decrease in the amount of bound label as a function of the concentration of antigen used to cause this decrease can be plotted, and the amount of antigen in an unknown solution can then be determined from the graph by a comparison of the decrease in bound label caused by the unknown solution to the decrease caused by known concentrations of pure antigen.

IMMUNOFLUORESCENCE

A fluorescent compound has the property of emitting light of a certain wavelength when it is excited by exposure to light of a shorter wavelength. Immunofluorescence is a method for localizing an antigen by the use of fluorescence-labeled antibodies. The procedure, originally described by Coons, employs antibodies to which fluorescent groups have been covalently linked without any appreciable change in antibody activity.

One fluorescent compound that is widely used in immunology is *fluorescein isothiocyanate (FITC),* which fluoresces with a visible greenish color when excited by ultraviolet light. FITC is easily coupled to free amino groups. Another widely used fluorescent compound is **tetramethyl rhodamine isothiocyanate (TRITC),** which fluoresces red-orange and is also easily coupled to free amino groups. Specially constructed microscopes permit visualization of fluorescent antibody on a microscopic specimen, and fluorescent antibodies are widely used to localize antigens on various tissues and microorganisms.

There are two important and related procedures that employ fluorescent antibodies: direct immunofluorescence and indirect immunofluorescence.

Direct Immunofluorescence

Direct immunofluorescence is primarily for detection of antigen and involves reacting the target tissue (or microorganism) with fluorescently labeled specific antibodies. It is widely used clinically for identifying lymphocytic subsets and for demonstrating the presence of specific protein deposition in certain tissues such as kidney and skin in cases of systemic lupus erythematosus (SLE).

Indirect Immunofluorescence

Indirect immunofluorescence involves first reacting the target with specific antibodies. This reaction is followed by subsequent reaction with fluorescently labeled anti-immunoglobulin.

The indirect immunofluorescence method is more widely used than the direct method, because a single fluorescent anti-immunoglobulin antibody can be used to localize antibody of many different specificities. Moreover, since the anti-immunoglobulins contain antibodies to many epitopes on the specific immunoglobulin, the use of fluorescent anti-immunoglobulins amplifies manyfold the fluorescent signal. An excellent example for the use of indirect immunofluorescence is the screening of patient's sera for anti-DNA antibodies in cases of SLE (see Chapter 18).

FLUORESCENCE-ACTIVATED CELL-SORTING ANALYSIS

A very powerful tool has been developed around the use of fluorescent antibody specific for cell-surface antigens. This is the technique of fluorescence-activated cell sorting (FACS). A cell suspension labeled with specific fluorescent antibody is passed through an apparatus that forms a stream of small droplets each containing one cell. These droplets are passed between a laser beam of ultraviolet light and a detector for picking up emitted fluorescence when a labeled cell is present in the droplet. This emitted signal is passed to an electrode that charges the droplet, leading to its deflection (Fig. 7.14) in an electromagnetic field. Thus as all droplets fall through they are collected and counted depending on whether they emit a signal. By sophisticated electronics the fluorescein-stained and unstained cells may be counted, as well as the intensity of fluorescence on each.

With this type of apparatus it is now possible to rapidly develop a profile of a pool of lymphocytes based on their differential expression of cell-surface molecules, the relative amount of cell-surface molecule expressed on each cell, and the

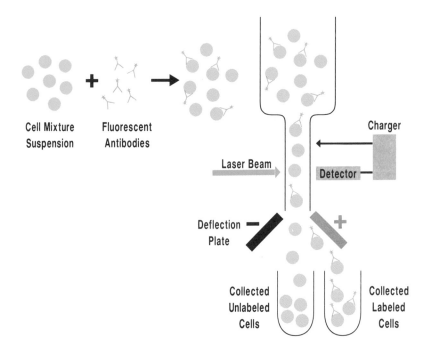

Figure 7.14.

A schematic representation of a fluorescence-activated cell sorter (FACS).

size distribution and numbers of each cell type. It is also possible to use the apparatus to sort a collection of cells stained with five or more different fluorescent labels and obtain a very homogeneous sample of a particular cell type.

A variation of this technique uses fluorescent antibodies coupled to magnetic beads to separate cell populations. Cells which bind to the fluorescent antibody can be separated from unstained cells by a magnet. Both FACS and magnetic bead separation methods have resulted in the isolation of very rare cells such as stem cells (see Chapter 8).

IMMUNOABSORPTION AND IMMUNOADSORPTION

Because of the specific binding between antigen and antibody, it is possible to "trap," or selectively remove, an antigen against which an antibody is directed from a mixture of antigens in solution. By the same token, it is possible to trap or remove selectively the antigen-specific antibodies from a mixture of antibodies, using the specific antigen.

There are two general methods by which this removal can be achieved. The methods are related, but, in one method, the absorption is done with both reagents in solution *(immunoabsorption);* in the second method, it is performed with one reagent attached to an insoluble support *(immunoadsorption).* Immunoadsorption is of particular value because the adsorbed material can be recovered from the complex by careful treatments that dissociate antigen–antibody complexes, such as lowering the pH (HCl-glycine or acetic acid, pH 2–3) or adding chaotropic ions. This enables one effectively to purify antigens or antibodies of specific interest.

MONOCLONAL AND GENETICALLY ENGINEERED ANTIBODIES

Monoclonal Antibodies

The specificity of the immune response has served as the basis for serologic reactions in which antibody specificity is used for the qualitative and quantitative determination of antigen. The discriminating power of serum antibody is not without limitations, however, because the immunizing antigen, which usually has many epitopes, leads to production of antisera that contain a mixture of antibodies with varying specificity for all the epitopes. Indeed, even antibodies to a single epitope are usually mixtures of immunoglobulins with different *fine specificities,* and therefore different affinities for the determinant. Furthermore, immunization with an antigen expands various populations of antibody-forming lymphocytes (see Chapter 11). These cells can be maintained in culture for only a short time (on the order of days), so it is impractical, if not impossible, to grow normal cells and obtain clones that produce antibodies of a single specificity

A quantum leap in the resolution and discriminating power of antibodies was provided in the 1970s with the development of methods for the generation of monoclonal antibodies by Milstein and Köhler, who shared the Nobel Prize for this development. *Monoclonal antibodies* are homogeneous populations of antibody molecules, derived from a single antibody-producing cell, in which all antibodies are identical and of the same precise specificity for a given epitope.

Milstein and Köhler took advantage of the properties of malignant plasma cells, which are "immortal" and can be maintained in culture for years. They selected a population of malignant plasma cells unable to secrete immunoglobulin and also deficient in the enzyme hypoxanthine phosphoribosyl transferase (HPRT) that would die unless HPRT were introduced. The malignant cells were then *fused* with antibody-producing cells, which have HPRT. The biotechnology for the production of *hybridomas*, developed by Köhler and Milstein, is illustrated in Figure 7.15. The fusion is generally accomplished by the use of *polyethylene glycol (PEG)* or by inactivated *Sendai virus*. The nuclei of the hybrids also fuse, and the hybridoma cells then possess both the capacity to manufacture immunoglobulins and the ability to survive in culture in a select medium such as that containing hypoxanthine, aminopterin, and thymidine (HAT). The enzyme

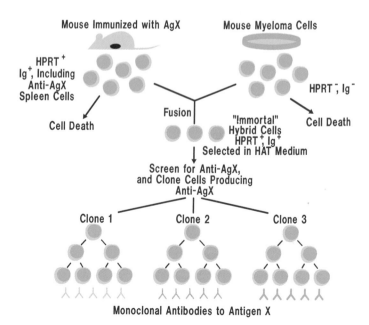

Figure 7.15.

A schematic representation of the production of monoclonal antibodies.

deficiency of the malignant cell results in its death in this medium unless that deficiency is corrected by the acquisition of the enzyme-producing genes derived from the antibody-producing cell. Thus, the hybrids can be separated from the contaminating malignant cells, which do not survive, because they have not acquired the enzyme.

Those hybrid cells synthesizing specific antibody are selected by some test for antigen reactivity and then *cloned* from single cells and propagated in tissue culture, each clone synthesizing antibodies of a ***single specificity***. These highly specific, ***monoclonal*** antibodies are used as reagents for numerous procedures, ranging from specific diagnostic tests to "magic bullets" in immunotherapy of cancer (see Chapter 21). In immunotherapy, various drugs or toxins are conjugated to monoclonal antibodies, which, in turn, "deliver" these substances to the tumor cells against which the antibodies are specifically directed (see Chapter 21).

Genetically Engineered Antibodies

To date most of the monoclonal antibodies are made in mouse cells. These are suitable for diagnostic and many other purposes. However, their administration into humans carries the complication that the patient will form antibodies to the mouse immunoglobulins. Attempts to develop in vitro human monoclonal antibodies are by and large quite difficult.

Human monoclonal antibodies are being currently produced by genetic engineering utilizing several approaches. One method utilizes the technology of recombinant DNA to produce a chimeric monoclonal antibody. This molecule consists of the constant region of human immunoglobulin and a variable region of a mouse immunoglobulin.

A more recent technology utilizes the polymerase chain reaction (PCR) to generate gene libraries of heavy and light chains from DNA obtained from hybridoma cells or plasma cells, joining at random numerous heavy and light chains and screening the resulting Fab clones for antibody activity against a desired antigen. With this technology it is now possible to produce millions of clones of different specificities, to rapidly screen them for the desired specificity and generate the desired monoclonal Fab constructs without immunization and without the difficulties encountered with the production of monoclonal antibodies, especially human monoclonal antibodies.

Although this chapter deals with antibodies, it seems appropriate to mention at this point that the hybridoma technology is not limited to the production of monoclonal immunoglobulins. In the late 1970s, methods for producing hybridomas were also developed for T cells, fusing lines of malignant T cells with nonmalignant, antigen-specific T lymphocytes whose populations have been expanded by immunization with antigen. T-cell hybridomas have been very useful for studying the relationship between T cells of a single specificity with their corresponding epitope.

SUMMARY

1. The reaction between an antibody and an epitope does not involve covalent forces; it involves weak forces of interaction such as electrostatic, hydrophobic, and van der Waals forces. Consequently, for a significant interaction, the antibody combining site and the epitope require a close steric fit like a lock and key.

2. Only the reaction between a multivalent antigen and at least a divalent antibody can bring about secondary antigen–antibody reactions that depend on cross-linking of antigen molecules by antibodies. These secondary reactions do not take place with haptens or monovalent Fab.

3. The interaction between a soluble antibody and an insoluble particulate antigen results in agglutination. The extent of agglutination depends on the proportions of the interacting antibody and antigen. At high antibody levels, excess agglutination may not occur. This is referred to as a prozone. The term _titer_ refers to the highest serum dilution at which agglutination still takes place and beyond which, at higher dilution, no agglutination occurs.

4. Because of the zeta potential, which precludes some antigenic particles from approaching each other closer than a certain distance, IgG antibodies may be incapable of causing agglutination. IgM antibodies, however, can bind such distant particles and agglutinate them.

5. The use of heterologous anti-immunoglobulin antibodies may bridge between antigenic particles that are bound to nonagglutinating antibodies, leading to agglutination. This sequence of events is the basis for the Coombs test.

6. Precipitation reactions occur on mixing, at the right proportions, of soluble multivalent antigen and (at least) divalent antibodies. The precipitation reaction may take place in aqueous media or in gels.

7. The reaction in gels, between soluble antigen and antibodies, may be used for the qualitative and quantitative analysis of antigen or antibody. Examples are gel diffusion tests, radial diffusion tests, and immunoelectrophoresis.

8. Radioimmunoassay is a test that is based on competitive inhibition of

nonlabeled and labeled antigen for antibody (in antibody deficiency). Antibody-bound antigen must be separated from nonbound labeled antigen. Separation is usually achieved by precipitation with anti-immunoglobulins.

9. Solid-phase immunoassay is a test that employs the property of many proteins to adhere to plastic and form a monomolecular layer. Antigen is applied to plastic wells, antibodies are added, the well is washed, and any antibodies bound to antigen are measured by the use of radiolabeled or enzyme-linked anti-immunoglobulins.

10. ELISA. This enzyme-linked immunosorbent assay is essentially a solid-phase immunoassay in which an enzyme is linked to the anti-immunoglobulin. Quantitation of enzyme-linked anti-immunoglobulins is achieved by colorimetric evaluation, after the addition of a substrate, which changes color on the action of the enzyme.

11. Immunofluorescence. In immunofluorescence, the antigen is detected by the use of fluorescence-labeled immunoglobulins. In direct immunofluorescence, the antibody to the antigen in question carries a fluorescent label. In indirect immunofluorescence, the antigen-specific antibody is not labeled; it is detected by the addition of fluorescently labeled anti-immunoglobulin.

12. Monoclonal antibodies are highly specific reagents consisting of homogeneous populations of antibodies, all of precisely the same specificity toward an epitope.

REFERENCES

Channing-Rodgers RP (1994): Clinical laboratory methods for detection of antigens and antibodies. In Stites DP, Terr AI, Parslow TG (eds): Basic and Clinical Immunology, 8th ed. Norwalk, CT: Appleton & Lange.

Harlow E, Lane D (1988): Antibodies: A Laboratory Manual. Cold Spring Harbor, NY: Cold Spring Harbor Laboratory.

Hudson L, Hay FC (1989): Practical Immunology, 3rd ed. Oxford: Blackwell Scientific Publications.

Johnstone A, Thorpe R (1987): Immunochemistry in Practice. Oxford: Blackwell Scientific Publications.

Mayforth RD (1993): Designing Antibodies. San Diego: Academic Press.

Mishell BB, Shiigi SM (eds) (1980): Selected Methods in Cellular Immunology. San Francisco: Freeman.

Rose NR, Friedman H, Fahey J (1986): Manual of Clinical Immunology, 3rd ed. Washington, DC: American Society for Microbiology.

Thompson KM (1988): Human monoclonal antibodies. Immunol Today 9:113.

Weir DM (ed) (1986): Handbook of Experimental Immunology, Vol 12, 4th ed. Oxford: Blackwell Scientific Publications.

REVIEW QUESTIONS

> For each question, choose the ONE BEST answer or completion.

1. A pregnancy test for human chronic gonadotropin (HCG) was performed by radioimmunoassay on a sample of urine, using standardized rabbit antiserum and radioactive HCG with specific radioactivity of 100,000 cpm/μg. The antiserum (0.1 ml), representing a slight antibody deficiency, and 1 μg of radioactive HCG were allowed to react together first. Analysis of antibody-bound HCG revealed 50,000 cpm bound. The urine (1.0 ml) was mixed with 1 μg of radioactive HCG and the mixture was reacted with 0.1 ml of the antiserum. Analysis of antibody-bound radioactivity revealed 25,000 cpm bound to antibody. The concentration (μg/ml) of HCG in the urine is
   A) 20 μg/ml
   B) 10 μg/ml
   C) 2 μg/ml
   D) 1 μg/ml
   E) 0.1 μg/ml

2. In a diagnostic laboratory a technician prepared plastic assay plates for ELISA by binding a certain antigen, gp120 (glycoprotein of molecular weight of 120 kDa) of HIV-1 (human immunodeficiency virus, the etiologic agent of AIDS), to the plastic surface. Several samples of serum from suspected infected individuals were tested for the presence of antibodies to gp120. When the assay was performed, all the test samples were positive, including control samples that were known not to contain anti-gp120 antibodies. What explanation best fits the facts?
   A) The technician forgot to "block" the plates with nonrelevant protein.
   B) The technician put too much antigen on the plates.
   C) The developing labeled anti-immunoglobulin was not added.
   D) The fluorescent labeling compound dissociated from the labeled antibody.
   E) None of the above are correct.

3. Which of the following reaction(s) require(s) multivalent antigens and divalent antibodies?
   A) precipitin
   B) radioimmunoassay using 33% saturated ammonium sulfate
   C) radioimmunoassay using anti-antibody
   D) the reaction between Fab and hapten
   E) only A and C are correct
   F) only B and D are correct

4. In the indirect immunofluorescent antibody test for syphilis, the reactants involved are
   A) patient's serum, fluorescein-labeled killed *Treponema pallidum*
   B) patient's penile exudate, fluorescein-labeled rabbit antihuman antibody
   C) fluorescein-labeled patient's serum, rabbit antihuman antibody, killed *Treponema pallidum*
   D) patient's serum, killed *Treponema pallidum*, fluorescein-labeled rabbit antihuman antibodies
   E) none of the above

5. The specificity of the reaction of antigen with antibody is usually highly dependent on
   A) molecular weight of the antigen
   B) charge of the antibody
   C) immunoglobulin isotype
   D) conformation of the reactants
   E) concentration of the reactants

6. Convalescence from bubonic plague is followed by performing agglutination reactions on sera. The following results were obtained:

   serum dilution

1:2	1:4	1:8	1:16	1:32	1:64	1:128	1:256
–	–	+	+	+	+	+	+

   Which of the following conclusions can be drawn?
   A) The test antigen is too concentrated.
   B) The patient's convalescence is satisfactory.
   C) The patient should be actively immunized against plague.
   D) The titer can not be determined.
   E) The test is not valid because there was no agglutination at high serum concentrations.

7. The forces involved in antigen–antibody interaction
   A) depend on the presence of complement
   B) involve covalent interactions
   C) operate between antigen in solution and antibody within the cytoplasm of plasma cells
   D) may involve electrostatic interactions
   E) involve disulfide bonds

8. A quantitative precipitin reaction between an antigen and serum was performed. No precipitate was formed between the reactants. The absence of precipitate may be due to the fact that
   A) the serum does not contain antibodies to the antigen
   B) the antigen is monovalent
   C) the proportions of the reactants are such that there is a great excess of antigen
   D) the pH of the reaction is too low
   E) only A and C are correct
   F) only B and D are correct
   G) all are correct

ANSWERS TO REVIEW QUESTIONS

1. **D** When antibody is present in limited quantity, the radioactive antigen and nonradioactive antigen compete for antibody. As stated, when a given amount of antibody (0.1 ml) is allowed to react with 1 μg of radioactive HCG (100,000 cpm) 50,000 cpm are bound to antibody (i.e., 0.5 μg). Premixing the nonlabeled sample with 1 μg of radioactivated HCG reduces the amount of radioactivity bound by the same amount of antibody (0.1 ml) to 25,000 cpm, because the mixture contains 2 μg of HCG (of which 1 μg is nonradioactive and 1 μg is radioactive; i.e., 2 μg with radioactivity of 100,000 cpm or 50,000 cpm/μg). The antibody is still capable of binding only 0.5 μg of antigen. However, this time the 0.5 μg of antigen is of specific radioactivity 50,000 cpm/μg. Thus the "unknown" sample contains a concentration of nonradioactive antigen identical to that of

the radioactive antigen (1 μg/ml) with which the antibodies are allowed to react.

2. **A** In any solid-phase immunoassay such as the ELISA, it is imperative that after coating the plastic well with antigen, one must again coat the well with large amounts of a nonrelated protein in order to "block" all available sites on the plastic from absorbing the test antiserum. The most likely explanation for all the test samples and the controls to turn out positive is that the plates were not adequately "blocked." Excess antigen on the plate usually does not affect the ELISA. When the developing labeled antiserum was added, it too was adsorbed to the plates, hence the positivity of the test. Dissociation of the label would have resulted in negative rather than positive outcomes.

3. **E** The precipitin reaction requires multivalent antigen and at least divalent antibodies *(A)*. A radioimmunoassay, in which antibodies bound to radioactive antigen are precipitated by anti-antibodies, also requires that the two sets of antibodies be more than univalent, so that they can generate a lattice of cross-linked complexes that is large enough to form a precipitate *(B)*. In contrast, 33% saturated ammonium sulfate causes precipitation of immunoglobulins. Under these conditions, the antibodies will precipitate in the salt solution, even if they are reacted with univalent antigens, which, when mixed with antibodies, do not precipitate because of their inability to cross-link antibody molecules. Similarly, Fab or haptens are univalent, cannot cross-link, and do not form precipitates.

4. **D** In the indirect method, the antibody to the antigen is not fluorescent. However, the anti-antibody (in this case, rabbit antihuman antibody) is fluorescent.

5. **D** The specificity of the reaction between antigen and antibody is highly dependent on a close fit between the epitope and the combining site on the antibody. This close fit is greatly dependent on the conformation of the reactants. It does not depend on concentration.

6. **D** A titer is defined as that dilution of serum beyond which no agglutination occurs. Since there is agglutination with a serum dilution of 1:256, and since it is impossible to tell whether the next dilution would result in agglutination, the titer of the serum cannot be determined from the data given. The absence of agglutination at high serum concentration represents the "prozone."

7. **D** From all the possibilities given, only **D**, namely that Ag–Ab reaction may involve electrostatic interactions, is correct. Ag–Ab interactions *do not* involve covalent bonds. The other possibilities are irrelevant for the interaction.

8. **G** No precipitation will occur if there are no antibodies with which antigen can react, or if the antigen is monovalent and incapable of cross-linking antibody molecules. Precipitation occurs maximally at the equivalence zone. Excess antigen will reduce precipitation, resulting in soluble complexes. Antigen–antibody complexes, whether soluble or not, dissociate at low pH.

BIOLOGY OF THE B LYMPHOCYTE

INTRODUCTION

In previous chapters we described the structural and genetic mechanisms by which the immune response is able to achieve its diversity (i.e., its ability to respond to many different antigenic determinants, or epitopes). We now consider the development of the cells responsible for several major characteristics of the immune response, which are:

Specificity: The ability to discriminate among different antigenic epitopes, and to respond only to those that necessitate a response rather than making a random response.

Memory: The ability to recall previous contact with a particular antigen, such that subsequent exposure leads to a more rapid and larger immune response.

Adaptiveness: The ability to respond to previously unseen antigens, which may never have existed before on earth.

Discrimination between "self" and "non-self": The ability to respond to those antigens that are not "self" but to avoid making responses to those antigens that are part of "self."

The most widely accepted theory that best explains these features of the immune system is the ***clonal selection theory*** (see Chapter 1). The postulates of this theory were originally developed for antibody-producing cells (B lymphocytes), since these cells were the first to be recognized as having antigen-specific receptors on their surface. We now know that the basic postulates of the theory apply to both B lymphocytes and T lymphocytes, the second set of cells which bears antigen-specific receptors. The essential features of the clonal selection theory may be summarized as follows:

1. B and T lymphocytes of all antigenic specificities exist *prior* to contact with antigen.

2. Each lymphocyte carries immunoglobulin or T-cell receptor molecules of only a *single* specificity on its surface.

3. Lymphocytes can be stimulated by antigen under appropriate conditions to give rise to progeny with *identical* antigenic specificity. In the case of B cells, but not T cells, the antigen-specific receptor—immunoglobulin—is secreted as a consequence of stimulation.

4. Lymphocytes potentially reactive with "self" are *deleted* or in some way *inactivated*. This ensures that no immune response is mounted against self components. (Lymphocytes reactive to "self" molecules that are not deleted or inactivated may give rise to autoimmunity.)

This chapter focuses primarily on the differentiation of B lymphocytes, the key cells in the production of antibody in antigen-specific responses. The subsequent chapter deals with the differentiation of T lymphocytes. However, before discussing this subject it is appropriate to describe how cells involved in the immune response are identified and characterized.

CELLS INVOLVED IN THE IMMUNE RESPONSE

In mammalian species, circulating blood cells have their common origin in a small cluster of cells that move from the primitive yolk sac to the fetal liver, and finally to the bone marrow, where they take up permanent residence. These cells are the ***hematopoietic stem cells,*** so called because they are the undifferentiated cells from which all the other specialized cells in blood develop (see Fig. 2.1 in Chapter 2).

The undifferentiated stem cells are characterized by an ability to proliferate throughout life as a self-renewing reservoir that replenishes the pool of more mature cells as they are used up during normal activity. These early stem cells are considered to be *pluripotent;* that is, they are capable of developing into any of the more differentiated lines of cells, under the influence of a variety of soluble factors that control both the extent and the direction of maturation. Isolation and characterization of these earliest hematopoietic and pluripotent stem cells have been facilitated by the recent identification on their surface of a molecule referred to as CD34. (The "CD" nomenclature is discussed below.) Expression of CD34 is quite specific for early progenitor cells (as well as endothelial cells).Once differentiation in any direction has occurred, the cells become committed to make only a single type of cell lineage; that is, they become *unipotent* and CD34 expression decreases.

One pathway of differentiation *(myeloid differentiation)* starts from a bone marrow stem cell that gives rise to differentiated precursors and culminates with erythrocytes, thrombocytes (platelets), and the various granule-containing cells of the granulocyte-monocyte series. The other pathway of differentiation *(lymphocytic differentiation)* leads to two distinct cell types called B and T lymphocytes.

IDENTIFICATION AND CHARACTERIZATION OF CELLS

Before describing lymphocyte differentiation, it is important to say a few words about how different cell types may be distinguished. Until comparatively recently, white blood cells could be distinguished only microscopically, for example, by size or ability to take up certain dyes with different patterns (thus: "basophils" and "eosinophils"). These techniques, however, were not helpful for discriminating between different populations of lymphocytes, since lymphocytes are relatively indistinguishable by light microscopy.

A major breakthrough was in defining reagents or markers that react with the surface of different cells. For example, the surface of the human T cell was found to react with sheep red blood cells to form "rosettes"; as this reaction was quite specific, it provided a convenient way to purify human T cells from other blood cells.

The development of monoclonal antibodies (see Chapter 7) gave an enormous impetus to the mapping of cell surface molecules. As vast numbers of monoclonal antibodies were produced in many laboratories, their nomenclature, as well as designation of the molecule they reacted with, became very complicated. An antibody produced in one laboratory specific for a particular epitope on a particular protein might be given one name, while another antibody made elsewhere to the same or different epitope on the same molecule would be called something else.

To overcome this confusion, a uniform system of nomenclature has been adopted in which all cell-surface markers are designated CD, followed by a number indicating the sequence of their acceptance. The acronym *CD (cluster determinant)* describes the cluster of antigens with which antibodies react, and the number indicates its order of discovery. Thus, anti-CD4 would designate any antibodies that could react with a particular cell surface protein called CD4 regardless of the epitope on the CD4 that they recognized. Cells that express a particular molecule such as CD19 at the cell surface are referred to as CD19$^+$. An added advantage of this nomenclature is that the same or similar molecules in many species bear the same CD designation; thus, CD4$^+$ cells have similar characteristics in human, mouse, sheep, and so on.

Many of these cell surface molecules have been detected by appropriate antibodies; to date, the list extends at least to CD130. Not all these 130 cell surface molecules defined by the panels of antibodies have a currently understood function. The prevailing view is that every molecule expressed at the cell surface has some natural ligand that binds to it, and thus the surface-expressed molecule plays some role in receiving a signal from outside the cell and transmitting it into the cell. The precise mechanisms by which this occurs for each cell surface molecule have not been defined.

It is also worth noting, however, that surface expression of a particular molecule may not be specific for just one cell or even for a cell lineage. Nonetheless, cell surface expression can be exploited for purification, as well as characterization, of cells. Appendix   (at the end of this book) lists the CD molecules mentioned in this book with their functions and known ligands.

ONTOGENY OF THE B LYMPHOCYTE

B cells are those cells concerned with the synthesis of antibody, and they owe their name to their historical origins. In early experiments with birds, it was found that the antibody-forming B cells developed in an organ called the *bursa of Fabricius,* an outpouching of the cloacal epithelium. Stem cells that migrated to this organ and developed into mature, antibody-forming cells were called bursal or B cells.

Mammals, in contrast, do not appear to have an organ analogous to the bursa; rather, in the early fetus, B-cell differentiation is first noted in the liver. Later in fetal development and throughout the rest of the life of the mammal, the bone marrow is the predominant site of B-cell differentiation. The bone marrow is therefore considered the primary lymphoid organ for B cell-differentiation in these species (see Chapter 2). Some further differentiation may also occur after migration of the B-cell precursors to lymphoid organs such as spleen, lymph node, and tonsils.

Our understanding of B-cell differentiation has been facilitated by studying different animals in which the early embryonic stages can be manipulated. For this reason, B-cell differentiation in chickens, as well as that in mammals, is particularly well characterized. Many of the differentiation steps are common to chickens, mice, and humans. In the paragraphs that follow we will focus on the stages of differentiation of mammalian B-cells (see Fig. 8.1); many of the gene rearrangement steps described in Chapter 6 define important stages in this pathway.

The first event in the development of B cells is the commitment of some of the bone marrow precursor stem cells to the B-cell lineage. The earliest distinguishable cell in the B lineage is known as a ***pro-B cell.*** At this stage, the pro-B cell starts to rearrange its heavy-chain genes, predominantly D_H to J_H gene segments (see Chapter 6), but no immunoglobulin product is made.

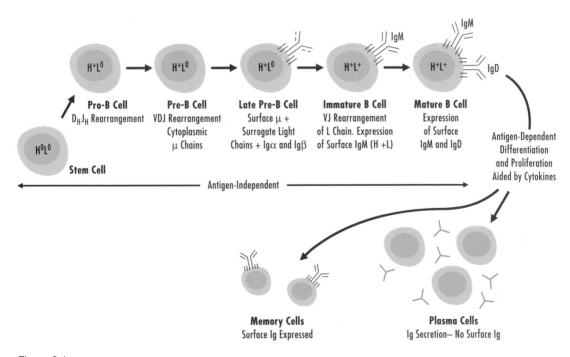

Figure 8.1.

Differentiation pathway of B lymphocytes. Heavy chain (H) and light chain (L) genes are designated H^0 or L^0 if in unrearranged or germ line configuration and H^+ or L^+ if rearranged.

In the next cell in the B-cell pathway, the ***pre-B cell,*** rearrangment of heavy-chain V, D, and J gene segments occurs, linking the VDJ unit to Cμ. Thus, the pre-B cell synthesizes a μ polypeptide. Until recently, it was believed that the μ chain made by the pre-B cell remained in the cytoplasm of the cell, since light-chain re-arrangement had not yet started. Recent research has indicated, however, that in some pre-B cells μ chains do reach the surface of the cell at low level, but in con-junction with the products of two nonrearranging genes, called Vλ5 and VpreB. These gene products are referred to as ***surrogate light chains*** and exclusively characterize the surface of the pre-B cell.

At the next stage of B-cell differentiation, light-chain genes start to rearrange and a light-chain polypeptide is synthesized. Surrogate light-chain synthesis is shut down and light chains now pair with μ chains to form monomeric IgM, which is inserted in the membrane. The cell bearing monomeric surface IgM ***(sIgM)*** only as its antigen-specific receptor is referred to as an ***immature B cell.*** It can recognize and respond to antigen, but this contact with antigen results in in-activation or deletion, rather than expansion and differentiation.

In the next stage of its maturation, a B cell expresses both IgM and IgD of identical antigenic specificities on its surface. (As described in Chapter 6, IgM and IgD are made from the alternative splicing of a single large nuclear RNA that con-tains a transcript of VDJ plus μ and δ genes.) This cell is now considered to be a ***mature B cell*** and fully capable of responding to stimulation by specific antigen.

It is important to note that all the maturation up to this point has taken place in the bone marrow and in the absence of specific antigen. The next stages in B cell development, however, are dependent on antigen, and occur primarily in the secondary lymphoid organs, the spleen and lymph node, and in specialized re-gions of the spleen and lymph nodes, known as ***germinal centers.*** Interaction with antigen triggers IgM$^+$IgD$^+$ B cells with the appropriate surface Ig receptor to enlarge (to become B-cell ***blasts***) and to proliferate. Several different events may occur after the initial stages of activation by antigen. Activated IgM$^+$IgD$^+$ B cells may differentiate further into ***plasma cells,*** which are the specialized end stage of B-cell development. Plasma cells synthesize and secrete antibody of the same antigenic specificity as that of the immunoglobulin on the surface of the B cell that was initially triggered by antigen. In the early stages of an immune response, plasma cells will secrete antibody of the IgM class.

If, however, antigen-activated IgM$^+$IgD$^+$ B cells receive appropriate signals from T cells, the B cells may differentiate along different pathways. ***Class*** or ***iso-type switching*** may occur. Under the influence of different T-cell-derived cy-tokines and T–B-cell-surface interaction, progeny of the IgM$^+$IgD$^+$ B cell that was involved in the initial response to antigen may switch to synthesis of IgG,

IgA, or IgE molecules. Whatever the isotype of the Ig produced, all the daughter cells have the same antigenic specificity.

The second major pathway after antigen activation is to become a ***memory B cell*** (see Fig. 8.1). These are B cells capable of being activated for a subsequent (secondary) and more rapid response to antigen. Memory B cells are nonproliferating, generally long-lived B cells that can be distinguished from other mature B cells by the differential expression of certain characteristics. Most importantly, memory cells express isotypes other than IgM and IgD on their surface. Memory cells also have distinct circulatory properties: they are found throughout secondary lymphoid tissue, and they express a high level of the molecule CD44 (a molecule that mediates "homing" of lymphocytes to tissues, as discussed in Chapter 9) on their surface. Thus, B cells activated in a primary response are distinct from B cells activated in a secondary or subsequent response. Although the precise stage at which memory cells develop is not clear, it is apparent that plasma cells do not become memory cells.

The generation of memory B cells is associated with class switch and somatic mutation (see Chapter 6). These processes occur in a specialized region of spleen and lymph node known as the germinal center, which consists predominantly of activated B cells, a few helper T cells and a small number of specialized cells known as follicular dendritic cells, which retain antigen on their surface and present it to B cells. The germinal center provides an environment where B cells with mutations for high affinity to the antigen are clonally selected. This results in the increase of high affinity antibodies, a process known as ***affinity maturation.*** B cells which are thus selected in the germinal center exit the lymphoid organ and make antibody of the appropriate class, or serve as memory cells for subsequent responses.

Interestingly, B cells with low affinity for antigen are selected against in the germinal center, and there is some evidence that these unselected cells die, by a process known as apoptosis or ***programmed cell death (PCD).*** It is noteworthy that the mechanisms of selection and apoptosis in the generation of a functional B-cell repertoire in the germinal center also operate during the development and generation of a functional T cell repertoire in the thymus, as we shall see in Chapter 9.

The overall result of the differentiation steps described above is that the individual builds up a continuously replenished library of diverse B-cell antigen specificities (a ***repertoire***) directed against a wide array of antigens. The development of a response to antigen therefore depends on the interaction of antigen with an existing B-cell clone contained in this library. It should be noted, however, that most B cells in the vast B-cell repertoire do not encounter antigen during their lifetime, but remain as resting unstimulated IgM$^+$IgD$^+$ cells.

One final point about the development of the repertoire is that ***mature B*** *cells are self-tolerant.* Since the early stages of B-cell differentiation occur in the absence of antigen, it is probable that some of the V–J and V–D–J rearrangements will lead by chance to the generation of an Ig molecule specific for a self-antigen, for example, generating a B cell with specificity for a protein found in the individual's liver or pancreas. To prevent this potential autoreactivity from developing, at some stage of ontogeny B cells with reactivity to self-antigens must be removed or functionally inactivated. Precisely how B-cell self-tolerance is achieved is currently not clear, nor is the anatomic location where this occurs. One mechanism of self-tolerance induction may be as a consequence of the interaction of immature IgM^+ cells with circulating self-antigens during the early development of the individual, resulting in cell inactivation or deletion.

B-CELL SURFACE MOLECULES

The key characteristic of B cells is their ability to synthesize antibody after antigenic stimulation. As we shall describe in more detail in subsequent chapters, production of antibody by B cells is a multistep process that generally requires the mutual interaction of B cells with T cells. In brief, after antigen has bound to Ig on a B cell, the B cell internalizes the antigen, partially degrades it, and subsequently presents a fragment of the degraded antigen on its surface to a T cell. The T cell becomes activated, leading in turn to B-cell activation, resulting in antibody synthesis and in class switching. In the next section, we will outline some of the B-cell molecules that play a key role in these interactions. These are shown diagrammatically in Figure 8.2.

Antigen-Binding Molecules: Surface Immunoglobulin (sIg)

The quintessential property of the B lymphocyte lineage is its expression of immunoglobulin molecules at the surface of the cell, with the concomitant ability to bind antigen. (It is noteworthy, however, that the pro-B cell, the most immature B cell, and the plasma cell, the end stage cell of B-cell differentiation that secretes Ig, do not express Ig on their surface.) The expression of surface Ig can thus be used to identify B cells, and to separate them from other lymphocytes and mononuclear cells.

Antibodies specific for different portions of the immunoglobulin molecule (i.e., anti-immunoglobulin antibodies) can be used for this purpose, and can serve to distinguish distinct subsets of B cells (e.g., B cells expressing only IgM or only

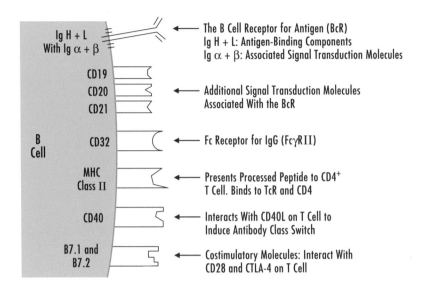

The B Cell Receptor for Antigen (BcR)
Ig H + L: Antigen-Binding Components
Ig α + β: Associated Signal Transduction Molecules

Additional Signal Transduction Molecules
Associated With the BcR

Fc Receptor for IgG (FcγRII)

Presents Processed Peptide to CD4⁺
T Cell. Binds to TcR and CD4

Interacts With CD40L on T Cell to
Induce Antibody Class Switch

Costimulatory Molecules: Interact With
CD28 and CTLA-4 on T Cell

Figure 8.2.

Important molecules on the surface of the mature B cell.

IgG). Certain anti-immunoglobulin antibodies may also act as triggers to activate B cells in the absence of any other antigen.

Signal Transduction Molecules Associated With Immunoglobulin Signaling

Recent findings indicate that Ig is noncovalently associated in the membrane of B cells with two other transmembrane molecules known as Ig α (CD79a) and Ig β (CD79b). One α and one β polypeptide are believed to associate with one Ig heavy chain. The cytoplasmic portions of α and β are, in turn, tightly linked to kinases inside the B cell. As a consequence of antigen binding to Ig on the external surface of the B cell, a signal is passed into the cell via the associated transmembrane Ig α and β molecules (which do not themselves bind antigen). This phenomenon is known as *signal transduction*. Inside the cell, the kinases associated with α and β phosphorylate several cellular proteins. As we shall see in Chapter 11, phosphorylation of these proteins leads to the transcription of different genes in the B cell and to B-cell activation.

Both α and β are found on all Ig-expressing cells, including pre-B cells, suggesting that even the Ig on the surface of the pre-B cell can signal to the interior of the cell.

Molecules on the B-cell surface (CD19, CD20, and CD21) have recently been shown to constitute other transduction molecules associated with immunoglobulins (Fig. 8.2). Molecules that play a similar signal transduction role in T cells, the CD3 complex, will be described in Chapters 9 and 11.

Molecules Involved in Isotype Switching: CD40

As we have mentioned previously, isotype switching by B cells is dependent on the presence of soluble factors, cytokines, released by T cells. Switching also requires the interaction of the B- and T-cell surfaces, specifically *CD40* on the B-cell surface (Fig. 8.2) and a molecule known as "CD40 ligand" on the T cell. The importance of this interaction is underscored by a condition known as human X-linked hyper-IgM syndrome. Boys who have a mutation in their CD40 ligand gene and thus whose T cells do not express the CD40 ligand make only IgM antibodies; their B cells cannot switch to any other isotype.

Molecules Involved in Antigen Presentation

As we shall see in Chapters 10 and 11 in detail, antigen must be presented by cells referred to as *antigen-presenting cells* or *APC*, to activate T cells. B cells, like many other cells in the body, act as APC for T cells, and B cells share several important characteristics with other APC. In common with other presenting cells, B cells express on their surface proteins referred to as *MHC class II molecules,* coded for by genes of the major histocompatibility complex (MHC). These proteins are essential for presenting antigen to a major set of T cells known as CD4$^+$ T cells (discussed more fully in Chapters 10 and 11). Unlike the expression pattern of many other cell types, B-cell expression of MHC class II molecules is *constitutive;* that is, the molecules are always expressed. Interestingly, MHC class II molecule expression on B cells can be further increased by exposure to certain cytokines. MHC class II expression is found on all cells of the B-cell lineage, starting with the pre-B cell (see Fig. 8.1).

Another crucial requirement for APC function is the expression of *costimulatory molecules.* These are surface molecules on B cells and other APCs that interact with surface molecules on T cells to send crucial positive signals to the T cell during antigen-specific stimulation. If the T cell does not receive these positive costimulatory signals, the T cell is turned off rather than on by contact with antigen (see Chapter 18). Several costimulatory molecules have recently been defined on the APC surface; the most prominent is known as B7, comprising at least two molecules B7.1 and B7.2 (CD80 and CD86, respectively). Both of these molecules can be expressed by B cells. An interesting point is that resting mature B cells are poor APC and express low levels of costimulatory molecules, whereas activated B cells express high levels of costimulatory molecules and are very efficient APCs.

Fc Receptor (FcR) (CD32)

Virtually all mature B cells express a low affinity receptor for the Fc portion of IgG, FcγRII or CD32. CD32 binds IgG when it aggregates in the absence of antigen (see Chapter 5), and when the IgG is in the form of antigen–antibody complex. Interestingly, if the Fc end of an antigen–antibody complex binds to CD32 on a B cell while the antigen end binds to Ig on the same cell, the B cell is inactivated. Thus, CD32 is believed to play a role in "antibody feedback," the inactivation of B cells by antigen in the presence of antibody.

Complement and EBV Receptor (CD21)

CD21 is a B-cell surface molecule involved in B-cell activation and is a receptor for a complement component, C3d (see Chapter 13). CD21 also acts as a receptor for Epstein–Barr virus (EBV), which is responsible for the conditions mononucleosis and in Africa, Burkitt's lymphoma. This is one important example of a pathogen using a normal cell-surface molecule to gain access to the cell. Other examples include human immunodeficiency virus (HIV) binding to CD4 on T cells and rhinovirus binding to ICAM-1 (CD54) on epithelial cells.

One useful result of EBV infection of B cells in vitro is that the infected cells proliferate continuously, becoming "immortalized." As a consequence, EBV-transformed cells provide a stable, continually replicating source of B cells derived from a normal individual, which can be used as antigen-presenting cells for activating T cells from the same donor.

Many other B-cell specific molecules have been described, some of which are receptors for hormones or T-cell products, while others represent differentiation antigens appearing and disappearing at various stages in the cell cycle.

SUMMARY

1. The differentiation of B cells occurs in the bone marrow throughout the life of an individual. The earliest recognizable cells in the B-cell lineage are the pro-B cell, followed by the pre-B cell. In these cells, the first stages of immunoglobulin gene rearrangement take place.

2. In the pro-B cell, a D_H gene segment rearranges to a J_H gene segment. In the pre-B cell, a V_H gene segment rearranges to the joined DJ segments to form a VDJ unit, which is thus put next to the $C\mu$ gene. The pre-B cell transcribes and translates the $VDJC\mu$ gene unit and thereby synthesizes a μ chain, which remains in the cytoplasm of the cell.

3. Later in the life of the pre-B cell, this μ chain can reach the surface of the cell in association with molecules referred to as "surrogate light chains."

4. When light-chain genes start to rearrange, surrogate light-chain synthesis is shut down and a κ or λ chain is formed that associates with the cell's μ chain. This results in the formation of an IgM molecule, which is expressed on the surface of the cell in the absence of IgD. This cell is referred to as an immature B cell: contact with antigen appears to shut down rather than activate the immature B cell.

5. The next step in B-cell differentiation is the expression of IgM together with IgD on the cell surface. The IgM and IgD expressed on a single cell have identical antigenic specificity. The cell expressing IgM and IgD is referred to as a mature B cell.

6. All these rearrangement events occur in the absence of antigen and define the cell as a B cell with a unique antigenic specificity.

7. Further development of the mature B cell occurs outside the bone marrow as a result of exposure to antigen. Activation of the B cell leads to proliferation and differentiation into a plasma cell, the end stage of B-cell differentiation. Plasma cells are B cells that synthesize and secrete antibody. In the primary response, predominantly IgM is synthesized.

8. In secondary responses, in which both B and T cells have been primed by antigen, B cells can differentiate further. They may (a) undergo class or isotype switch, that is, produce antibody of different isotypes or (b) develop into memory B cells. These differentiation events occur in specialized regions of secondary lymphoid organs, the germinal centers. In these areas, somatic mutation of antibody molecules also takes place, enhancing the affinity of antibody for the stimulating antigen.

9. Isotype switching involves a rearrangement mechanism unique to B cells. In the presence of antigen and cytokines released by T cells, the VDJ heavy-chain unit that was joined to the $C\mu$ and $C\delta$ genes rearranges to join another C-region gene, such as $C\gamma$, $C\alpha$, or $C\epsilon$. The B cell that was synthesiz-

ing IgM and IgD can now synthesize antibody of a different isotype (IgG, IgA, or IgE) but with the same antigenic specificity.

10. Expression of surface immunoglobulin is a characteristic unique to B cells. B cells also express an array of molecules on their cell surface, which play a vital role in the B cell's interactions with other cells. These include molecules important in B-cell interactions with T cells, such as MHC class II molecules, B7, and CD40.

REFERENCES

Kincade PW, Lee G, Pietrangeli CE, Hayashi SI, Gimble JM (1989): Cells and molecules that regulate B lymphopoiesis in bone marrow Annu Rev Immunol 7:111.

Möller G (1993): The B-cell antigen receptor complex. Immunol Rev 132:5.

Nossal GJV (1994): Negative selection of lymphocytes. Cell 76:229.

Pfeffer K, Mak T (1994): Lymphocyte ontogeny and activation in gene targeted mice. Annu Rev Immunol 12:367.

Reth M (1994): B cell antigen receptors. Curr Opinion Immunol 6:3.

Weissman IL, Cooper MD (1993): How the immune system develops. Sci Am 269:64.

REVIEW QUESTIONS

For each question, choose the ONE BEST answeror completion.

1. The earliest stages of B-cell differentiation
   A) occur in the embryonic thymus
   B) require the presence of antigen
   C) involve rearrangement of κ-chain gene segments
   D) involve rearrangement of surrogate light-chain gene segments
   E) involve rearrangement of heavy-chain gene segments

2. Which of the following is *not* expressed on the surface of the mature B lymphocyte?
   A) CD40
   B) MHC class II molecules
   C) surrogate light chains
   D) CD19
   E) IgM and IgD

3. Which of the following statements is *incorrect*?
   A) antibodies in a secondary immune response generally have a higher affinity for antigen than antibodies formed in a primary response

B) somatic mutation of V region genes may contribute to changes in antibody affinity observed during secondary responses

C) synthesis of antibody in a secondary response occurs predominantly in the blood

D) isotype switching occurs in the presence of antigen

E) IgM antibody will be produced in the primary response

4. Immature B lymphocytes
   A) produce only μ chains
   B) are progenitors of T as well as B lymphocytes

C) express both IgM and IgD on their surface

D) are at a stage of development where contact with antigen may lead to unresponsiveness

E) must go through the thymus to mature

5. Antigen binding to the B-cell receptor
   A) transduces a signal through the four-chain Ig molecule
   B) invariably leads to B-cell activation
   C) transduces a signal through the Ig α and β molecules
   D) results in macrophage activation

ANSWERS TO REVIEW QUESTIONS

1. *E* The earliest events in B-cell differentiation take place in bone marrow and fetal liver and bone marrow in the adult and involve rearrangenment of heavy-chain V, D, and J gene segments.

2. *C* Surrogate light chains are expressed only on the surface of pre-B cells. The other molecules are expressed on the mature B-cell surface.

3. *C* Antibody synthesis in secondary responses occurs predominantly in lymph nodes, not blood.

4. *D* In immature B cells, which express only IgM, contact with antigen leads to unresponsiveness rather than activation.

5. *C* The molecules associated with the surface Ig molecule, Ig α and β, transduce a signal following antigen binding to surface Ig.

BIOLOGY OF THE T LYMPHOCYTE

INTRODUCTION

In the preceding chapters we have described how the specificity of the immune response is derived from the presence of millions of different lymphocytes, each with a slightly different receptor able to interact with a particular antigenic epitope. Thus far, we have focused on one set of lymphocytes, the B lymphocytes and their receptor for antigen, immunoglobulin.

We now turn to the second major set of lymphocytes, known as T lymphocytes, or more simply T cells. T cells play a central role in the response to protein antigens. Since nearly all infectious organisms contain protein, T cells are prominently involved in the immune response to almost every antigen and pathogen (bacterial lipopolysaccharides are an exception, consisting of carbohydrate but without protein).

Why are there two major sets of lymphocytes? We believe it is because antibodies, the products of B cells, play a critical role in interacting with antigens when they are found *outside* cells, such as occurs when viruses are encountered in blood. Once an antigen gets into a cell, however, antibodies do not generally have access to it and so antibodies are ineffective in dealing with antigens *inside* cells. Thus, T cells probably evolved to deal with the crucial phase of the response to pathogens such as viruses, bacteria, and parasites that invade cells and live inside them.

The fact that T cells respond to antigens only when the antigens are inside or on the surface of cells indicates that T-cell recognition of antigen is fundamentally different from B-cell recognition of antigen. As we shall describe in this and subsequent chapters, T cells also have on their surface a receptor for antigen, known as the T-cell receptor (TcR), which shares several similarities with the receptor for antigen on B cells, immunoglobulin (Ig). The key difference between Ig and TcR recognition of antigens, however, is that Ig can interact with antigen directly, even in solution. In contrast, TcR recognition of antigen occurs only when the antigen is on the surface of a cell, and more precisely when the antigen is bound to cellular proteins known as MHC (major histocompatibility complex) molecules. Thus, as we shall describe in greater detail in Chapter 10, MHC molecules are critically involved in the presentation of antigen and hence the triggering of T cells.

The consequences of antigen recognition by B and T cells are similar but differ in fundamental ways. Thus, after antigen stimulation both B and T cells become activated, proliferate, and may differentiate into memory cells. The end product of B cell activation, however, is Ig secretion. In contrast, T cells have two major functions as a result of antigenic stimulation: (1) they produce a series of nonimmunoglobulin soluble mediators called *cytokines*, which influence many different cells, and (2) they may kill the cell that contains the foreign antigen.

In this chapter we will examine the fundamental biology of the T cell receptor for antigen and compare and contrast its characteristics with those of the B-cell receptor for antigen. We will also describe how T cells differentiate and some of the molecules they express.

NATURE OF THE ANTIGEN-SPECIFIC T-CELL RECEPTOR

As with B cells, each T cell bears on its surface a clonally distributed receptor (i.e., each clone of T cells expresses a different receptor) that interacts with antigen. This is known as the *T-cell receptor* (TcR) (Fig. 9.1). The TcR is a disulfide-linked two-chain molecule or heterodimer. Two different types of TcR are found. The first is known as $\alpha\beta$ and the second as $\gamma\delta$. α, β, γ, and δ are all distinct polypeptides with molecular weights varying between 40 and 60 kDa. An individual T cell can express either $\alpha\beta$ or $\gamma\delta$ as its receptor, never both. (By "express" we mean that in this particular cell these specific genes are being transcribed and

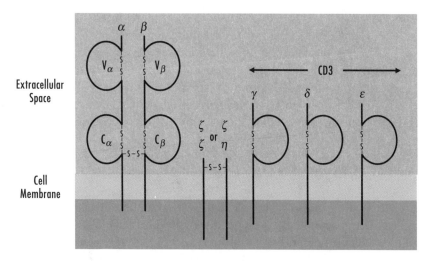

Figure 9.1

The structure of the T-cell receptor (TcR) complex, showing the antigen-binding chains α and β and the associated signal transduction complex, CD3 plus ζ or η.

translated, as described in Chapter 6. A cell expressing the gene of interest is referred to as "+", and a cell not expressing this gene is "–". Thus, a T cell may be either $\alpha\beta^+\gamma\delta^-$ or $\alpha\beta^-\gamma\delta^+$ but never $\alpha\beta^+\gamma\delta^+$.) The role of the $\alpha\beta$ and $\gamma\delta$ heterodimers is to interact with antigen.

There are striking similarities in organization of the genes as well as the structure of the proteins for immunoglobulin and the TcR. These similarities or *homologies* between the TcR and Ig (and, indeed, many other molecules expressed at the cell surface) suggest that they have evolved from a common ancestral gene. These genes are said to belong to the ***immunoglobulin gene superfamily***, and the molecules are referred to as members of the ***immunoglobulin superfamily.***

A complete TcR has not yet been crystallized (although a β chain was crystallized recently), and so structural details are not as complete as for Ig molecules. Nonetheless, several features are known (see Fig. 9.1). Like Ig, the TcR is a transmembrane molecule with a short cytoplasmic tail. The extracellular portion of the TcR comprises both variable and constant regions, with the constant region containing a domain structure homologous to an Ig domain. Antigen binding occurs at the V regions of the TcR, analogous to antigen binding to the V regions of an immunoglobulin molecule on a B cell.

There are fewer V-region genes in the germ line able to code for TcR chains than there are V-region genes able to code for immunoglobulin H and L chains. Nonetheless, as we shall describe later in the chapter, there is as much diversity in an individual's TcR repertoire as in her immunoglobulin repertoire. Individual TcR V regions have been given numbers, e.g., $V\alpha2$ or $V\beta7$. Interestingly, the usage of certain TcR V regions is associated with the response to particular antigens. This has been shown in the response to *superantigens*, discussed in Chapter 11, as well as in some autoimmune disorders which show restricted TcR V-gene usage.

The T-Cell Receptor Complex

The TcR is expressed on the surface of T cells only in noncovalent association with a complex of transmembrane polypeptides (see Fig. 9.1). Three of these TcR-associated molecules comprise a molecule known as *CD3*, which is T-cell specific. CD3 is made up of three distinct polypeptides known as γ, δ, and ϵ, molecular weights 25, 20, and 20 kDa, respectively. The precise number of each CD3 chain in the complex is currently not clear. The CD3 and TcR polypeptides are also tightly associated at the cell surface with another molecule comprising two identical ζ *(zeta)* chains, molecular weight 16 kDa. ζ is not T-cell specific; it is also associated with the high affinity Fc receptor for IgE on mast cells. The ζ chain also exists in an alternatively spliced form know as η *(eta),* molecular weight 22 kDa, which can form a heterodimer with ζ. The majority of T-cell receptors are associated with $\zeta\zeta$.

CD3 and ζ (or η) are present on all T cells, both $\alpha\beta^+$ and $\gamma\delta^+$. The entire set of molecules at the cell surface, comprising the antigen-binding heterodimer $\alpha\beta$ (or $\gamma\delta$) plus the CD3 γ, δ, and ϵ polypeptides in addition to $\zeta\zeta$ or $\zeta\eta$, is referred to as the *T-cell receptor complex*. CD3 γ, δ, and ϵ polypeptides are evenly distributed across the membrane of the T cell (their extracellular regions have an immunoglobulin-like domain), but the ζ polypeptide is almost totally intracellular, with only 9 amino acids outside the cell. Each of the CD3 and ζ chains is linked to a kinase inside the cell.

CD3 and ζ polypeptides do not bind antigen. When antigen binds to the V regions of the $\alpha\beta$ or $\gamma\delta$ molecules, however, some change occurs in the closely linked CD3 and ζ molecules that activates the associated kinases; we know that as a consequence of this binding the ζ chains are phosphorylated on tyrosine residues and the γ, δ, and ϵ chains of CD3 are phosphorylated on both serine and tyrosine residues. These phosphorylations set off a cascade of intracellular events leading to changes in transcription of different genes in the nucleus of theT cell.

Thus CD3 and ζ play a crucial role as *transducer* molecules for transferring a signal into the T cell after antigen binding to the TcR. CD3 molecules are analogous to the Ig-associated α and β molecules on B cells described in Chapter 8.

CD4 AND CD8

As we have described in the two preceding sections, both αβ and γδ TcR molecules are associated on their surface with the CD3 and ζ proteins. Those T cells that use αβ as their TcR also express another transmembrane molecule that is also closely but noncovalently linked to the TcR, and is referred to as an ***accessory*** or ***coreceptor*** molecule. This accessory molecule can be one of two molecules on the mature αβ expressing cell, ***either CD4 or CD8.*** (Both CD4 and CD8 are members of the Ig superfamily.) Accessory molecule expression divides the αβ$^+$ T cell population into one of two major subsets, either CD4$^+$CD8$^-$ or CD4$^-$CD8$^+$. Only immature αβ$^+$ T cells at a specific stage of differentiation in the thymus are CD4$^+$CD8$^+$. Indeed, the majority of cells in the thymus of a young mammal express both CD4 and CD8. Some γδ T cells express CD8, but very few express CD4; it is not clear whether γδ T cells have other types of accessory molecules or simply do not use them.

The functions of CD4 and CD8 are at least twofold. First, the extracellular portions of ***CD4 and CD8 bind to MHC molecules*** on the surface of cells that present antigen to T cells. Thus, CD4 and CD8 act as ***adhesion molecules*** that help to tighten the binding of T cells to antigen-presenting cells. This is believed to be very important because the binding of antigen plus MHC molecules to the TcR is of low affinity, and thus the binding of the accessory molecule on the T cell to MHC tightens this crucial interaction. As we shall describe in more detail in the next chapter, CD4 binds to what is referred to as the ***invariant*** portion of the MHC class II molecule and CD8 to the invariant portion of the MHC class I molecule.

The second major function of CD4 and CD8 is to act as ***signal transducers*** in T cells; the intracellular portions of CD4 and CD8 are linked to specific kinases. Thus, because CD4 and CD8 are associated with the TcR in the membrane of the T cell, CD4 and CD8 are also phosphorylated as a consequence of antigen binding to the αβ T cell receptor.

A unique characteristic of the CD4 molecule, which we shall describe later in more detail (see Chapter 18), is that it binds to the human immunodeficiency virus (HIV), allowing the virus to enter T cells expressing CD4, eventually leading to the disease AIDS.

GENES CODING FOR TcR

The organization of the human gene coding for the α, β, and δ T-cell receptor chains is shown in Figure 9.2. (Because of its complexity, the organization of γ genes is not shown.) Several features are noteworthy:

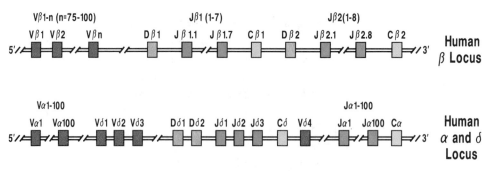

Figure 9.2

Organization of the α, β, and δ genes coding for the T-cell receptor. The organization of the γ-gene locus of the TcR is not shown because of its complexity.

1. α and γ chains are constructed from V and J gene segments, like Ig light chains.

2. β and δ chains are constructed from V, D, and J gene segments, like Ig heavy chains.

3. Genes for β and γ are each found on different chromosomes, while α and δ genes are found on the same chromosome. Genes coding for the δ-chain are flanked on both the 5' and 3' sides by genes coding for the α-chain.

4. There are many more Vα and Vβ genes (50–100) than Vγ and Vδ genes (5–10) in the germ line.

The same fundamental principles of gene rearrangement, as described in Chapter 6 for Ig apply for the T-cell receptor. ***Recombinases*** and ***joining sequences*** are used to link up a VJ or a VDJ unit to fix the variable region specificity of a particular TcR polypeptide chain. The same enzymes are probably involved in the recombination events in both B and T cells. As described in Chapter 6, two genes known as RAG-1 and RAG-2 have been shown to play a crucial role in activating the recombinase genes in both early B and T cells. T-cell receptor genes also show ***allelic exclusion***, just like Ig, ensuring that a single T cell makes a receptor with only a single antigenic specificity.

The generation of diversity in T-cell receptors is thus very similar to the generation of diversity in the B-cell receptor, immunoglobulin. As in the generation of Ig diversity, TcR diversity is generated by (1) multiple V genes in the germ line, (2) random combination (at least of TcR α and β chains), and (3) junctional and insertional variability (see Chapter 6).

As described earlier in the chapter, there are fewer V genes in the germ line for the TcR than for Ig. Despite the smaller number of V genes for TcR, however, the repertoire of different TcRs is believed to be at least as large as the repertoire of Ig molecules. There are two reasons for this. First, there are more J-gene segments coding for the TcR α and β molecules than for Ig. Second, there is far greater junctional variability in the generation of both $\alpha\beta$ and $\gamma\delta$ TcRs than in the generation of Ig molecules. Interestingly, unlike immunoglobulin, T-cell receptors do not appear to somatically mutate after antigenic stimulation.

$\gamma\delta$ T CELLS

T cells using either $\alpha\beta$ or $\gamma\delta$ as their TcR differentiate in the thymus. It is known that the $\alpha\beta$ and $\gamma\delta$ lineages diverge early in intrathymic development. That apart, little is known about the differentiation steps involved in generating T cells that use $\gamma\delta$ as their TcR ("$\gamma\delta$ T cells"). Furthermore, the functions of $\gamma\delta$ T cells are still poorly understood: in general, $\gamma\delta$ T cells do not respond to a wide range of protein antigens.

Some important properties of $\gamma\delta$ T cells are as follows:

1. They are found at much lower numbers than $\alpha\beta$ cells in normal adult humans, but they are present in all mammalian species at some level.

2. They appear in the thymus before $\alpha\beta$-bearing cells.

3. Generally, they lack the CD4 accessory molecule found on $\alpha\beta$-expressing T cells. Some $\gamma\delta$ cells do express CD8.

4. They are at least two subpopulations of $\gamma\delta$ cells, defined by different Vγ-gene usage. The subpopulations migrate to different sites: skin or, alternatively, epithelial areas, such as lung and intestine.

5. They are capable of producing the same cytokines as $\alpha\beta$ TcR cells, and may exhibit other functions associated with $\alpha\beta$ T cells such as cytotoxicity.

6. Some $\gamma\delta$ T cells have been found to be activated by mycobacterial anti-

gens and some γδ T cells respond to heat-shock proteins (proteins that form in cells when they are heated or stressed in different ways). Unlike αβ T cells, some γδ T cells may not respond to complexes of peptide and MHC molecules.

From this sparse information, it has been suggested that γδ TcR cells are involved in forming a line of defense against common antigens of some bacterial pathogens. Recent information also suggests that γδ T cells may play a role in the defense against infectious agents such as the malarial parasite, *Plasmodium yoelii.* More information about the role of γδ T cells in immune responses will doubtless emerge, particularly from studies of "knockout" mice lacking either γδ or αβ T cells.

T-CELL DIFFERENTIATION IN THE THYMUS

The thymus is absolutely required for the differentiation of immature precursor cells into cells with the characteristics of T cells: children born without a thymus (DiGeorge's syndrome, discussed in Chapter 18) or mice genetically lacking a thymus (known as "nude" mice because they also lack hair) do not have mature T cells. T-cell differentiation in the thymus occurs throughout the life of the individual but diminishes significantly after puberty. The size of the thymus itself decreases with the onset of puberty in mammals ("thymic involution"), presumably because of the accompanying synthesis of steroid hormones at this time. In some species, in particular the mouse, if the thymus is removed within 4 days after birth the animal has a drastically depleted mature T-cell population. Indeed, these were the pioneering observations of Jacques Miller, who established the crucial role of the thymus in T-cell responses. Removing the thymus later in the development of the animal has much less impact on the mature T-cell population.

In the thymus the rearrangement events occur that determine whether a T cell expresses αβ or γδ as its receptor, as well as determine the specificity of the particular TcR for an antigenic epitope. Thus, as described in Chapter 2, the thymus is the primary lymphoid organ for the development of T cells, analogous to the bone marrow as the primary organ for mammalian B-cell differentiation. As we shall discuss later in this chapter, there are two other major consequences of differentiation in the thymus. Firstly, mature T cells emerge recognizing antigen only when it is associated with "self"-MHC molecules; that is, ***T cells are self-MHC restricted.*** Secondly, mature T cells emerge that do not respond to self components; that is, ***T cells are self-tolerant.***

T-cell differentiation in the thymus is a complex multistep process (see Fig.

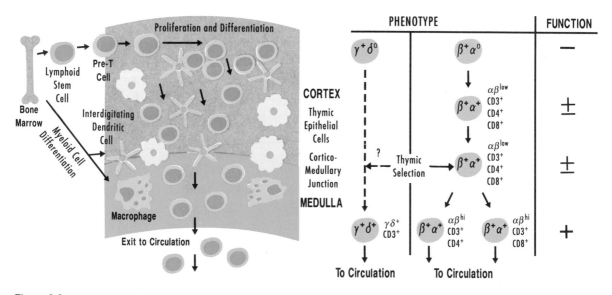

Figure 9.3

The developmental pathway of T cells in the thymus. Genes coding for the α, β, γ, or δ chains of the T-cell receptor are designated as α^0, β^0, γ^0, or δ^0 if not rearranged and α^+, β^+, γ^+, δ^+ if rearranged.

9.3). It has been easiest to study in the embryo where the sequence of events can be determined from the very earliest stages. In brief, the steps involved in the differentiation of the T cell are as follows. Precursor cells with no T-cell characteristics enter the thymus and start to rearrange their T-cell receptor genes *(pre-T cells)* in the **thymic cortex**. Cells that express $\gamma\delta$ as their TcR separate from the sublineage of cells expressing $\alpha\beta$ at an early stage in intrathymic differentiation. (Many of the details of $\gamma\delta$ T-cell differentiation in the thymus are incompletely understood, and more is known about $\alpha\beta$-expressing T cells.) The differentiating T cells *(thymocytes)* trickle down through the mesh formed by the stromal cells of the thymus (described below) into the **thymic medulla**. As the thymocytes progress from cortex to medulla they become more mature, characterized not only by the expression of a TcR and CD3 but also by the ordered appearance and loss of several other molecules found on the T-cell surface. The most mature cells leave the thymus and enter the circulation, forming the repertoire of T cells able to respond to foreign antigen.

At every stage of thymic maturation, from precursor to mature T cell, the developing lymphocytes are in contact with, and interact with, nonlymphoid stromal cells of the thymus. The most important stromal cells are (1) *thymic epithelial cells* and (2) bone-marrow-derived *interdigitating dendritic cells*, analogous to the antigen-presenting dendritic cells described in Chapter 11.

SEQUENCE OF TcR GENE REARRANGEMENTS

The order of T-cell receptor gene rearrangements in the thymus is highly regulated. The earliest cell entering the thymus has its TcR genes in an unrearranged or germ line configuration. Both γ and β TcR chain genes then start to rearrange, more or less simultaneously (see Fig. 9.3). If the γ-chain genes rearrange successfully, then δ-chain genes also start to rearrange. If both γ and δ genes rearrange functionally, that is, if they can be transcribed and translated into polypeptides, no further rearrangement occurs and the cell remains a $\gamma\delta$ T cell. For this reason, T cells bearing $\gamma\delta$ appear earlier in development than $\alpha\beta$-expressing T cells. If, however, γ and/or δ rearrangements are not functional, β-gene rearrangement continues followed by α-gene rearrangement. If α- and β-gene rearrangements are nonfunctional, however, a receptor is not expressed and the cell line dies. This ordered array of gene rearrangements for TcR genes is highly analogous to the ordered rearrangement of immunoglobulin genes during B-cell development; in that case, κ is tried before λ.

Selection of T Cells in the Thymus

One of the key intermediate cells in the differentiation of $\alpha\beta$ cells in the thymus (see Fig. 9.3) is a relatively immature cell that expresses low levels of $\alpha\beta$ ($\alpha\beta^{lo}$) on its surface in association with CD3. One of the unique features of this cell is that it co-expresses the molecules CD4 and CD8, a situation not found in mature T cells outside the thymus. This $\alpha\beta^{lo}$ CD3$^+$CD4$^+$CD8$^+$ thymocyte, referred to as a CD4$^+$CD8$^+$ T cell, is found in the thymic cortex, and forms the majority of thymocytes in a young mammalian thymus. The CD4$^+$CD8$^+$ thymocyte undergoes the process known as *selection.* Whether $\gamma\delta^+$ T cells undergo a similar selection process is currently not clear.

Thymic selection for $\alpha\beta^+$ T cells is divided into two phases, known as *positive selection* and *negative selection.* The immature CD4$^+$CD8$^+$ cell is in contact with and interacts with the stromal cells of the thymic cortex. The crucial interactions appear to be between *MHC molecules* expressed by the thymic stromal cells and the CD4 and CD8 molecules expressed by the developing T cell. The role of MHC molecules in the immune response is discussed more fully in Chapters 10 and 11.

In the first stage, *positive selection,* it is believed that the TcR, CD4 and CD8 of a developing T cell are "screened" by the MHC molecules of the cortical epithelial cells of the thymus. Only $CD4^+CD8^+$ T cells that bind with a certain critical affinity to the epithelial cells' MHC molecules survive the selection. If, however, the affinity of interaction between the developing thymocyte and the thymic epithelial cell is either too high or too low, the cell is not positively selected and the thymocyte dies, by a process known as apoptosis or programmed cell death, discussed in more detail later in this chapter.

Experimental evidence strongly suggests that positive selection of a T cell on the MHC molecules expressed in the thymus leads to expansion of that particular T-cell clone. An important consequence of this interaction and expansion is that the T cells become "*educated*" to the MHC molecules expressed by the thymic structural cells. This means that for the rest of the life of the T cell, even as a mature cell when it leaves the thymus, it will respond to antigen only when the antigen is bound to the type of MHC molecules that the developing T cell encountered in the thymus. This crucial phenomenon is known as *MHC restriction of T-cell responses*, and emphasizes again the critical importance of MHC in T-cell responses, as we will see in more detail in the next chapter.

Cells that survive positive selection in the thymus are potentially able to respond to peptides derived from self as well as foreign-antigens. Allowing cells with reactivity to self antigens to leave the thymus and circulate would result in autoimmunity, a highly undesirable situation. To prevent this potential reactivity to self, it is believed that the developing $CD4^+CD8^+$ cell undergoes a second selection step, *negative selection,* which probably occurs at a stage when the thymocyte is moving from the thymic cortex to the medulla as a consequence of interactions with the interdigitating dendritic cell at the cortico-medullary junction. As a result, cells that express T-cell receptors with reactivity to self antigens are removed or functionally inactivated, leaving intact only T cells with reactivity to foreign antigens.

Accompanying these selection processes, the surviving $CD4^+CD8^+$ cells downregulate the expression of one or other of the co-receptor molecules they express and become either $CD4^+CD8^-$ or $CD4^-CD8^+$. These cells also upregulate the expression of their $\alpha\beta$ TcR molecules. The resultant cells, expressing either $\alpha\beta^{hi}CD3^+CD4^+$ or $\alpha\beta^{hi}CD3^+CD8^+$, are the end point of the complex differentiation pathway in the thymus. These cells leave the thymus and comprise the peripheral (i.e., outside the thymus) mature $CD4^+$ and $CD8^+$ T-cell lineage.

As a consequence of the steps in intrathymic differentiation of T cells a repertoire of antigen-recognizing $\alpha\beta$ TcR-expressing T cells is constructed. These T cells have two general characteristics: (1) *they are MHC-restricted*; they react to peptides derived from foreign antigens only when these peptides are associated with MHC molecules that were expressed in the thymus in which the T cells developed and (2) *they are self-tolerant*; T cells expressing receptors for self antigens are eliminated or functionally inactivated. A repertoire of T cells is created that responds only to foreign antigen.

Apoptosis

In early life the thymus is one of the most active sites of cell proliferation in the whole body. However, many more cells are produced by multiplication in the thymus than actually leave it or can be accounted for in the circulation. In fact, it is estimated that as many as 90% of the developing T cells produced in the thymus die there. This can occur at several stages of differentiation in the thymus; the most prominent are (1) when a precursor fails to rearrange successfully the genes needed to code for either an $\alpha\beta$ or a $\gamma\delta$ TcR, (2) when a precursor is not positively selected on the MHC molecules of thymic structural cells, and (3) when a cell is eliminated at the negative selection stage because it expresses a receptor specific for a self antigen.

In all these cases, cells are removed by a process known as *apoptosis* or *programmed cell death.* The major characteristic of apoptosis is that as a consequence of a signal to the cell, new genes are turned on that lead to the cell's destruction. It may be compared to the cell being induced to commit suicide. Interestingly, apoptosis is common to many different cell types, including T cells and B cells (in Chapter 8 we referred to apoptosis as the fate of mature B cells that failed to produce high-affinity mutations during stimulation in the germinal center). It is also worth nothing that the consequence of activatory events in the immune response is the death of most of the stimulated cells, presumably by a process akin to apoptosis. Put another way, if all the B and T cells that resulted from antigen-specific stimulation were to survive indefinitely the body would quickly become filled with lymphocytes. This does not occur: only a small fraction of the activated cells survive and become memory cells; the fate of the majority of activated cells is death. The precise mechanisms involved in determining which cells will survive and which will die are currently poorly understood.

OTHER T-CELL SURFACE MOLECULES

There are many molecules on the surface of T cells that are up- or downregulated during different stages of T-cell development. Activation of mature T cells, for example, leads to the expression of multiple surface molecules. Many of these molecules play a key role in regulating interactions with other cells. Some of these molecules are involved in the adhesion of the activated T cell to other cell types, and yet others are involved in the homing of the T cell to appropriate tissue. It is noteworthy that some of these molecules can perform more than one of these functions. The T-cell surface molecules which we consider important are described below. They are shown diagrammatically in Figure 9.4, which also shows the molecules associated with the TcR of an $\alpha\beta^+$ T cell.

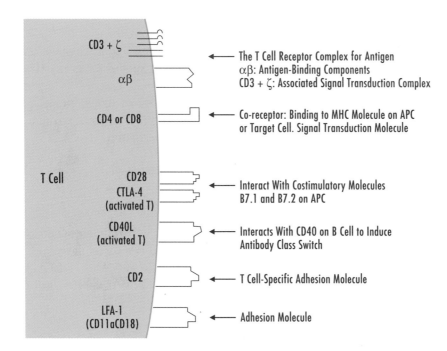

Figure 9.4

Important molecules on the T cell surface.

MOLECULES INVOLVED IN COSTIMULATION

We now recognize that the interaction of peptide bound to MHC on the antigen-presenting cell (APC) surface with the TcR of a T cell is generally not a sufficiently strong signal by itself to activate the T cell. In most circumstances, additional *costimulatory signals* are required for full T-cell activation. These signals involve the interaction of molecules on the APC and T-cell surfaces. The best-characterized costimulatory pair is *CD28* on the T cell interacting with *B7* on the APC. This interaction appears to be crucial in the generation of IL-2 following the stimulation of resting, unprimed T cells.

CD28 is a transmembrane molecule, and a member of the Ig supergene family, expressed on a large percentage of human peripheral T cells (and some activated B cells). It is not associated on the cell surface with the T-cell receptor. It interacts with B7, now recognized to consist of at least two molecules, B7.1 and B7.2 (CD80 and CD86, respectively), which are expressed on APC such as activated B cells, dendritic cells, and activated macrophages (discussed in Chapters 8 and 11). The interaction of the CD28-B7 costimulatory pair transduces a signal into the T cell that enhances the signal transmitted by the peptide-MHC-TcR interaction. As a result, IL-2 is synthesized by the T cell.

A T-cell surface molecule very closely related to CD28, known as *CTLA-4*, is expressed on activated T cells. CTLA-4 interacts with the same B7 ligands on the APC as CD28, namely B7.1 and B7.2. Recent research suggests that the B7-CTLA-4 interaction may be a negative signal to the activated T cell, serving to turn off the production of IL-2 and thus limiting the extent of the immune response. Doubltess, other costimulatory pairs of molecules will be characterized in the reaction of APC with T cells in distinct stages of differentiation.

ADHESION MOLECULES

CD2, like the molecules CD4 and CD8 described previously, is found almost exclusively on T cells and plays a role in adhesion. Its ligand is a molecule named *LFA-3 (CD58)*, which is found on many cells. The interaction of CD2 with LFA-3 enhances the binding *(adhesion)* of T cells to other cells. In the development of human T cells, CD2 is one of the first T-cell-specific molecules expressed. Expression of CD2 persists throughout the life of the T cell.

One other important adhesion molecule on the T-cell surface, but whose expression is not confined to T cells, is *leukocyte function associated antigen-1 (LFA-1), or CD11aCD18.* LFA-1 is a two-chain protein that binds to a molecule known as *intercellular adhesion molecule-1 (ICAM-1 or CD54)* on other cells. As a result of the interaction between the adhesion molecules on T cells and other cells, the binding of T cells to these other cells is considerably enhanced.

CD40 LIGAND (CD40L OR gp39)

CD40L is a 30–39 kDa glycoprotein expressed predominantly on activated T cells. Evidence suggests that the interaction between CD40L on the T cell and CD40 on the B cell is required for B-cell switching from IgM to other isotypes, such as IgE (class switching; see Chapter 8). Children with mutations in their CD40L make only IgM antibodies.

LYMPHOCYTE TRAFFICKING TO TISSUES

The ability of lymphocytes to leave the circulation and to enter tissues is a central feature of the immune system, allowing lymphocytes to reach the site of exposure to antigen, no matter where it occurs. This rapid redistribution of lymphocytes from blood to tissues is particularly vital when the effects of the antigen result in damage to the tissue: lymphocytes, as well as other leukocytes, play a key role in the inflammatory response in the damaged tissue.

One of the most interesting aspects to emerge from studies in this area is the understanding that different lymphocytes traffic to different tissues, a phenomenon known as *homing.* Some of the molecules involved in the phenomenon of lymphocyte homing are described below.

A further major point to emerge from studies of lymphocyte trafficking is that this selective entry into tissues involves multiple paired adhesive interactions between surface molecules on the circulating lymphocytes and those on endothelial cells at the boundary of the tissue. It is important to note that these adhesive interactions occur in the absence of antigen and do not involve the TcR. To date, no absolutely tissue-specific homing molecules have been defined; for example, there is no molecule that specifies a lymphocyte to leave the circulation in the brain or lung. It is presumed that a specific combination of adhesion interactions in conjunction with locally released cytokines or chemokines may be responsible for tissue entry.

One major difference in lymphocyte homing is between naive and antigen-activated cells: *naive T cells home to peripheral nodes,* where they may come in contact with antigen and become activated. In contrast, *activated and memory cells move to sites in the skin and mucosa* and not to peripheral nodes. The homing interaction of naive T cells and high endothelial venules (HEV), a specialized region of endothelium at the boundary of the peripheral nodes, is well characterized. A molecule expressed on the T-cell surface, referred to as *L-Selectin* or

MEL-14 (CD62L), binds to a carbohydrate ligand on the HEV. The interaction of this pair allows further paired lymphocyte–HEV interactions to occur, including *LFA-1 (CD11aCD18)* on the T cell binding to *ICAM-1 (CD54)* on the HEV. The effect of all these adhesion interactions is to enhance the tightness of the binding of the lymphocyte to the HEV. As a consequence, the T cell can squeeze through adjacent endothelial cells (a process known as diapedesis) and enter the node. If the naive T cells are stimulated by antigen in the node, they downregulate expression of CD62L, exit from the node and home to sites in the skin and mucosa. As CD62L expression is high on naive cells and low or absent on activated and memory cells, CD62L is referred to as a *"homing receptor"* for T lymphocytes. The nature of the adhesion interactions that allow activated and memory cells to home to distinct sites are not so well understood.

A further major point to stress is that lymphocyte redistribution from blood to tissue in response to an inflammatory stimulus shares many of the characteristics described above for the homing of T cells into tissues. The key interactions in both phenomena involve a similar set of adhesion events, mediated by the T cell and endothelial cell surface. It is also worth noting that other leukocytes, such as neutrophils, use fundamentally similar processes to leave the circulation and move into inflamed tissue. The array of cell-surface adhesion molecules expressed on other leukocytes, however, may differ from those expressed on lymphocytes.

SUMMARY

1. The role of T cells in the immune response is to deal with the protein components of foreign antigens that enter cells of the body. T cells use two major mechanisms to achieve this goal: (a) they release soluble factors, cytokines, which influence the function of multiple cell types and (b) they can kill the cell that has been penetrated by the antigen.

2. As with B cells, the individual has millions of different T cells. Each T cell bears a unique, clonally distributed receptor for antigen, known as the T-cell receptor (TcR). The same rearrangement strategies and recombinase machinery are used to generate a repertoire of T cells with different TcRs as are used by B cells to generate immunoglobulin diversity. As with the generation of the Ig repertoire, the development of the TcR repertoire takes place in the absence of antigen.

3. The part of the TcR that binds antigen is a two-chain molecule: $\alpha\beta$ on the majority of T cells, or a different two-chain structure, $\gamma\delta$, on a minor population of T cells.

4. All T cells—both those using $\alpha\beta$ and those using $\gamma\delta$ as their receptor—are expressed on the surface of the cell in association with CD3 and ζ, a multimolecular complex that acts as a signal transduction unit after antigen binding to the receptor.

5. The $\alpha\beta$-expressing cells, but generally not $\gamma\delta$-expressing T cells, also have accessory or coreceptor molecules associated with the TcR. On mature $\alpha\beta^+$ T cells the coreceptor is either CD4 or CD8, dividing T cells into two subsets: either $\alpha\beta^+CD4^+$ or $\alpha\beta^+CD8^+$. The function of these coreceptor molecules is to (a) bind MHC (major histocompatibility complex) molecules on an antigen-presenting cell (discussed in the next chapter) and (b) act as signal transduction molecules after antigenic stimulation.

6. The TcR is initially expressed on the T-cell surface during differentiation in the thymus. The differentiation pathways of T cells using $\alpha\beta$ as their receptor and those cells using $\gamma\delta$ as their receptor diverge in the thymus.

7. A key feature of thymic differentiation is the interaction of developing $\alpha\beta^+$ T cells with the stromal cells of the thymus. The interaction of the TcR of the developing T cell with MHC molecules expressed by the thymic stromal cells results in thymic selection. Thymic selection ensures that the mature $\alpha\beta^+$ T-cell population that leaves the thymus is (a) self tolerant, that is, will not interact with molecules normally expressed on cells of an individual, and (b) MHC restricted, that is, the mature T cell will interact subsequently only when foreign antigen is presented by a cell that expresses the same MHC molecules that the T cell interacted with during differentiation in the thymus.

8. Ig and the TcR have the following similarities: (a) each has only one antigenic specificity per cell, (b) each is composed of variable and constant regions, (c) each undergoes similar pathways of gene rearrangement, and (d) each is associated in the membrane of the cell with signal transduction molecules.

9. Ig and TcR have the following differences: (a) Ig is a four-chain antigen-binding molecule, whereas the TcR is a two-chain antigen-binding structure; (b) Ig can undergo somatic mutation to increase diversity, but the TcR

does not; and (c) in antigen recognition, Ig, the B-cell receptor for antigen, can interact directly with antigen. In contrast, αβ-expressing T cells interact with antigen only when the antigen is presented on the surface of a cell, and bound to a MHC molecule (discussed in detail in the following chapter).

REFERENCES

Bevilacqua MP (1993): Endothelial cell-leukocyte adhesion molecules. Annu Rev Immunol 11: 767.

Haas W, Pereira P, Tonegawa S (1993): Gamma/delta cells. Annu Rev. Immunol 11:637.

Janeway CA Jr (1993): How the immune system recognizes invaders. Sci Am 269:73.

King LB, Ashwell JD (1993): Signaling for death of lymphoid cells. Curr Opinion Immunol 5:368.

Kruisbeek AM (1993): Development of alpha beta T cells. Curr Opinion Immunol 5:227.

Marrack P, Kappler JW (1993): How the immune system recognizes the body. Sci Am 169:81.

Robey E, Fowlkes BJ (1994): Selective events in T cell development. Annu Rev Immunol 12:675.

Springer TA (1994): Traffic signals for lymphocyte recirculation and leukocyte emigration: the multistep paradigm. Cell 76:301.

von Boehmer H (1992): Thymic selection: a matter of life and death. Immunol Today 13:742.

REVIEW QUESTIONS

For each question, choose the ONE BEST answer or completion.

1. Which of the following is not a function of T cells?
   A) production of cytokines
   B) direct cellular killing of target cells
   C) involvement in response to viral and bacterial proteins
   D) induction of B-cell isotype switching
   E) antibody directed cytotoxicity (ADCC)

2. Considering development of CD4$^+$ T cells, which of the following is *incorrect*?
   A) their antigen specificity is determined prethymically
   B) they are derived from CD8$^+$CD4$^+$ precursors
   C) they undergo negative selection in the thymus

D) they are positively selected on thymic stromal cells

E) cells potentially reactive to self antigens are functionally inactivated

3. Which of the following statements is correct?

A) the αβ receptor transduces a signal into a T cell

B) a cell depleted of its CD4 molecule would be unable to recognize antigen

C) T cells with fully rearranged α and β receptors are not found in the thymus

D) T cells expressing the γδ receptor are found only in the thymus

E) Immature CD4⁺CD8⁺ T cells form the majority of T cells in the thymus

4. Which of the following cell types is found in the thymus?

A) αβ⁺γδ⁺ CD3⁺ CD4⁻ CD8⁻

B) αβ⁺ CD3⁺ CD4⁻ CD8⁺

C) γδ⁺ CD3⁺ CD4⁺ CD8⁺

D) αγ⁺γδ⁺ CD3⁺ CD4⁻ CD8⁻

E) αβ⁺ CD3⁻ CD4⁺ CD8⁺

5. CD8

A) binds to an invariant portion of MHC class II molecules

B) binds to an invariant portion of MHC class I molecules

C) binds directly to peptide antigen

D) binds to adhesion molecules on the target cell surface

E) binds to the peptide-binding site of MHC class I

6. Which of the following statements is *incorrect* concerning the TcR and Ig?

A) in both B- and T-cell precursors, multiple V-, D-, J-, and C-region genes exist in an unrearranged configuration

B) rearrangement of both TcR and Ig genes involves specific recombinase enzymes that bind to specific regions of the genome

C) both Ig and TcR are able to switch C-region usage

D) both Ig and TcR exhibit allelic exclusion

E) both Ig and the TcR use combinatorial association of V, D, and J genes and junctional imprecision to generate diversity

ANSWERS TO REVIEW QUESTIONS

1. *E* ADCC is not a property of T cells. It is mediated by natural killer (NK) cells and other cells expressing an Fc receptor (discussed in Chapter 2).

2. *A* The antigenic specificity of a T cell is determined by the acquisition of the T-cell receptor for antigen, which takes place in the thymus.

3. *E* CD4⁺CD8⁺ T cells, poorly responsive to antigen, form the majority of cells in the thymus.

4. **B** $\alpha\beta^+$CD3$^+$CD4$^-$CD8$^+$ T cells are found in the thymus. These are cells that have undergone selection and will emerge from the thymus to make up the mature CD8$^+$ T-cell population in the periphery. The expression patterns described in the other parts of the question do not occur in the T-cell lineage.

5. **B** CD8 expressed on T cells binds to an invariant or nonpolymorphic region of all MHC class I molecules.

6. **C** The ability to change the heavy-chain constant region while retaining the same antigen specificity is a property unique to Ig. The other features are common to both the TcR and Ig.

THE ROLE OF THE MAJOR HISTOCOMPATIBILITY COMPLEX IN THE IMMUNE RESPONSE

INTRODUCTION

In the previous chapter, we referred several times to the key functions of molecules coded for by the major histocompatibility complex (MHC) in the development of T cells and in T-cell responses. Indeed, the centrality of MHC molecules to T cells is referred to as the ***MHC restriction of T-cell responses.*** As we shall describe in more detail in this chapter, the role of molecules coded for by the MHC is to bind to peptide fragments derived from protein antigens, allowing them to be recognized by antigen-specific T cells. Since this binding of MHC molecules to peptide is ***selective***, that is, MHC molecules bind to only certain peptides, ***MHC molecules may be viewed as a third set of recognition molecules for antigen in the immune response, in addition to the antigen-specific T-cell and B-cell receptors, TcR and immunoglobulin (Ig).***

Originally, however, as its name implies, the MHC was recognized by its major influence on transplantation rejection (see Chapter 20). Since it was unlikely that a system as complex as the MHC evolved merely to thwart the effort of transplant surgeons, the normal function of the MHC became the focus of intense investigation. Only within the last 20 years has the relevance of MHC molecules to "everyday" responses within an individual been understood.

We shall describe first the variability of MHC genes, and then focus on the structure and function of MHC gene products, which play such a central role in the control of the immune response.

ORGANIZATION AND STRUCTURE OF MHC GENES AND PRODUCTS

The MHC is a set of genes present in all vertebrate species. It is referred to as a "complex" because the genes are closely linked and inherited as a unit. The two best-studied are the murine MHC, H-2, located on chromosome 17, and the human MHC, HLA (human leukocyte antigens), located on chromosome 6. Over the last fifteen years, the MHC regions of mouse and human have been mapped by molecular biological approaches and an understanding of the true complexity of the regions is still emerging. Each MHC complex contains about 40 genes and pseudogenes (i.e., long stretches of DNA that have some defect that prevents them from being transcribed or translated). The chromosomal organization of the various gene loci (i.e., the positions of the genes on the chromosome) that constitute the mouse and human MHC complexes is shown in Figure 10.1. We shall first discuss MHC class I and MHC class II molecules because of their key function in cellular interactions, and then describe the other genes in this region and their products.

MHC Class I Molecules

In the human there are three independent MHC class I loci (A, B, C). The mouse also has three class I loci (K, D, L) that occupy somewhat different chromosomal positions within the complex (see Fig. 10.1). There is a high degree of homology between the molecules coded for by the murine K, D, and L loci and the human A, B, and C loci, indicating a common ancestral origin. MHC class I molecules are members of the immunoglobulin superfamily, and contain Ig-like domains.

Each MHC class I locus codes for a transmembrane polypeptide of molecu-

HUMAN HLA COMPLEX

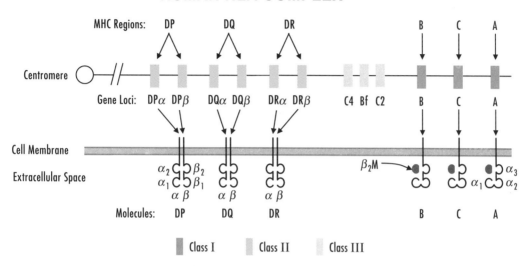

MOUSE H-2 COMPLEX

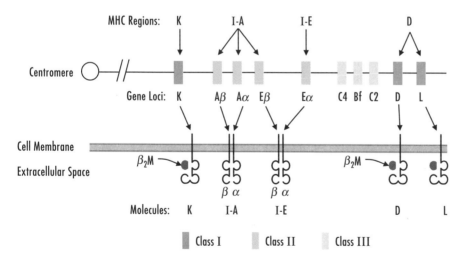

Figure 10.1.

Top) The human major histocompatibility complex (HLA). Bottom) The murine major histocompatibility complex (H-2).

lar weight 43 kDa containing three extracellular domains, called α_1, α_2, and α_3. Each MHC class I molecule is expressed at the surface of a cell in noncovalent association with an invariant small polypeptide called β_2-*microglobulin* (β_2*m*, molecular weight 12 kDa), which is coded for on another chromosome. β_2m has a structure homologous to a single Ig domain, and indeed, β_2m is also a member of the Ig superfamily. Thus, the cell surface complex of MHC class I and β_2-microglobulin appears like a four-domain molecule, with the α_3 domain of the class I molecule and β_2m juxtaposed closest to the membrane.

MHC class I molecules are expressed on almost every nucleated cell in the body. Their expression is *coordinate*, in that all three MHC class I molecules are expressed on the cell surface at the same time. The level of MHC class I expression at the cell surface is similarly coordinately up- or downregulated by different stimuli; for example, in the mouse the cytokine interferon γ (IFN-γ) enhances expression of all MHC class I molecules.

A key point to note is that different individuals within a species have slightly different forms, *alleles*, of each MHC class I gene; that is, at a single locus, different individuals can have different genes. Thus, different individuals express distinct MHC molecules. This phenomenon of having multiple stable forms of one gene in the population is known as *genetic polymorphism.* In other words, genetic polymorphism is the strategy for generating diversity of MHC molecules. It contrasts with the unique strategy of gene rearrangement for generating diversity of antigen-specific T- and B-cell receptors, discussed in Chapters 6 and 9. As a consequence of rearrangement strategies, each lymphocyte within an individual expresses a slightly different Ig or TcR. In contrast, every cell in one individual expresses the same MHC molecules, but as a consequence of genetic polymorphism, the MHC molecules expressed by genetically distinct individuals are different.

The MHC is the most highly polymorphic gene system in the body; for example, about 50 distinct alleles of the HLA-B gene have been described to date. In humans, different alleles are given numbers, such as HLA-B15 or 27, whereas in mice alleles are given superscripted small letters such as H-2K^b or K^d. From sequencing different MHC class I (and class II molecules) it became apparent that different allelic forms of the molecule are very homologous; for example, the sequences of H-2K^b and K^d molecules are over 90% identical. Sequence differences between the molecules are confined to a limited region, found in their extracellular α_1 and α_2 domains. Thus, an individual class I molecule can be divided into a *nonpolymorphic* or *invariant* region (similar in all class I allelic forms) and a *polymorphic* or *variable* region (sequence unique to that allele). The T cell molecule CD8 binds to the invariant region of all MHC class I molecules (see Fig. 10.2A).

One further point worth noting is that MHC molecules (both class I and II) are *codominantly* expressed; that is, each cell expresses MHC proteins which are transcribed from both maternal and paternal chromosomes. (This again contrasts with the formation of Ig and TcR molecules, described in Chapter 6 and 9, where only one chromosome is used, the unique phenomenon of allelic exclusion.) As a consequence of codominant expression of MHC molecules, each cell within one individual therefore expresses six different MHC class I molecules: HLA-A, B and C proteins encoded by the paternal chromosome, and HLA-A, B and C proteins encoded by the maternal chromosome. Thus, for example, all the cells in one individual may express the molecules HLA-A2 and A5, HLA-B7 and B13, and HLA-C6 and C8 on their surface. Cells in another individual may express six completely different HLA class I molecules. This extensive polymorphism of MHC genes therefore makes it very unlikely that two random individuals will express identical sets of MHC molecules. As we shall describe in Chapter 20, this polymorphism is the basis for rapid graft rejection between genetically different individuals.

DETAILED STRUCTURE OF MHC CLASS I MOLECULES. One of the most important findings of the last 10 years has been the crystallization of a number of human and mouse MHC class I molecules (and more recently MHC class II molecules), initiated by the efforts of Don Wiley and colleagues. We now have a clear picture of the three-dimensional structure of several MHC molecules. This structural information has had an enormous impact on our understanding of the biology of the MHC.

All MHC class I molecules from mouse and human have the same general structure, depicted in Figures 10.1 and 10.2. The most striking feature is that the part of the molecule furthest from the membrane contains a deep groove or cleft. This cleft is made up of parts of the α_1 and α_2 domains. *All the evidence points to this cleft as the unique peptide-binding site for the MHC class I molecule.* As shown in Figure 10.2B, peptide bound in this cleft and parts of the MHC class I molecule interact with the variable regions, Vα and Vβ, of a T-cell receptor. The cleft resembles a basket with an irregular floor made up of 8 β-pleated sheets and each surrounding wall forming an α-helix. The cleft appears closed at both ends and can fit peptides 8–9 amino acids long in a linear array. When the structure of different MHC class I molecules is compared, it is found that amino acid differences between the alleles are confined primarily to the region of this cleft, while

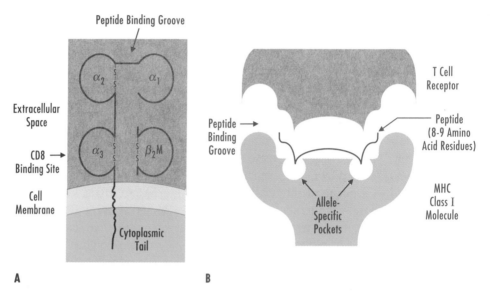

Figure 10.2.

Two views of an MHC class I molecule on the cell surface showing A) the association of an MHC class I molecule with β_2-microglobulin and B) how a T-cell receptor interacts with the MHC class I molecule and peptide bound in the peptide binding groove. [After Rammensee, Falk, and Rötzschke (1993): Curr Op Imm 5:35.]

the rest of the molecule is relatively constant. Comparing clefts between different MHC class I molecules, the floor of each is different, consisting of a number of ***allele-specific pockets.*** The shape and charge of these pockets at the bottom of the cleft help to determine which peptides bind to a particular MHC molecule. The pockets also help to secure peptides in a position in which they can be recognized by specific T-cell receptors.

A single MHC class I molecule can bind to a variety of peptides but binds preferentially to peptides with certain ***motifs***, specific amino acids at certain positions in the 8 or 9 amino acid sequence. Thus, for example, the peptides which bind to mouse MHC class I molecule K^b have the amino acids phenylalanine or tyrosine at position 5, and leucine at position 8, whereas the human class I molecule HLA-A2 binds peptides with leucine at position 2 and valine at position 9. The other positions on the peptide can be occupied by a variety of different amino acids, indicating that there is a great deal of flexibility in the peptides that can be bound by any one MHC molecule.

MHC Class II Molecules

In this section we will focus on the organization of genes coding for MHC class II molecules (shown in Fig. 10.1). (This region also codes for several other important genes that we shall describe subsequently.) In the human, the MHC class II region (originally named the D region) contains three sets of genes—DP, DQ, and DR—each of which codes for a two-chain cell surface glycoprotein. DP, DQ, and DR each contains an α gene and a β gene, coding for an α and a β chain (molecular weights 35,000 and 28,000 daltons), respectively. Thus, the genes DPα and DPβ, DQα and DQβ, and DRα and DRβ code for the surface molecules DP, DQ, and DR respectively. Recent evidence indicates that there is more than one functional β gene in the DP, DQ, and DR regions. Because the DRα chain can pair with the products of each of the different DRβ genes, more than one DR$\alpha\beta$ molecule can be expressed. Similarly, more than one DP$\alpha\beta$ and DQ$\alpha\beta$ molecule may be expressed.

In the mouse, the MHC class II region was originally named the I region, and its products were known as Ia molecules, standing for Immune associated. The mouse MHC class II region contains only two sets of genes—A and E—each coding for a two-chain α plus β-cell surface glycoprotein, homologous to the human MHC class II molecules DP and DR molecules, respectively. Thus, humans express three different types of MHC class II molecules at their cell surface: DP$\alpha\beta$, DQ$\alpha\beta$, and DR$\alpha\beta$, and the mouse expresses just two, A$\alpha\beta$ and E$\alpha\beta$. Some mouse strains are unable to synthesize E molecules, and thus cells from these mice express only MHC class II A molecules at their cell surface.

MHC class II molecules, like MHC class I molecules, are transmembrane molecules with extracellular Ig-like domains and cytoplasmic tails. MHC class II molecules are also members of the immunoglobulin superfamily.

Like MHC class I genes, MHC class II genes also exhibit polymorphism, with multiple allelic forms expressed in the human and mouse populations. Allelic variants of human MHC class II genes are given numbers such as HLA-DR4 or HLA-DR7, whereas alleles in the mouse are given superscripts, such as A^d or A^k.

As was described with MHC class I molecules, MHC class II molecules also comprise variable or polymorphic regions (differing between alleles) and invariant or nonpolymorphic regions (common to all alleles). ***The T cell molecule CD4 binds to the invariant portion of all MHC class II molecules*** (Fig. 10.3A).

MHC class II molecules also exhibit codominant expression. Thus, a diploid murine cell may express four different MHC class II molecules (as well as six different MHC class I molecules) on its surface. Because of the variability in DP$\alpha\beta$,

DQ$\alpha\beta$, and DR$\alpha\beta$ described above, a human cell can express between 10 and 20 different MHC class II molecules on its surface. Like class I molecules, class II molecules also constitute strong transplantation antigens, which, because of their polymorphism, differ among various individuals and are responsible for a rapid and vigorous graft rejection (see Chapter 20).

MHC class II molecules have a somewhat more limited distribution than class I molecules: they are expressed *constitutively* (i.e., under all conditions) only on B lymphocytes, dendritic cells, and thymic epithelial cells. Nonetheless, many other cells such as macrophages and endothelial cells may be *induced* to express MHC class II molecules by activating factors such as IFN-γ. (Interestingly, human but not mouse T cells can be induced to express MHC class II molecules following antigen stimulation.) It is also worth noting that MHC class II molecules, like class I molecules, are coordinately expressed and regulated. In summary, in the absence of inducing factors such as IFN-γ, most cells express MHC class I molecules without expressing MHC class II molecules. Certain cells, such as B cells, constitutively express both MHC class I and II molecules. In contrast, very few, if any, cells express MHC class II in the absence of MHC class I.

DETAILED STRUCTURE OF MHC CLASS II MOLECULES. The MHC class II molecule, HLA-DR1, was recently crystallized by a group led by Don Wiley. Several characteristics are strikingly similar to the fine structure of MHC class I molecules. As shown in Figure 10.3B, the key feature is a peptide-binding groove or cleft at the top of the molecule, analogous to the MHC class I groove, in the region between the α_1 and β_1 domains. The floor of the class II groove comprises 8 β-pleated sheets, with the α_1 and β_1 domains each contributing four. In contrast to the class I groove, however, the class II groove is open at both ends, allowing larger peptides to bind. As we shall discuss in a subsequent section, MHC class II molecules preferentially bind peptides varying from 12 to 25 amino acids in length, indicating that peptides binding to class II have their ends outside the groove. Peptide bound in the groove of the MHC class II molecule, and parts of the MHC class II molecule, interact with the variable regions, Vα and Vβ, of a T-cell receptor (Fig. 10.3B).

The most striking difference between the fine structure of the class II molecule and the structure of the class I molecule is that the class II crystal consists of a pair of class II molecules or "dimer of dimers." The functional significance of this finding remains to be clarified, since a class II dimer has not been observed at the cell surface. It may relate to the ability to cross-link two T-cell receptor molecules, leading to T-cell activation (as we shall see in Chapter 11).

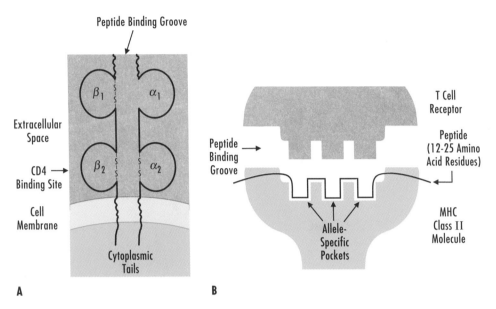

Figure 10.3.

Two views of an MHC class II molecule on the cell surface showing A) the structure of the two-chain molecule and B) how a T-cell receptor interacts with the MHC class II molecule and peptide bound in the peptide binding groove. [After Rammensee, Falk, and Rötzschke (1993): Curr Op Imm 5:35.]

OTHER GENES WITHIN THE MHC

As described in the introduction to this chapter, the genetic complexity of the MHC region has been appreciated only in recent years with the advent of molecular biological techniques. The function of many of these genes awaits clarification. Why all these genes are linked in a complex with genes coding for crucial cell interaction molecules is currently not known.

As shown in Figure 10.1, the MHC class III region contains genes coding for serum complement components (C2, C4, and factor B; see Chapter 13). The region between class I and class III genes in the human contains several different genes: two cytokines [tumor necrosis factor (TNF) α and β], two heat-shock proteins (hsp 70-1 and 70-2), and an enzyme involved in the hydroxylation of steroids. Additional murine human MHC class I genes (HLA-E, F, G, and H) and murine MHC class I genes (Qa and TLa) have been identified which are not variable like other class I genes. The function of products coded for by these class I genes is poorly understood.

The MHC class II region includes genes other than those coding for the cell-surface molecules described earlier in the chapter. These include genes known as M and O in the mouse, and DM, DN, and DO in the human class II regions. The precise function of their gene products is not clear, although DM is now believed to play a role in the pathway of MHC class II molecule movement through the cell, which is described later in the chapter. Genes coding for the peptide transporter molecules TAP-1 and TAP-2, whose function will be discussed below, are also found in the MHC class II region.

FUNCTION OF MHC MOLECULES

As we have mentioned previously, pathogens such as bacteria and viruses can penetrate and infect the cells of the body. To deal with these infections, T cells are required to mount an immune response against the cell harboring the invading organism. T cells must therefore be able to distinguish between infected and noninfected cells. The T cell's ability to discriminate between infected and non-infected cell is achieved by displaying peptides derived from the foreign antigen on the surface of the host cell in which they were generated. ***Only those cells displaying "foreign" peptides trigger a T-cell response.*** In a sense, the foreign peptides that reach the cell surface are a representative sampling of all the peptides derived from the pathogen inside the infected cell. In this way, T cells are able to recognize the difference between an infected and a noninfected cell.

The events involved in the generation of peptides from proteins inside cells and the display of such peptides at the cell surface is known collectively as ***antigen processing and presentation.*** MHC molecules play a central role in the phenomena of antigen processing and presentation because they bind to selected peptide fragments inside the cell and transport them to the cell surface. This complex of peptide and MHC molecule on the surface of the "target" or antigen-presenting cell may now be recognized by a T cell with the appropriate receptor. In this way, T-cell responses are said to be MHC-restricted.

In the paragraphs which follow we will describe these events in more detail.

ANTIGEN PROCESSING AND PRESENTATION

Determining how protein antigens activate T cells has been the subject of intense study for several years. Early experiments in the field suggested that antigens had to be ingested by specialized cells such as macrophages, and then broken down to peptide fragments before T cells would respond. In which part of the cell and how this occurred were not understood. Tracing the fate of antigen inside the cell was difficult because it became apparent that only a tiny fraction of the input antigen generated an immune response; the vast majority of the antigen was broken down to very small fragments that were not immunogenic. It was thus not possible to follow the intracellular fate of that crucial portion of the antigen that generated a T-cell response. Furthermore, although the immunogenic antigenic moieties were suspected to be on the surface of the macrophage, they could not be detected by antibodies specific for the protein.

The involvement of MHC molecules in processing and presentation was also suggested by a key early finding: antibody specific for MHC molecules was able to block macrophage presentation of antigen to T cells. Since the antibody directed at MHC molecules presumably sterically blocked the interaction of MHC on the APC with the T-cell receptor, this finding strongly suggested that MHC molecules and antigen were closely associated on the surface of the APC.

Several findings over the last 10 years have revolutionized our understanding of the nature of antigen processing and presentation, as well as the role of MHC molecules in these phenomena. One of the most important changes was to study the immune response to small protein antigens whose complete sequence was known, (rather than complex multimeric proteins) for example, cytochrome c and lysozyme molecules obtained from a variety of animals. In conjunction with advances in the in vitro culture of T cells using growth factors, it was determined that a single T cell was able to respond to a specific linear peptide region of the molecule. Generally these peptides are 10–20 amino acids long. Another key finding was that many different cells have the machinery to process and present antigen to T cells, and so it is now recognized that cells such as B cells, epithelial cells, and dendritic cells—and not macrophages alone—have the ability to act as antigen-presenting cells for T cells.

A further finding with crucial impact was that MHC molecules purified from the cell surface could bind selectively to peptides in vitro. This finding established the role of MHC molecules as selective peptide binders. Initially, this was shown with MHC class II molecules, but more recently it has also been shown for MHC class I molecules.

Several general rules have now become apparent concerning antigen processing and MHC binding of peptides:

1. To activate the T-cell response to any foreign protein, the protein must be broken down to peptides, at least one of which must bind to an MHC molecule. A

peptide which does not bind to an MHC molecule does not activate a T-cell response. If an entire antigen fails to generate a single peptide able to bind to an MHC molecule, the individual would not mount a T-cell response to that particular antigen. This kind of unresponsiveness to an entire antigen can occur, for example, in the response of certain strains of mice to synthetic polymers of amino acids that contain a very limited number of epitopes, but is very rare in the response to naturally occurring pathogens. Thus, even though there is only a limited number of different MHC class I molecules (6) and MHC class II molecules (10–20 in the human, 6 in the mouse) per cell, it is likely that the processing of a protein will generate at least *one* peptide with a motif that can bind to at least one of the MHC molecules expressed. It is therefore highly probable that a protein antigen will trigger a T-cell response in almost any individual.

2. The association of MHC molecules and processed peptides is selective. Only a limited number of peptides derived from a single protein bind to one MHC molecule; stated another way, different MHC molecules bind distinct peptides generated from a single protein. This selectivity in peptide binding arises from the structure and charge of the peptide-binding groove of the MHC molecule.

To give one example of this selectivity, 10 different peptides may result from the processing of an influenza protein in the cells of an individual who expresses HLA-DP2,DP3; DQ4,DQ5; and DR4,DR7: one of the peptides may bind only to HLA-DR4, another peptide to HLA-DP2, and the remaining eight peptides may not bind to any of the class II molecules (see Fig. 10.4). Thus, in this individual, the peptides binding to HLA-DP2 and to HLA-DR4 constitute the epitopes that trigger the T-cell response to the influenza protein, and these epitopes are referred to as ***immunodominant*** for this antigen in this individual. (The remaining peptides are probably rapidly degraded and do not trigger an immune response.) In contrast, another individual who expresses a completely different set of MHC class II molecules may bind to two other, distinct peptides from the 10 generated by processing the same influenza protein. (It is generally felt that the cleavage events involved in processing are the same in different people; that is, that the set of peptides generated from one protein is the same in different individuals.) Thus, both individuals are making an immune response to the same influenza protein; because of differences in the MHC molecules between these individuals, however, the individuals respond to different portions of the molecule. Thus, different regions of a protein are immunodominant in individuals with differing MHC molecules.

In summary, it is crucial that every individual mount a response to one or a few peptides derived from a single, foreign protein, but these peptides may differ in individuals expressing different MHC molecules.

3. MHC class I molecules preferentially bind peptides of 8 or 9 amino acids, whereas MHC class II molecules preferentially bind peptides of much more variable length, between 12 and 25 amino acids in length. These binding differences are due to the ends of the class I groove being closed, and the ends of the class II groove open so that larger peptides may "flop over" the ends of the groove.

4. MHC class I molecules preferentially bind to peptides derived from molecules that arise in the cytoplasm of the cell; MHC class II molecules preferentially bind to peptides derived from proteins that have come from outside the cell and end up in acid vesicles inside the cell (see the following section and Fig. 10.5).

5. The affinity of peptide binding to an MHC molecule approaches that of an antigen–antibody interaction. Generally, a single peptide would bind with high affinity to some allelic forms but not to others (Fig. 10.4).

6. The interaction of peptide and MHC occurs slowly, but once formed, the complex of MHC and peptide dissociate slowly, indicating that the complexes are stable for several hours.

7. MHC molecules can bind "self" peptides. It has been found that peptides

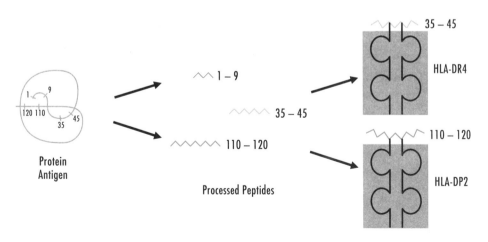

Figure 10.4

Selective binding of processed peptides by different MHC alleles. The numbers refer to positions of amino acids in the sequence of the protein antigen.

purified from MHC molecules at the cell surface are components of various normal cellular constituents, such as ribosomal proteins or even other MHC molecules. These self components do not generally result in T-cell activation. Either these components are present at too low a number to activate T cells, or the T cells have been made tolerant (see Chapters 9 and 12) to this combination of MHC and peptide. (As discussed in Chapter 9, most T cells reactive to self antigens are removed during differentiation in the thymus, so that the mature T cells are depleted of reactivity to self antigens.) Thus, as described above, if a peptide does not bind to an MHC molecule it does not trigger a T-cell response. However, even if a peptide *does* bind to an MHC molecule, it does not invariably lead to a T-cell activation.

This binding of peptides derived from self components raises an interesting issue, because it indicates that MHC molecules do not discriminate self from nonself peptides. Since an individual's cells are bathed in an ocean of self proteins, which they are continually processing and binding to their MHC molecules, how can the individual respond to a tiny amount of foreign protein? The answer appears to be that a very small number of MHC–foreign peptide complexes is all that is required at the surface of the APC to generate an immune response. It is believed that as few as 80–100 MHC–foreign peptide complexes on the surface of a cell (which may express about 10^5 total MHC molecules on its surface) is sufficient to trigger a T-cell response.

Cell Biology of Antigen Processing and Presentation: What Determines Whether an Antigen Elicits an MHC Class I or Class II Restricted Response?

As we have seen, the structural features of MHC class I and class II molecules that bind and present peptides to T cells are very similar. We have recently begun to understand the processes that occur inside a cell to determine how a particular protein antigen is processed and presented by either class I or class II molecules.

The evidence suggests that protein breakdown into peptides takes place in two compartments: (1) within acid vesicles and (2) within the cytoplasm and endoplasmic reticulum. In brief, ***peptides generated in acid vesicles bind to MHC class II whereas peptides generated in the cytoplasm and endoplasmic reticulum bind to MHC class I*** (illustrated diagrammatically in Fig. 10.5).

We will deal first with the set of antigens known as ***exogenous antigens.*** Exogenous antigens are taken into cells by endocytosis if the antigen is soluble or by phagocytosis, in specialized cells such as macrophages, if the antigen is particulate (see Fig. 10.5). These exogenous antigens include bacteria, viruses taken up

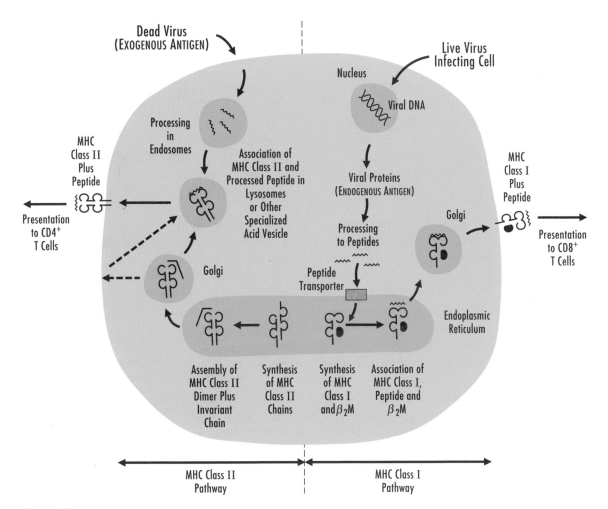

Figure 10.5

Differential processing of antigens in the MHC class II pathway (left) or MHC class I pathway (right). Dotted lines: "empty" class II molecules may move to the cell surface and cycle back to acid vesicles.

by macrophages, and potentially harmless foreign proteins, such as ovalbumin or sheep red blood cells.

Once internalized, the antigen is contained in an intracellular vesicle that then fuses with existing endosomal or lysosomal vesicles. The endosomal and lysosomal vesicles are highly acidic (pH ~4.0) and contain an array of degradative enzymes, including proteases and peptidases. Some regions of the antigenic protein are thus catabolized to single amino acids, but at least some portions of the protein seem less sensitive to degradation and remain as peptides for a finite period. These peptides (12–25 amino acids long) constitute the discrete epitopes to which the T cells subsequently make their response. Generally, a complex protein gives rise to only a few such epitopes. As described previously, the small number of fragments that lead to T-cell activation are referred to as the ***immunodominant*** peptides of this antigen in this particular individual.

MHC class II molecules synthesized on ribosomes of the rough endoplasmic reticulum (RER) traffic via the Golgi and trans-Golgi network to the cell surface. At some stage in this intracellular movement, vesicles containing MHC class II molecules intersect with acidic vesicles containing peptides. Exactly where this occurs in the cell is not completely understood although it is believed to occur in a specialized compartment. If a peptide binds to an MHC class II molecule, the peptide–MHC complex moves to the cell surface, where it is available for recognition by $CD4^+$ T cells expressing the appropriate TcR.

Proteins that generate peptides able to bind MHC class I molecules follow a different pathway of processing. These antigens (generally viral or parasitic in origin) are ***endogenous*** in that they are generally synthesized within the cell. Their processing occurs in the cytosolic compartment or endoplasmic reticulum (not in acid vesicles). Peptide fragments generated by processing in the cytoplasm are selectively transported into the endoplasmic reticulum by the products of two "transporter" genes, known as TAP-1 and TAP-2. In the endoplasmic reticulum, peptides can bind to newly synthesized MHC class I molecules, associated with β_2-microglobulin. Binding of peptide to MHC in this milieu is selective, and is based on the physicochemical properties of the peptide and the particular MHC class I allele. Complexes of peptide, β_2m, and MHC class I move to the surface of the cell, where they can be recognized by the $CD8^+$ T cell.

Since newly synthesized MHC class II (as well as MHC class I) molecules are also found in the endoplasmic reticulum, why do peptides derived from endogenous proteins not bind to the MHC class II molecules? The reason appears to be that when MHC class II α and β chains are synthesized in the ER they associate rapidly into a complex with a third molecule known as ***invariant chain*** (Ii, CD74), which prevents peptide binding (see Fig. 10.5). This complex of Ii and MHC class II α plus β chains is broken down in the cell's acid vesicles. In these vesicles, Ii is removed and peptides derived from exogenous antigens may now bind to the MHC class II molecule. Other molecules, known as ***chaperones***, are involved in regulating distinct stages of the association of peptide with both MHC class I and II molecules, as well as in the transport of peptide–MHC molecules from compartment to compartment within the cell.

It is worth noting that current research favors the view that peptide binds to newly synthesized MHC class I and II molecules on their way to the cell surface, but cannot exclude that some peptide binding may take place with MHC molecules that are recycling from the membrane of the cell (shown by a dotted line in Fig. 10.5). It is also possible that peptide may bind to some MHC molecules at the cell surface, either to MHC molecules not containing peptide or by displacing previously bound peptide.

In summary, a protein antigen needs to be proteolytically cleaved (processed) before it is presented either via MHC class I or class II molecules, but the outcome is dependent on the pathway it takes through the presenting or target cell. Thus, if a viral antigen is taken up by macrophages, for example, as may occur when a noninfectious viral particle is presented in a vaccine, processing occurs in acid vesicles and peptides are presented on MHC class II molecules to $CD4^+$ T cells. If, however, the same viral antigen is synthesized following the infection of a cell, processing will occur in the cytoplasm or ER of the cell and peptides will associate with MHC class I molecules for presentation to $CD8^+$ T cells. Thus, as a consequence of these distinct processing pathways of a single protein, $CD4^+$ and $CD8^+$ T cells in the same individual may respond to different epitopes on the same antigen.

Over the last few years we have come to realize that the phenomena of antigen processing and presentation are aspects of normal cell physiological pathways. Thus, a great deal of recent attention has focused on understanding basic cellular physiology, including how normal cellular proteins move through the cell to its surface, how long they remain on the cell surface, and what happens to them after they leave the cell surface; in short, to try and gain an understanding of the dynamic aspects of intracellular traffic and turnover.

MHC RESTRICTION

In the foregoing section we described how $CD4^+$ T cells interact with peptide antigen when it is associated with an MHC class II molecule. $CD8^+$ T cells interact with antigen only when it is bound to an MHC class I molecule. We therefore say that ***T-cell responses are MHC-restricted***, and we refer to the responses of $CD4^+$ T cells as being restricted by MHC class II molecules, and $CD8^+$ T cells by MHC class I molecules.

It is important to note that this T-cell response to antigen occurs only if antigen is presented by self MHC. Self MHC is the allelic form of MHC molecule that the T-cell precursor is exposed to on thymic structural cells during intrathymic differentiation (Chapter 9). Nonself MHC is by definition any other MHC allele that the developing T cells have not been exposed to during differentiation in the thymus. Peptide-specific responses do not occur if the peptide is presented by nonself MHC molecules. More strictly, we should say that *T-cell responses are self-MHC-restricted.* In this sense, MHC molecules define what is self and what is nonself for an individual's immune system.

DIVERSITY OF MHC MOLECULES

In this chapter, we have described the extensive polymorphism of MHC genes and molecules. We have indicated that such polymorphism is a great impediment to the acceptance of tissue between individuals, because it is highly unlikely that two random individuals are genetically identical (discussed more fully in Chapter 20). Since nearly every vertebrate species has developed a similarly diverse array of MHC genes and molecules, it suggests that the maintenance of MHC diversity must have some major benefit to be so widespread.

It is likely that this diversity is a mechanism that the species uses to protect itself from potentially lethal infectious agents. To illustrate this point, imagine the situation if there were only one MHC molecule in the population and a new pathogen emerged that did not produce an epitope able to bind to the single MHC molecule. In this extreme case, no T-cell response would be mounted and the entire species could be wiped out. Thus, maintaining a large number of MHC genes and molecules in the species would greatly reduce the risk of one pathogen having such a negative effect.

ASSOCIATION OF DISEASE WITH MHC TYPE

In the preceding section we described the potential advantage to the species of maintaining a highly diverse array of MHC genes in the face of surrounding pathogenic organisms. Indeed, it has been shown that the possession of certain MHC alleles may confer protection against infectious diseases such as malaria. In contrast, it has also been recognized for many years that individuals with certain allelic HLA genes have a higher risk of contracting certain diseases (Table 10.1), especially those of an autoimmune nature. One of the most dramatic examples of all HLA-associated diseases is *ankylosing spondylitis* (an inflammatory disease that leads to stiffening of the vertebral joints of the spine). Over 90% of people with the disease carry one particular HLA allele (the B27 allele), but not everyone carrying the B27 allele gets the disease, indicating the need for other factors, such as environment or infection.

TABLE 10.1   Association of HLA Types and Disease

Disease	HLA allele	Relative risk factor[a]
Hashimoto's thyroiditis	DR5	3
Rheumatoid arthritis	DR4	6
Dermatitis herpetiformis	DR3	56
Goodpasture's syndrome	DR2	13
Multiple sclerosis	DR2	5
Ankylosing spondylitis	B27	87
Reiter's disease	B27	37
Postgonococcal arthritis	B27	14
Psoriasis vulgaris	C6	13
Myasthenia gravis	B8	4

[a]The risk of contracting the disease for an individual who possesses the HLA allele compared to the risk of an individual who does not.

For almost all known cases of association of a disease with a particular HLA genotype, the explanation is complicated by the fact that the causative agent is unknown. Many of the diseases appear to have an immunologic component, probably of autoimmune origin (see Chapter 17), and many are also suspected of being viral in origin. The following hypotheses have been proposed to account for these associations of HLA type and disease:

1. MHC molecules serve as *receptors* for the attachment and entry of pathogens into the cell. Thus, individuals with a certain HLA type could be more susceptible to an infection by a particular virus that uses that HLA molecule as a receptor.

2. Serendipitous *resemblance* between the antigenic determinants of the pathogen and the MHC molecule of the host (molecular mimicry) may either prevent an immune response, because the pathogen is seen as "self" and no response is made, or, in the event of an immune response to the pathogen, lead to destruction of tissue in an autoimmune reaction.

3. Since antigens are recognized in combination with products of the MHC, it is possible that the antigens of some pathogens, in combination with particular molecules of the MHC, cannot be recognized by T cells. Such a combination would thus be ignored by the host and slip through a "hole in the repertoire" of the host's T cells.

4. It is possible that an allele in the MHC itself is not responsible for the disease, but rather that some other genetic locus closely linked to the MHC causes the disease.

Whatever the explanation for the association between HLA and disease, there is great practical value in studying it to identify individuals at risk, to make more precise diagnoses, and to protect the course of the disease.

SIMILARITIES AND DIFFERENCES BETWEEN MHC CLASS I AND CLASS II MOLECULES

Similarities:

1. *Function:* Both (a) are critical cell interaction molecules, as a consequence of their ability to bind peptides, and to present bound peptide at the surface of an antigen-presenting cell to T-cell receptors and (b) are strong transplantation antigens (see Chapter 20).

2. *Structure:* Both (a) are two-chain transmembrane proteins, (b) have a single peptide-binding site in the extracellular region that is unique to that particular allele, and (c) have a polymorphic region (which includes the peptide-binding region) and a nonpolymorphic region.

3. *Expression:* Both are codominantly expressed.

4. *Diversity:* Both show genetic polymorphism, with multiple alleles in the population.

Differences:

1. Cells expressing MHC class I + peptide interact with $CD8^+$ T cells; cells expressing MHC class II + peptide interact with $CD4^+$ T cells.

2. MHC class I molecules bind peptides of 8–9 amino acids derived from endogenous antigens; MHC class II molecules bind peptides of 12–25 amino acids derived from exogenous antigens.

3. MHC class I molecule expression is constitutive on nearly all nucleated cells; constitutive MHC class II expression is more limited.

4. MHC class II heterodimer coded for entirely within MHC, MHC class I molecule includes β_2-microglobulin coded for outside MHC.

SUMMARY

1. The function of MHC molecules is to bind selected peptides generated inside a cell during the processing of protein antigens. The complex formed between an MHC molecule and peptide moves to the cell surface, where the MHC molecule is inserted into the membrane of the cell with peptide on the outside. The peptide–MHC complex on the cell surface can now be recognized by a T cell with an appropriate receptor.

2. The MHC codes for two major categories of cell surface molecules: MHC class I molecules consist of a single polypeptide chain associated with a molecule known as β_2-microglobulin on the surface of nearly all nucleated cells. MHC class II molecules consist of two polypeptide chains (α and β) and have a more limited cellular distribution.

3. The outer region of every MHC class I and class II molecule contains a deep groove that functions as the peptide-binding site.

4. MHC class I molecules preferentially bind peptides 8–9 amino acids long, derived predominantly from proteins processed in the cytoplasm and endoplasmic reticulum of the cell. Bacteria and viruses that have infected cells generate peptides via this *"endogenous pathway"* of antigen processing. In contrast, MHC class II molecules bind peptides 12–25 amino acids long, derived predominantly from proteins processed in the acid compartments of the cell (endosomes and lysosomes). Peptides are generated in this compartment following the uptake of antigens from the outside of the cell (the *"exogenous pathway"* of antigen processing).

5. Within one individual, the MHC class I and II molecules expressed are the same on all cells of the body. An individual expresses only a limited number of different MHC class I molecules (6) and class II molecules (10–20 in the human) per cell.

6. Different individuals express a distinct array of MHC class I and class II molecules. This diversity comes about because different individuals within a species have a range of slightly different forms, *alleles*, of MHC class I and class II genes. Because of the extensive polymorphism of MHC genes, every individual has an almost unique array of inherited MHC genes.

7. The binding of peptides to MHC molecules is selective. Each MHC class I or class II molecule binds peptides with a particular *motif.* Since complex proteins usually generate at least one peptide able to bind to an MHC molecule, however, a T-cell response to at least some part of a foreign antigen is more or less assured.

8. **T-cell responses are MHC-restricted:** T-cell receptors on CD4$^+$ helper T cells recognize and respond to antigen only when bound to an MHC class II molecule on the surface of an antigen-presenting cell. Antigen-specific receptors on CD8$^+$ cytotoxic T cells recognize antigen only in association with MHC class I molecules. Thus, CD4$^+$ T cells are restricted by MHC class II, and CD8$^+$ T cells by MHC class I molecules.

9. **MHC molecules expressed on the structural cells of the thymus play a key role in the development of T cells in the thymus.** The set of MHC alleles that T-cell precursors are exposed to during their differentiation in the thymus is referred to as "self MHC." T-cell responses are thus referred to as "self-MHC-restricted." The response of a mature T cell to peptide occurs only when the peptide is presented by self MHC class I or class II on the surface of an antigen-presenting cell.

10. **Many human diseases are associated with particular MHC alleles.**

REFERENCES

Cresswell P (1994): Assembly, transport and function of MHC class II molecules. Annu Rev Immunol 12:259.

Engelhard VH (1994): Structure of peptides associated with MHC class I molecules. Curr Opinion Immunol 6:13.

Germain RN, Margulies DH (1993): The biochemistry and cell biology of antigen processing and presentation. Annu Rev Immunol 11:403.

Madden DR, Gorga JC, Strominger JL, Wiley DC (1992): The three dimensional structure of HLA-B27 at 2.1A resolution suggests a general mechanism for tight peptide binding to MHC. Cell 70:1035.

Monaco JJ (1993): Structure and function of genes in the MHC class II region. Curr Opinion Immunol 5:17.

Neefjes JJ, Momburg F (1993): Cell biology of antigen presentation. Curr Opinion Immunol 5: 27.

Rammensee H-G, Falk K, Rötzschke O (1993): MHC molecules as peptide receptors. Curr Opinion Immunol 5:35.

Rötzschke O, Falk K (1994): Origin, structure and motifs of naturally processed MHC class II ligands. Curr Opinion Immunol 6:45.

REVIEW QUESTIONS

For each question, choose the ONE BEST answer or completion.

1. All the following are characteristics of both MHC class I and class II molecules *except*:
   A) they are expressed codominantly
   B) they are expressed constitutively on all nucleated cells
   C) they are glycosylated polypeptides with domain structure
   D) they are involved in presentation of antigen fragments to T cells
   E) they are expressed on the surface membrane of B cells

2. MHC class I molecules are important for which of the following:
   A) binding to CD8 molecules on T cells
   B) presenting exogenous antigen (e.g., bacterial protein) to B cells
   C) presenting viral protein to antigen-presenting cells such as macrophages
   D) binding to CD4 molecules on T cells
   E) binding to Ig on B cells

3. Which of the following is *incorrect* concerning MHC class II molecules?
   A) B cells may express six different MHC class II molecules on their surface
   B) they are synthesized in the endoplasmic reticulum of antigen-presenting cells

C) their expression can be induced on some cells by treating them with cytokines
D) they are associated with β_2-microglobulin on the cell surface
E) they control the level of response to a particular epitope

4. Certain HLA genes are linked to diseases such as ankylosing spondylitis. This linkage has all the following characteristics *except*:
   A) it is related primarily to the D and B loci
   B) it may be the result of closely linked genes
   C) it may be the result of cross-reactivity between self antigen and infectious agent
   D) it carries no increased risk for a specific disease for those individuals with the gene
   E) it may be the result of an MHC molecule serving as an attachment site for an infectious agent

5. Which of the following is *incorrect* concerning endosomal antigen processing of a bacterial protein?
   A) it results in production of potentially immunogenic peptides that associate with MHC class II molecules
   B) it may lead to the activation of $CD4^+$ T cells
   C) it may result in the formation of peptide–MHC class II complexes but not lead to T-cell activation
   D) it may lead to the activation of $CD8^+$ T cells

ANSWERS TO REVIEW QUESTIONS

1. ***B*** MHC class I molecules are expressed on all nucleated cells, but the constitutive expression of MHC class II molecules is more limited (B cells, dendritic cells, and thymic epithelial cells). MHC class II expression can be induced on other cell types (such as macrophages, endothelial cells, and human T cells) by cytokines.

2. ***A*** As described in Chapters 9 and 10, the interaction of CD8 on the T cell and an invariant region of MHC class I molecule is crucial in the triggering of CD8$^+$ T cells.

3. ***D*** The MHC class I molecule associates with β_2-microglobulin. MHC class II molecules at the cell surface are heterodimers of an α and a β chain.

4. ***D*** Individuals who carry specific HLA genes *are* at increased risk of developing autoimmune diseases. For example, HLA-B27-expressing individuals are over 80 times likely to develop ankylosing spondylitis as individuals who are not HLA-B27-positive.

5. ***D*** CD8$^+$ T cells are generally not activated by peptides generated in endosomes. Endosomal processing of exogenous antigens in acid compartments within the cell results in the selective association of peptides with MHC class II molecules, rather than MHC class I molecules. Peptide–MHC class II complexes are recognized by a CD4$^+$ T cell with the appropriate receptor. Recognition of these complexes, however, does not guarantee T-cell activation.

ACTIVATION OF T AND B CELLS BY ANTIGEN

INTRODUCTION

The interaction of antigen with antigen-specific receptors on T and B cells initiates a cascade of events that results in the proliferation and differentiation of both sets of cells. The intracellular events that follow activation of the antigen-specific receptor by antigen are very similar in both B and T cells following receptor triggering at the cell surface. As a result of antigenic stimulation, both B and T cells differentiate into *effector cells,* and a small fraction of both populations becomes *memory cells.*

As we have described in Chapters 8–10, however, antigen recognition by B and T cells is distinct and the consequences of B- and T-cell activation (i.e., their effector functions) are different. In the case of B cells, antigen-driven differentiation results in antibody production, and to the generation of antibody of distinct isotypes. In contrast, antigen-driven T-cell activation leads to the generation of subsets of cells that may produce cytokines or alternatively act as cytotoxic T cells.

In this chapter we will describe in more detail how T and B cells are activated, emphasizing the mutual interaction of T and B cells in the immune response, and pointing out both the similarities and the differences between T- and B-cell activation.

ACTIVATION OF CD4⁺ T CELLS

Specialized Cells Present Antigen to T Cells

Antigen can enter the body via several different routes; for example, through the skin, via the airways or by injection. Specialized *antigen-presenting cells (APC)* are found at all these distinct antigen entry sites as well as in lymphoid organs. The function of these APC is to take up antigen, process it, and present it to T cells; in particular, to present antigen to CD4$^+$ T cells that play a central role in responses to protein antigens.

Bone marrow-derived APC of the myeloid type, and *dendritic cells* in particular, are extremely efficient at initiating *primary responses,* i.e., of *unprimed* or *naive T cells,* due to their constitutive and high level of expression of MHC class II molecules, as well as costimulatory and adhesion molecules. [These peripheral dendritic cells, depicted in Figure 2.1, are in the same family of cells as the interdigitating dendritic cells of the thymus which play such a crucial role in thymic selection (Chapter 9).] Once lymphocytes have interacted with antigen they are said to be *primed*. Subsequent responses of primed lymphocytes are referred to as *secondary* or *memory responses*. B cells can also act as very efficient APC, especially in responses in which both CD4$^+$ T cells and B cells have already been primed by antigen. B cells are not likely to have a central role as APC in primary T-cell responses, since T cells in humans with B-cell deficiencies and animals lacking B cells can be primed by antigens. The role of the B cell as antigen-presenting cell is discussed further in the section on T–B interactions below.

In general, induction of T-cell responses occurs in the secondary lymphoid organs, especially lymph nodes. For example, antigen that enters via the skin is taken up by specialized skin APC known as *Langerhans cells* (which belong to the macrophage/dendritic cell family of cells), and these antigen-bearing cells circulate via the lymph to lymph nodes draining the skin area. In the nodes, antigen-bearing cells interact with specific T cells that have entered the node via high endothelial venules. As we have described in Chapters 2 and 9, the ability of T cells to leave the circulation and enter the node is dependent on "homing" interactions between adhesion molecules on the surface of T cells and endothelial cells. T cells are retained in the so-called T-cell area of the node. Here, the antigen-bearing APC can interact with antigen-specific T cells, to initiate the cascade of events outlined below. The interaction of primed T cells and B cells takes place in specialized areas of the node, the follicles, and the production of antibody in distinct areas known as germinal centers, as discussed in Chapters 6 and 8.

MHC Class II Plus Peptide Engages the Antigen-Specific TcR

As described in Chapter 10, the variable regions, Vα and Vβ, of the antigen-specific receptor (TcR) on a CD4$^+$ T cell expressing the appropriate receptor interacts with the complex formed by the immunogenic peptide bound in the cleft of an MHC class II molecule. This recognition of peptide–MHC complex on the surface of the APC by the T cell's TcR is crucial in initiating the series of events that results in T cell activation. Interaction between the peptide–MHC complex on the APC and the TcR on the T cell is necessary, however, but generally not sufficient by itself to lead to T-cell activation. In part, this may be due to the low affinity of the interaction between the TcR and peptide–MHC complex. For this reason other cell interaction molecules are needed for cell activation to occur, as described below and illustrated in Figure 11.1.

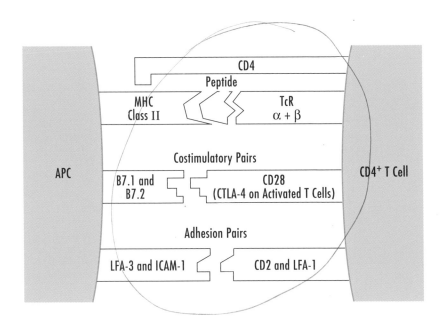

Figure 11.1

Cell surface molecules involved in T-cell activation.

Function of Coreceptor and Other Adhesion Molecules

The affinity of TcR and MHC–peptide interaction is increased by the binding of the accessory or coreceptor molecule, CD4, on the T cell to an invariant or non-polymorphic region of the MHC class II molecule (Fig 11.1). In this way, CD4 enhances the binding of cells expressing MHC class II molecules to $CD4^+$ cells, and thus functions as an adhesion molecule for APC–T-cell interactions. As we shall discuss below, when the APC and T cell interact, the CD4 molecule also acts as a signal transduction molecule, sending signals into the T cell. Thus, this interaction of CD4 and MHC class II also constributes to antigen-specific activation.

Molecules with similar coreceptor function are also found associated with the antigen receptor of $CD8^+$ T cells. The cell surface molecule CD8 plays a similar dual role as a coreceptor on the set of T cells expressing CD8; that is, CD8 enhances the binding of $CD8^+$ T cells to MHC class I expressing cells, and also acts as a signal transduction molecule. On B cells, the molecules CD19, CD20, and CD21 have been suggested to play a similar coreceptor role for the B cell antigen receptor, immunoglobulin.

In addition to the coreceptor molecules, other pairs of adhesion molecules, such as CD2 and LFA-1 on T cells, which bind to LFA-3 and ICAM-1, respectively, on the APC, further enhance T-cell–APC interactions. Thus, by a combination of antigen-specific and nonspecific interactions, antigen-specific receptors are engaged with sufficient avidity to initiate T-cell activation.

Nature of Costimulatory Signals

Binding of the T cell's TcR to the peptide–MHC complex on the APC constitutes what is referred to as the first signal for activation of T cells. Additional signals, known as *costimulatory* or *second signals*, are required to complete the process of T-cell activation (Fig. 11.1). Costimulatory interactions are believed to be vital in activating unprimed, resting T cells but are probably less important for the activation of primed or memory T cells.

Currently, the best understood of the costimulatory molecules is the B7 family of molecules [B7.1 (CD80) and B7.2 (CD86)] on the surface of the APC, which interacts with molecules known as CD28 and CTLA-4 on the T-cell surface. Interaction of the B7–CD28 costimulatory pair, in conjunction with the signal transmitted through the TcR, is crucial for production of the cytokine interleukin 2 (IL-2) by naive T cells. In the absence of the costimulatory signal, little or no IL-2 is produced. As we shall describe subsequently, CTLA-4 is induced after T-cell activation. The interaction of CTLA-4 with B7 molecules is believed to constitute a signal that turns off the synthesis of IL-2.

As we have described in Chapter 10, many cells can express MHC class II molecules. It appears, however, that not all cells that express MHC class II molecules express costimulatory molecules and hence not all MHC class II⁺ cells are effective APC; for example, dendritic cells constitutively express the costimulatory molecule B7, whereas resting B cells do not. This pattern of costimulator expression correlates with their relative effectiveness as APC. When B cells are activated, however, cell-surface B7 expression is induced and thus activated B cells function effectively as presenting cells.

Intracellular Events in Lymphocyte Activation

COMMON FEATURES OF T- AND B-CELL ACTIVATION. The earliest studies of T- and B-lymphocyte cell activation showed that stimulating resting cells with antigen, or with polyclonal activators (described later in the chapter), resulted within hours in increased cell size (T- or B-cell *"blasts"*), followed hours or days later by the proliferation and differentiation of the cell. More recent work has focused on identifying the sequence of events starting with the initiating antigenic signal at the surface of B and T cell and results in changes in the nucleus of the cell.

A complex and as yet incomplete picture has emerged. In brief, after antigen binds to the antigen receptor, a series of defined events occurs over a period of several hours. The earliest events (within seconds) are the phosphorylation of certain cellular proteins, especially proteins associated with the receptor (CD3 and ζ in the T cell and Ig α and β in the B cell), and the breakdown of membrane phospholipids. As a result of these phosphorylations, a cascade of protein activation occurs in a regulated sequence. Membrane phospholipids are broken down, and intracellular calcium levels rise. Within a few minutes, transcription factors are activated to enter the nucleus of the cell, and the transcription of formerly nontranscribed genes occurs. In T cells, some of the important genes activated include cytokines and cytokine receptors, whereas B cells will start to transcribe immunoglobulin genes. After about 48 hours, DNA is synthesized and the cells undergo division.

INTRACELLULAR EVENTS IN T-CELL ACTIVATION. Evidence suggests that after the peptide–MHC complex binds to the extracellular variable regions Vα and Vβ of the surface TcR, a change occurs in the TcR molecule that is transmitted via the tightly associated CD3 and ζ molecules into the interior of the cell. (It is thought that the peptide–MHC complex "cross-links," i.e., brings together multiple molecules of the TcR in the membrane of the responding cell.) The cytoplasmic domains of the CD3 and ζ chains interact with two different families of phosphotyrosine kinases, enzymes that phosphorylate their protein substrates on tyrosine residues inside the cell. Thus, one of the first intracellular events after antigen binding is the phosphorylation of the cytoplasmic tails of CD3 and ζ chains by a kinase. This phosphorylation results in the attachment of a T cell-specific kinase, ZAP-70, to the complex of proteins at the T-cell surface. ZAP-70 also phosphorylates chains of the TcR complex. As we mentioned previously, the coreceptor molecule CD4 enhances binding of the T cell to the APC by binding to the MHC class II molecule on the APC. Because CD4 is also linked inside the cell to a kinase known as lck, the triggering of the TcR results in phosphorylation by lck as well as the other phosphorylases. In this way, CD4 acts as a signal transduction molecule. It is also worth noting that at least one cell membrane phosphatase, CD45, is involved in the regulation of the phosphorylating enzymes that are activated as a consequence of T-cell triggering. This molecule appears to have an important role in T-cell activation, since cells lacking CD45 show defective responses to antigen.

All these phosphorylation events result in the activation of intracellular proteins. One of the major cellular proteins activated in the sequence of phosphorylations is phospholipase C, which is involved in the breakdown of membrane phospholipids, as well as generating increased intracellular calcium levels. This, in turn, leads to the activation of other proteins, including molecules known as protein kinase C, calcineurin, and Ras. As a consequence, different transcription factors are activated that move to the nucleus of the cell and activate gene transcription by binding to the control sites of specific genes. One important example is the transcription factor known as NF-AT, which enters the nucleus, binds to control sites on the IL-2 gene, and thus activates IL-2 gene transcription. At later times, genes for cytokine receptors are transcribed into mRNA and translated into protein. In particular, T-cell activation results in the transcription of one chain of the IL-2 receptor, IL-2Rα. Within 24 hours the cell enlarges and IL-2 protein is secreted from the cell. The IL-2 can then bind to its receptor on the same or different T cell and the cell proliferates (Fig. 11.2).

As we have pointed out previously, little, if any, IL-2 is made by an unprimed T cell in the absence of an interaction between the costimulatory pair B7 on the APC and CD28 on the T-cell surface. Thus, CD28 also transduces signals into the T cell, which result in increased IL-2 production. As described in Chapter 9, CTLA-4, a surface molecule which is closely related to CD28, is induced by T-cell activation. This molecule also interacts with the costimulatory ligands B7.1 and B7.2 on the APC. It is believed, however, that the interaction between CTLA-

4 and B7 is a negative, rather than a positive, signal to the T cell. It appears to turn off the production of IL-2, limiting the extent of the immune response, and leading to the differentiation of T cells into memory cells. T-cell activation also results in the expression of CD40L, which as we shall describe below, plays an important role in T cell-mediated isotype switching in B cells.

In addition to the events described, activated T cells stop expressing the "homing" receptor L-Selectin (CD62L), which allowed resting T cells to enter the node (see Chapter 9). Consequently, activated T cells can leave the node and move to sites of infection in the body where antigen is present. Trafficking of the activated T cell is also enhanced by induction of expression of the cell surface molecule, VLA-4 (CD49d), which binds to molecules on the surface of endothelial cells in an infected tissue. In this way, the activated T cell changes its pattern of circulation so that it can migrate to and be effective in an area away from the node in which it was activated (also see Chapter 9).

Cytokine Production

Activation of T and B cells by antigen results in completely different effector functions. B-cell activation results in the release of the antigen-specific receptor, Ig, which binds to free antigen. T-cell activation, on the other hand, does not result in the release of the antigen-specific receptor: it results in the secretion of a number of antigen-nonspecific soluble factors known as *cytokines.*

Every cytokine has a specific cell surface receptor, expressed on a variety of different cell types. Thus, the cytokines released as the result of primed CD4$^+$ T-cell activation affect the function of multiple cell types. Some of the cytokines produced, such as IL-2 and IL-4, have profound effects on the proliferation and differentiation of T cells, as well as other cells, such as B cells. Other cytokines produced in the response influence the activation and growth of different cell types, including macrophages and bone marrow precursor cells.

A summary of the most important properties of different cytokines and their receptors is included at the end of this chapter.

Subsets of CD4$^+$ T Cells

The predominant cytokine synthesized after the activation of naive or unprimed CD4$^+$ T cells is IL-2. Further stimulation of primed CD4$^+$ T cells results in the synthesis and secretion of a vast array of cytokines. Studies in the mouse indicate that CD4$^+$ T cells can be divided into subsets based on the different cytokines they produce. In the human, the existence of nonoverlapping subsets of T cells, i.e., synthesizing completely distinct cytokines, is less clear but is gaining acceptance.

One CD4$^+$ subset, known as Th1, synthesizes IL-2 and interferon γ (IFN-γ), but not IL-4 or IL-5. Antigenic stimulation of naive CD4$^+$ T cells in the presence of IL-12 and IFN-γ is thought to drive T cells toward the Th1 subset. The IL-12 and IFN-γ that drive this T-cell differentiation step are most likely derived from viral or bacterial stimulation of natural-killer (NK) cells and macrophages.

A second subset of CD4$^+$ T cells, Th2, synthesizes IL-4 and IL-5, but not IL-2 or IFN-γ. Th2 cells develop if antigenic stimulation occurs in the presence of IL-4. Mast cells may be the source of this IL-4 in the early phases of an immune response, before T cells are activated. Both Th1 and Th2 sets synthesize several cytokines in common, including IL-3 and granulocyte-macrophage colony stimulating factor (GM-CSF). In addition to Th1 and Th2, a third set of T cells, Th0, has been described that can make IL-2, IFN-γ, and IL-4. Th0 may be the precursors of both Th1 and Th2 subsets.

Since different cytokines affect distinct target cells, the result of activating Th1 rather than Th2 cells, or vice versa, is to activate different types of immune responses. *Thus, Th1 cells produce IL-2 and IFN-γ, which activate CD8$^+$ T cells, NK cells, and macrophages, whereas Th2 cells secrete IL-4 and IL-5, which activate B cells and switch antibody synthesis to IgE.* This functional dichotomy in cytokine production may have some clinical relevance in humans. Disease conditions have been described in which there is a preponderance of the Th1 cytokines, IL-2 and IFN-γ. These diseases include the responses to most viruses, and in delayed-type hypersensitivity, described in Chapter 16. In contrast, in allergy and as a consequence of parasitic infection, "Th2 cytokines" such as IL-4 predominate. It has also been suggested that the onset of AIDS is accompanied by a bias toward Th2 cytokine production.

It is also noteworthy that cytokines produced by one subset of CD4$^+$ cells can inhibit the function of the other subset, reinforcing the functional differentiation of Th1 and Th2 subsets. Thus, IFN-γ produced by Th1 cells inhibits the generation of Th2 cells, and IL-10 produced by Th2 cells inhibits the generation of Th1 type cells. Interestingly, pathogens have evolved to take advantage of this: Epstein–Barr virus (EBV) synthesizes a protein with strong homology to IL-10. It is thought that the viral protein acts like IL-10, namely, to inhibit the generation of Th1 cells. Since the host uses Th1 cytokines IFN-γ and IL-2 to activate antiviral responses, this strategy allows the pathogen to subvert a key element of the immune response directed against it.

T–B CELL COOPERATION IN ANTIBODY PRODUCTION

It has long been recognized that one of the key functions of CD4⁺ T cells is to co-operate with B cells in the production of antibody to the major class of antigens referred to as **thymus-dependent (TD).** For this reason, the set of CD4⁺ T cells which participates in antibody production is referred to as **helper T cells**. The production of antibody to a thymus-dependent antigen requires that both B *and* T cells be activated and interact.

We described earlier in the chapter the events which occur as a consequence of the activation of CD4⁺ T cells by antigen bound to APC: in addition to the induction of cell surface molecules such as adhesion molecules, CD40 ligand (CD40L), and CTLA-4, the CD4⁺ T cell proliferates and secretes cytokines. Many of the cytokines secreted by the activated T cell also activate B cells.

To activate the B cell, an antigen-specific B cell with the appropriate receptor must also bind antigen via its receptor, namely, surface immunoglobulin. For T–B cooperation to occur, the B and T cells respond to epitopes which are physically linked in the same antigen. The B and T cells may respond to different epitopes on that antigen, but these epitopes must be physically linked in order to produce antibody. Thus, the phenomenon of T–B cell cooperativity is also known as **linked recognition.** This is shown in Figure 11.2. As a consequence of direct antigen binding and the effects of T cell-secreted cytokines, the B cell is activated to proliferate and then differentiates to produce antibody. The nature of the cytokine secreted by the T cell determines which immunoglobulin isotype the B cell switches to. The importance of T-cell involvement in B cell antibody production can be gauged from findings with antigens which do not use T-cell help, so-called T-independent (TI) antigens, discussed later in the chapter. These TI antigens do not induce memory B cells and B cells cannot switch from IgM isotype.

In the primary response, T-cell activation results predominantly in IL-2 synthesis, which appears to be necessary for B-cell activation and proliferation. This results in B-cell secretion of IgM. In secondary responses, IgG, IgA, and IgE antibodies are produced as a consequence of the phenomenon known as **class** or **isotype switch.**

As we have described earlier in the chapter, in the primary response T cells are most effectively activated by antigen processed and presented by dendritic cells or other so-called "professional" antigen-presenting cells, such as macrophages. To produce antibody in this response, it is unlikely that all three types of cells (T, B, and professional APC) are present at the same time and in the same location, as shown in Figure 11.2. It is more likely that activation of T cells by APC may occur first and that the released cytokines subsequently trigger an

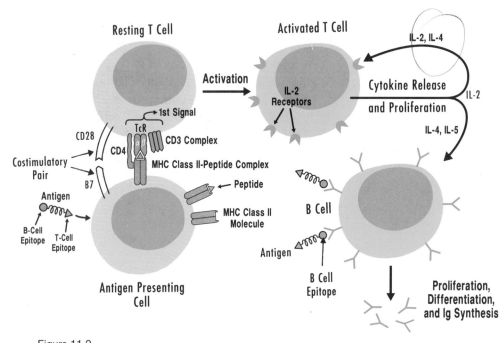

Figure 11.2

The interaction between an antigen-presenting T cell and B cell leading to T- and B-cell activation in a primary response.

antigen-activated B cell, which may not be in direct contact with the T cell, but in close proximity to it.

In secondary responses, both the relevant B and T cells have been previously activated and expanded by antigen, and in contrast to primary responses, very efficient T–B cooperation is thought to be achieved between B and T cells *only*, with no requirement for a dendritic cell or macrophage. This is depicted in Figure 11.3. In this response, the B cell captures antigen by binding it to its specific immunoglobulin receptors. Following antigen binding at the B-cell surface, the complex of antigen and immunoglobulin is taken into the cell (internalized) and then degraded in acid compartments which also contain MHC class II molecules. Some of the peptides formed by the degradation of antigen bind to MHC class II molecules and return to the B-cell surface where the combination of peptide plus MHC class II molecule is presented to a CD4$^+$ T cell with the appropriate TcR.

Antigen presentation by the B cell is accompanied by paired interactions at the surface of the B and T cells and cytokine secretion by T cells. The most important of these interactions are shown in Figure 11.3. These include the interac-

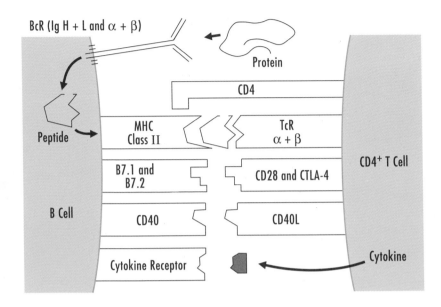

BcR (Ig H + L and α + β)

Protein

CD4

MHC Class II

TcR α + β

Peptide

B7.1 and B7.2

CD28 and CTLA-4

CD4+ T Cell

B Cell

CD40

CD40L

Cytokine Receptor

Cytokine

Figure 11.3
T- and B-cell interactions.

tion of B7 costimulatory molecules, induced on the B-cell surface by activation, with CD28 on the T cell. Induction of B7 expression enhances the ability of the B cell to act as an effective antigen-presenting cell to T cells. (As described earlier in the chapter, interaction of B7 with the homologous molecule CTLA-4 is believed to signal to the T cell to shut off the synthesis of IL-2.) Paired adhesion molecules such as LFA-1 with ICAM-1, shown in Figure 11.1, also contribute to strengthening the T–B interaction. A further key interaction is between CD40 on the B cell and its ligand CD40L on the activated T cell. This interaction promotes B-cell proliferation and is required for the B cell to switch the class of antibody that it can synthesize. In the absence of this CD40–CD40L interaction, only IgM is made. This is demonstrated in humans with nonfunctional CD40L, a clinical condition known as hyper-IgM syndrome, and in so-called "CD40L knockout mice." IgM antibody, but no other isotype, is made at normal levels in these two examples.

In addition to the CD40–CD40L interaction, class switching by the B cell in the secondary response also requires T cell-derived cytokines. The nature of the cytokine produced by the primed T cell determines which class of antibody is produced by the B cell. Thus, if the T cell makes IL-4, the B cell will switch to producing predominantly IgE, whereas if the T cell produces IFN-γ, the B cell will switch to producing IgG subtypes. This is of great biological importance because certain antigens such as parasites and allergens induce T-cell production of

IL-4 and hence B-cell production of IgE. In contrast, viruses generally induce T-cell synthesis of IFN-γ and thus IgG synthesis by B cells.

As the foregoing paragraphs demonstrate, the interaction of B and T cells in a secondary or primed response results in T-cell activation leading to cytokine synthesis, as well as B-cell activation which results in proliferation and antibody secretion.

The Carrier Effect

One final point should be made about B and T cell epitope recognition in primary and secondary responses. To achieve linked recognition, it is important that the B cell epitope and the T cell epitope be the same in both primary and secondary responses. If primary immunization is given with a B cell epitope linked to one T cell epitope, but the secondary immunization is given with the same B cell epitope linked to a different T cell epitope, no secondary response is generated. This is because the second immunization does not prime a sufficient number of T cells specific for the "new" T cell epitope to allow effective cooperation with B cells specific for the B cell epitope. This phenomenon was originally observed in the secondary response to *haptens,* a set of small molecules which by themselves cannot induce immune responses (described in Chapter 3). Secondary antibody responses to a hapten could be generated only if the hapten were linked to the same large protein or *carrier* in both primary and secondary immunizations. For this reason, the phenomenon is known as the *carrier effect.* The carrier effect has present application in the immunization of individuals with peptide vaccines. In such vaccinations, it is crucial to use the peptide linked to the same carrier in both and primary and secondary immunizations.

B-CELL ACTIVATION

Intracellular Pathways in B-Cell Activation Through Surface Immunoglobulin

Earlier in the chapter, we described the series of events that occurs inside the cell as a consequence of the activation of the T-cell receptor at the T-cell surface. A very similar activation cascade appears to occur in B cells after triggering the B-cell antigen-specific receptor, immunoglobulin. When antigen binds to the V_H and V_L regions of the four-chain Ig molecule at the cell surface, a signal is transmitted into the cell through the tightly associated Ig α and β. The antigen also induces receptor cross-linking, thus bringing together more than one Ig receptor molecule in the cell membrane. The short intracellular regions of the Ig molecule are not believed to play a role in signal transduction. Thus, Ig α and β play the same role in signal transduction for the B-cell receptor as CD3 plays for the T-cell receptor.

Ig α and β are associated with a phosphotyrosine kinase, syk, which is found almost exclusively in B cells. (B cells do not appear to express the T cell-specific kinase ZAP70, which is important in T-cell activation.) Phosphorylation of substrates inside the cell by syk and other kinases results in phospholipase C activation, leading to phospholipid breakdown and elevations in intracellular calcium. The B-cell surface molecules CD19, CD20, and CD21, discussed in Chapter 8, also play a role in signaling after antigen binding, by enhancing the signal transmitted through Ig. CD45, a surface phosphatase, is also associated with the Ig molecule of B cells and is believed to regulate the activity of B-cell phosphokinases. As was described previously, CD45 also associates with the TcR in T cells and plays a similar role in regulating T-cell activation.

As a result of this sequence of early activation events, transcription factors such as NF-AT and NF-κB enter the nucleus of the B cell and promote the transcription of specific genes, the most important of which are immunoglobulin and cyokine receptor genes. Around 12 hours after antigenic stimulation, the B cell increases in size (becoming a *B-cell blast*) and if it receives the appropriate signals, generally from T helper cells, the B-cell blast proliferates and differentiates into a cell that synthesizes and secretes immunoglobulin *(a plasma cell)*.

ACTIVATION OF CD8⁺ CYTOTOXIC T CELLS

In the sections above we have described the function of one of the major sets of T cells, CD4⁺ T cells, which produce a plethora of cytokines and thus interact with a vast array of cells. We now turn our attention to the other major population of T cells, CD8⁺ T cells. The major function of CD8⁺ T cells is to kill cells which have been infected by pathogens, such as bacteria and viruses. For this reason, CD8⁺ T cells are frequently referred to as "T killer" or "cytotoxic T cells" (Tc). CD8⁺ T cells are also involved in killing transplanted foreign cells during graft rejection ("allo-specific" cytotoxic cells; see Chapter 20). CD8⁺ T cells also synthesize cytokines, but a more limited spectrum than CD4⁺ T cells. CD8⁺ T cells can produce IFN-γ, which regulates certain viral and bacterial infections, as well as TNF-β, which as we shall describe below, plays a role in target cell killing.

We have also previously described how the TcR of a CD4⁺ T cell recognizes the combination of an MHC class II molecule with peptide bound in its groove. In contrast, the TcR of a CD8⁺ T cell recognizes a combination of peptide in association with an MHC class I molecule on the surface of an APC or target cell. These two statements form the core of ***MHC restriction of T-cell responses*** that we referred to in Chapters 9 and 10. ***Recognition of a peptide–MHC class I complex by the TcR of a CD8⁺ T cell results in activation of the CD8⁺ cell, leading to the killing of the APC or target cell presenting the foreign peptide.***

The sequence of events involved in the activation of a virus-specific CD8⁺ T cell and killing of an infected target cell is depicted in Figure 11.4. The precise steps involved in the activation of CD8⁺ T cells are not completely worked out. A key requirement, however, is that a CD8⁺ T cell bearing an appropriate TcR must interact with the target cell expressing an MHC class I molecule bound to a peptide derived from the infecting virus. [Viral proteins are synthesized in the cytoplasm of the infected cell. Peptides derived from the virus interact with MHC class I molecules in the endoplasmic reticulum (ER), as described in Chapter 10.]

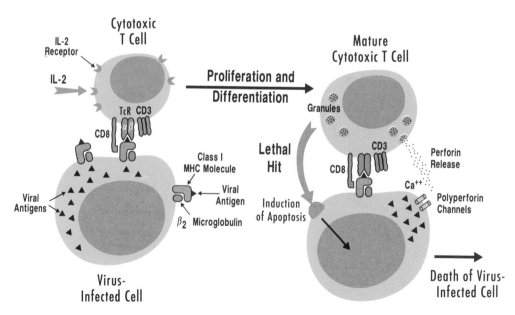

Figure 11.4

Recognition and killing by CD8⁺ cytotoxic T cells.

Activation also requires IL-2 to interact with IL-2 receptors expressed on the the CD8$^+$ T cell, allowing the cells to proliferate and differentiate. Other cytokines may also be required for cytotoxic T-cell activation.

It is currently not clear if IL-2 required for these activatory events is generated by the CD8$^+$ T cell itself, or alternatively must be supplied by antigen-activated CD4$^+$ T cells. In this latter pathway, viruses taken up by APC such as macrophages or B cells can initially activate CD4$^+$ helper T cells via viral peptides presented in association with MHC class II molecules. Activation of the CD4$^+$ T cell results in IL-2 synthesis, which in turn activates the CD8$^+$ T cell. Once activated, this CD8$^+$ T cell kills infected cells expressing viral peptides associated with MHC class I molecules. Thus, when IL-2 is provided by the activation of CD4$^+$ T cells, the viral epitope which activates the CD4$^+$ T cells need not be the same as the viral epitope on the surface of the infected cell which is recognized by CD8$^+$ T cells. The responses to some viruses at least appear dependent on IL-2 production by CD4$^+$ T cells, while the responses to other viruses do not appear to require such help from CD4$^+$ cells.

Killing of Target Cells by Cytotoxic T Cells

As shown in Figure 11.4, the activated Tc initiates killing by attaching to the target cell via its TcR, as well as adhesion molecules, described in Chapters 9 and 10, to enhance binding to the target. Killing by cytotoxic T cells appears to occur by two major pathways. The first pathway involves the action of cytotoxic substances in the granules of T cells, which produce lesions in the membranes of target cells, similar to those produced by the attack complex of complement (see Chapter 13). After attaching to the target cell, the killer cell mobilizes its granules directionally toward the target, and finally by exocytosis releases the contents of these granules onto the target cell (Fig. 11.4). One of the major constituents of these granules is the monomeric form of a species of molecules called *perforins.* In the presence of Ca^{2+} they bind to the target–cell membrane and polymerize to form ring-like transmembrane channels similar to the action of C9. The resulting increase in permeability of the cell membrane leads to eventual cell death. This mode of cell killing is not only common to cytotoxic T cells and complement but may also be used by other granulated cells such as natural killers (NK), as described in Chapter 2. Cells that function in antibody-dependent cellular cytotoxicity (ADCC) mediated by Fc receptor binding to IgG-coated target cells probably also use the same mechanism (discussed in Chapters 7 and 22). As described above, the CD8$^+$ T cell may also release the cytokine TNF-β, which has cytotoxic properties.

The second major pathway of target cell killing shown in Figure 11.4 is the induction of ***apoptosis,*** or ***programmed cell death,*** as described in Chapter 9. In this pathway, the interaction of the killer and target induces gene expression in the target which results in the death of the target. In a sense, the target cell is induced to commit suicide. Since death by apoptosis does not result in the release of the cell's contents, killing by this pathway may prevent the spread of infectious virus into other cells. The cytotoxic T cell may then detach from the target cell to attack additional target cells while the cell that was first attacked dies.

Activation of $CD8^+$ T cells and killing of the target cell are separable events. This can be demonstrated by preparing cytotoxic T cells from an individual who has been infected with a virus. These virus-specific cytotoxic cells are able to kill virus-infected targets outside the body (shown on the right hand side of Fig. 11.4). In vitro killing of the infected target does not require the addition of any further factors. Killing can be measured in a four-hour assay by the release of ^{51}Chromium from radiolabeled target cells; target cells killed by the cytotoxic T cells release the radioactive label, whereas viable cells do not. This assay is routinely used to assess the generation of allo-specific killer T cells generated in transplantation responses (see Chapter 20).

It is worth repeating that ***the killing of a target cell by a virus-specific Tc occurs via the recognition of a specific combination of viral peptide associated with a particular MHC molecule.*** This means that a $CD8^+$ Tc specific for a flu virus peptide and isolated from an individual expressing HLA-A2 will kill a target cell that expresses HLA-A2 that has bound the flu-derived peptide. However, uninfected or normal cells from the same individual expressing HLA-A2 in the absence of the flu peptide are not killed. Furthermore, this virus-specific $CD8^+$ T cell will not kill targets expressing different combinations of peptides plus MHC molecules, such as a measles virus-derived peptide bound to HLA-A2 or even the same flu peptide bound to HLA-B3. These findings, by Rolf Zinkernagel and Peter Doherty, established the concept of ***MHC restriction of T-cell responses, indicating that T cells recognize the combination of antigen plus MHC molecule rather than antigen alone.***

It is also worth noting that the recognition of peptide–MHC class I by a $CD8^+$ T cell occurs irrespective of the expression of any MHC class II molecule on the APC or target cell. In other words, the target cell need not express *any* MHC class II molecule to be killed by a $CD8^+$ T cell. This is a finding of enormous biological importance; we have described previously how MHC class I molecules are expressed on almost every cell in the body. Now we can see the biological relevance of this ubiquitous MHC class I expression: since an infectious pathogen (such as a virus, parasite or bacterium) may infect *any* nucleated cell in the body, the pathogen will generate foreign peptides in its cytoplasmic or endo-plasmic reticulum compartment able to associate with MHC class I molecules. Expression of these foreign peptide–MHC class I complexes at the cell surface leads to recognition by CD8$^+$ T cells, followed by the killing of the infected cell. Thus, killing by CD8$^+$ T cells provides a mechanism to eliminate *any* cell in the body that becomes infected with a pathogen. Clearly, elimination of the pathogen does result in the destruction of host cells, but this is the bearable price the indi-vidual pays to remove the source of infection.

CD8$^+$ T cells almost invariably function as cytotoxic T cells in both mouse and human. In humans, however, a considerable proportion of CD4$^+$ T cells also display cytotoxic function. As might be expected from our foregoing discussion of MHC restriction, these cytotoxic human CD4$^+$ T cells are activated to kill by the recognition of peptide–MHC class II complexes on the APC or target cell. The mechanisms used by CD4$^+$ and CD8$^+$ to kill targets appear to be very similar.

It is also worth repeating that *only antigens that infect cells and generate peptides that reach the cell's cytoplasmic or ER compartment routinely evoke responses from CD8$^+$ T cells.* This set of antigens includes viruses, parasites, and some bacteria. For these organisms and viruses in particular, elimination of in-fected cells by CD8$^+$ T cells is of major importance. Not all antigens, however, give rise to responses involving CD8$^+$ T cells. "Harmless," noninfectious anti-gens, such as hen egg lysozyme, trigger only CD4$^+$ T cell and antibody responses, because these antigens are brought into the cell in acid compartments; if such antigens, however, are artificially introduced into the cytoplasm, they can gener-ate CD8$^+$ T-cell responses.

OTHER WAYS TO ACTIVATE UNPRIMED T CELLS

In the preceding sections, we focused on how peptide–MHC complexes on APC activate T cells via the latter's antigen-specific receptor, the TcR. Since T cells ex-pressing any one particular TcR are rare, approximately 1 in 10^4 T cells, only a small fraction of the total T-cell pool is activated by any one peptide–MHC com-plex. Detecting the response to antigen of those rare antigen-specific cells in the total population of 10^9 T cells has thus proved difficult. (The number of T cells re-sponding to a particular antigen can obviously be expanded, however, by priming and boosting in vivo followed by in vitro cloning. Ultimately, the T-cell popula-tion that emerges should respond exclusively to only one antigen plus MHC com-bination.)

Naive or unprimed T cells can be activated in a number of different ways, however, allowing us to measure the function of more than just a rare subpopulation of antigen-specific T cells. In general, the consequences of activation via these alternative pathways result in similar consequences, most notably cytokine production and cell proliferation. A few of these alternative ways of activating the population of unprimed T cells are described below.

Superantigens

Superantigens (SAg) are a class of antigen that activate T cells expressing a specific Vβ segment, such as Vβ3 or Vβ11, as a component of their TcR, irrespective of the Vα molecule used by the TcR. Since individual Vβ segments may be expressed in up to 10% of the T-cell population, a high percentage of T cells of various antigenic specificities may become activated by the interaction of superantigens with the T-cell population.

There are several unique aspects of SAg interactions with T cells. SAg bind more or less exclusively to the Vβ region of the TcR and not to the Vα region. SAg are presented by class II MHC molecules of APC, but are not bound in the peptide groove. They are not believed to be processed by APC. The intracellular pathways following SAg activation may also be different from those following peptide–MHC complex activation of the TcR.

More importantly, there are several clinically relevant features of SAg. The first is that several disease-causing organisms produce SAg. These include staphylococci, some of which are responsible for food poisoning and toxic shock, and viruses such as rabies. In the case of *Staphylococcus aureus*, the bacterial toxin acts as a superantigen, and activates a large percentage of T cells. It is believed that the massive release of cytokines following SAg action results in injury to the host.

Plant Proteins and Antibodies to T-Cell Surface Molecules

Several naturally occurring materials have the ability to trigger the proliferation and differentiation of many if not all clones of T lymphocytes. These substances are referred to as *polyclonal activators* or *mitogens,* because of their ability to induce mitosis of the cell population. The plant glycoproteins *concanavalin A (Con A)* and *phytohemagglutinin (PHA)* are particularly potent mitogens for T cells. These molecules are *lectins,* molecules that bind to carbohydrate moieties on proteins. Both Con A and PHA are thought to act through the TcR. Another plant lectin, *pokeweed mitogen,* activates both T and B cells. As we shall also describe later in the chapter, certain substances such as bacterially derived lipopolysaccharide are specifically mitogenic for mouse B cells.

Interestingly, certain antibodies specific for CD3 have the ability to activate T cells. Since CD3 is expressed on all T cells in association with the T-cell receptor, anti-CD3 thereby induces all T cells to proliferate.

It is also worth noting that other antibodies directed against certain molecules on the T-cell surface such as CD2 and CD28 may induce the cell to proliferate, either acting alone or in conjunction with other activation signals. Using antibodies in this way has led to the identification of a number of cell surface molecules that are important in T-cell activation.

T-INDEPENDENT RESPONSES: B-CELL ACTIVATION IN THE ABSENCE OF T-CELL HELP

Although the majority of antigens involved in immune responses are proteins that require help by T cells in order to provoke a response (i.e., they are *T-dependent antigens*), a few antigens are capable of activating B cells to produce antibody in the absence of T cells or cytokines produced by T cells. These antigens, referred to as *thymus-independent or TI antigens,* share a number of common properties, in particular, they (1) are *large polymeric molecules* with multiple, repeating, antigenic determinants, for example, polysaccharides and (2) frequently have some poorly defined *mitogenic properties;* at high concentrations they are able, in a nonspecific fashion, to activate B-cell clones to proliferate and to produce antibody. Such antigens are called *polyclonal activators.*

The combination of these properties is apparently sufficient to allow these TI antigens (such as *lipopolysaccharide, dextran,* and *ficoll*) to trigger B cells to proliferate and produce antibody. The polyclonal activation of B cells by TI antigens such as lipopolysaccharide, derived from the cell walls of gram-negative bacteria, may therefore be considered analogous to the activation of T-cell responses by mitogens such as Con A.

It appears that the B cell becomes activated as a consequence of the cross-linking of its surface receptors by the multivalent antigen, which results in the movement of these antigen-bound receptors into *"patches"* on the cell membrane that then move to one area of the cell surface *("capping")*. A second, mitogenic signal leads to differentiation and immunoglobulin secretion (Fig. 11.5).

There are two biologically relevant features of TI responses. First, unlike responses involving T-dependent antigens, responses to TI antigens generate primarily *IgM* and they *do not give rise to memory.* In other words, a second injection of a TI antigen leads to the same level of production of IgM as the first, with no increase in level, speed of onset, or class switch. This finding reinforces the importance of T cell-derived cytokines in the development of memory cells and

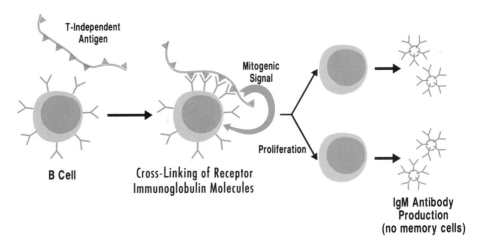

Figure 11.5

The induction of IgM antibody synthesis by a T-independent antigen.

B-cell isotype switch. Second, a protective immune response can still be made against TI antigens even if an individual lacks T cells. Thus, patients with T-cell immune deficiencies can still make protective IgM responses against extracellular bacteria, even if they cannot make significant responses to viruses which are T cell-dependent.

CYTOKINES

As we have described throughout the chapter, the activation of B and T cells requires several signals, some of which are provided by cell–cell contact, such as the interaction of CD40 with CD40 ligand, while others are provided by cytokines released by a variety of cells.

Although we have focused on the important role of T cells and CD4$^+$ T cells in particular in synthesizing cytokines, it is important to note that few cytokines are made exclusively by T cells; IL-2, for example, is considered to be synthesized exclusively by T cells, but IL-4 can be made by mast cells as well as Th2 CD4$^+$ T cells. Cytokines produced by one type of leukocyte and that affect other leukocytes are referred to as ***interleukins.***

Cytokines have several features in common. They are nonantigen-specific glycoproteins, which are generally synthesized and rapidly secreted in response to a stimulus; thus, they are usually not stored within the cell that makes them. Most cytokines have very short half-lives; consequently, cytokine synthesis production and function occurs in a burst.

Cytokines can act over both short and long range, with consequent systemic effects. ***Cytokines thus play a crucial role in the amplification of the immune response***, because the release of cytokines from just a few antigen-activated cells results in the activation of multiple different cell types, which are not necessarily located in the immediate area. This is apparent in a response such as delayed-type hypersensitivity, discussed in detail in Chapter 16, in which the activation of rare antigen-specific T cells is accompanied by the release of cytokines. As a consequence of cytokine effects, monocytes are recruited into the area in great numbers, dwarfing the originally antigen-activated T-cell population. It is also worth noting that the production of too high a level of cytokines by a powerful stimulus can trigger deleterious systemic effects: one example is the toxic-shock syndrome, which may result from staphylococcal enterotoxin stimulation of T cells using certain Vβ segments as their TcR. Similarly, macrophage release of high levels of TNF-α may also lead to septic shock.

One cell may make many different cytokines. Moreover, one cell may be the target of many cytokines, each binding to its own cell-surface receptor. Consequently, one cytokine may affect the action of another, which may lead to either an additive or an antagonistic effect on the target cell.

It is also common for cytokines to have overlapping functions; for example, both IL-6 and IL-1 induce fever and several other phenomena. This is known as the redundancy of cytokine function. Nonetheless, cytokines such as IL-1 and IL-6 that share functional characteristics also have properties that are unique. One reason for this functional overlap is now understood: ***several cytokines share at least one chain of a common multichain receptor***. For example, the cytokine IL-3, 5, and GM-CSF use a shared chain of the cell-surface receptor as a signal transduction molecule. Cytokines are a crucial link between cells of the immune system and other systems in the body; for example, IL-2 acts on T cells as well as on osteoclasts, the bone-forming cells. TGF-β similarly acts on many cells, including connective tissue fibroblasts, as well as T cells and B cells.

Cytokine Receptors

Understanding how cytokines affect their target cells has been the subject of a great deal of recent study. Clinically, knowledge about cytokine–cytokine receptor interactions may be useful in devising strategies to prevent the action of cytokines involved in inflammatory responses, such as rheumatoid arthritis, or in responses such as transplantation rejection.

It is now apparent that the *receptors for cytokines can be divided into several sets or families*. The *first set* includes the *receptor for IL-1*; these receptors contain the domain structure of the typical member of a member of the immunoglobulin superfamily. The *second set* is known as the *hematopoietin receptor family*. Some of the receptors in this set have multiple chains; for example, the IL-2 receptor (IL-2R) comprises three separate chains, IL-2Rα, β, and γ. This family of receptors also includes the IL-3Rα chain, IL-4R, IL-7R, and IL-13R. One very interesting feature of this family of receptors is that the IL-2Rγ chain, which is involved in signal transduction, is common to several members of the family (IL-2, 4, 7, 9, 13 receptors). Recently a defect in the common IL-2Rγ chain was been shown to cause a profound immune deficiency in boys: the activatory effects of multiple cytokines were inhibited by this defect.

The *third family of cytokine receptors* is known as the *TNF receptor family*. The members of this family include not only TNF but also the molecules CD40 and Fas, both of which play crucial roles in cell–cell surface interaction. The fourth family of receptors is known as the *chemokine receptor family*. *Chemokines* are low-molecular-weight proteins that play an important role in the inflammatory response by inducing leukocyte populations to migrate into areas of infection. The chemokines include molecules known as IL-8, MCP-1, RANTES, and MIP-1 α and β. Some of these chemokines specifically attract neutrophils or monocytes into infected tissue.

The list of cytokines continues to grow, the number of interleukins now reaching to IL-15. (Less is known about the more recently discovered interleukins, with higher numbers.) The major cytokines that play a role in the immune response and a brief description of their functions are listed in Table 11.1.

TABLE 11.1   Cytokines and Their Functions

Cytokine	Produced by	Major functions
Interleukin-1 (IL-1)	Monocytes, many other cell types	Produces fever, stimulates acute-phase protein synthesis, promotes proliferation of Th2 CD4$^+$ T cells
Interleukin-2 (IL-2)	Th0 and Th1 CD4$^+$ T cells	T-cell growth factor
Interleukin-3 (IL-3)	Primarily T cells	Growth factor for hematopoietic stem cells and mast cells
Interleukin-4 (IL-4)	Th2 CD4$^+$ T cells and mast cells	Growth factor for B cells and Th2 CD4$^+$ T cells; promotes IgE and IgG synthesis; inhibits Th1 CD4$^+$ T cells
Interleukin-5 (IL-5)	Th2 CD4$^+$ T cells	Stimulates B-cell growth and Ig secretion; growth and differentiation factor for eosinophils

TABLE 11.1 *Continued*

Cytokine	Produced by	Major functions
Interleukin-6 (IL-6)	T cells and many others	Induces acute-phase protein sythesis, T-cell activation, and IL-2 production; stimulates B-cell Ig production and hematopoietic progenitor cell growth
Interleukin-7 (IL-7)	Fibroblasts, endothelial and some T cells	Growth factor for pre-T and pre-B cells
Interleukin-8 (IL-8)	Many cell types	Chemotactic for neutrophils and granulocytes
Interleukin-9 (IL-9)	T cells	Mast-cell activation
Interleukin-10 (IL-10)	Th2 CD4$^+$ T cells and macrophages	Inhibits production of Th1 CD4$^+$ T cells and macrophage function
Interleukin-11 (IL-11)	Fibroblasts	Stimulates megakaryocyte (platelet precursor) growth
Interleukin-12 (IL-12)	B cells and macrophages	Activates NK cells and promotes generation of Th1 CD4$^+$ T cells
Interleukin-13 (IL-13)	T cells	Shares characteristics with IL4 such as Ig switch to IgE sythesis, but does not affect T cells; growth factor for human B cells
Interleukin-14 (IL-14)	T cells	Involved in the development of memory B cells
Interleukin-15 (IL-15)	T cells and epithelial cells	T-cell growth factor, similar to IL-2
Interferon-gamma (IFN-γ)	Th1 CD4$^+$ T cells	Activates NK cells, macrophages, and killer cells; inhibits Th2 CD4$^+$ T cells; induces expression of MHC class II on many cell types
Transforming growth factor β (TGF-β)	T cells and monocytes	Enhances production of IgA; inhibits activation of monocytes and T-cell subsets; active in fibroblast growth and wound healing
Tumor necrosis factors (TNF-α)	Monocytes	Involved in inflammatory responses; activates endothelial cells and other cells of immune and nonimmune systems; induces fever and septic shock
TNF-β (lymphotoxin)	T cells	Involved in inflammatory response; also plays a role in killing of target cells by CD8$^+$ T cells
Colony-stimulating factors	T cells and monocytes	Growth and differentiation of immature hematopoietic cells
Granulocyte-monocyte-stimulating factor (GM-CSF)		Promotes growth of granulocytes and macrophages; growth of dendritic cells in vitro
Granulocyte-stimulating factor (G-CSF)		Promotes granulocyte growth
Macrophage-stimulating factor (M-CSF)		Promotes macrophage growth

SUMMARY

1. In primary responses to thymus-dependent antigens, antigen is initially processed and presented by MHC class II$^+$ antigen-presenting cells, such as dendritic cells, to resting, unprimed CD4$^+$ T cells. This occurs in T-cell areas of secondary lymphoid organs, such as lymph nodes.

2. Binding of MHC class II plus peptide to the TcR of the CD4$^+$ T cell, in conjunction with the interaction of costimulatory and adhesion pairs of molecules on the surface of the APC and the T cell, leads to T-cell activation.

3. T-cell activation involves a cascade of events inside the cell after initiation at the cell surface. The earliest activation events include the phosphorylation of intracellular proteins, phospholipid breakdown, and increases in intracellular calcium. As a consequence of these early intracellular changes, changes occur in the nucleus of the T cell. This results in the transcription of specific genes in the nucleus. Among the important genes transcribed as a consequence of T-cell activation are genes coding for cytokines, such as IL-2, and cytokine receptors. Ultimately, the activation of these genes results in the proliferation and differentiation of the T cell.

4. As a consequence of activation by antigen, CD4$^+$ T cells secrete cytokines, soluble factors that affect T cells, B cells, and many other cell types. Subsets of CD4$^+$ T cells have been defined by the range of cytokines they produce. Th1 cells secrete IL-2 and IFN-γ, but not IL-4 or IL-5. Cytokines produced by Th1 cells activate other T cells, NK cells, and macrophages. In contrast, Th2 cells secrete IL-4 and IL-5, but not IL-2 or IFN-γ. Cytokines produced by Th2 cells predominantly affect B cells.

5. The generation of antibody in the response to T-dependent antigens (the vast majority of responses to proteins) requires antigen, CD4$^+$ T cells, and B cells. This T–B cell cooperation involves (a) interaction between pairs of molecules on the surface of the CD4$^+$ T cell and the B cell, resulting in mutual activation and (b) cytokine secretion by T cells. A further requirement for antibody to be generated by T–B cooperation is _linked recognition_: the antigenic epitope that the T cell responds to and the epitope that the B cell responds to must both be on the same molecule. T and B cells may, however, respond to different epitopes on the same antigen.

6. Class or isotype switching to IgG, IgA, or IgE requires the interaction of CD40 on the B cell with its ligand CD40L on the T cell. The cytokine produced by the T cell determines the isotype of antibody synthesized by the switched B cell.

7. **CD8⁺ T cells kill cells infected by microorganisms, such as bacteria or viruses. The TcR of a CD8⁺ T cell interacts with peptide derived from the pathogen bound to an MHC class I molecule on the surface of an infected cell. This interaction results in killing of the infected cell, as a result of (a) release of cytotoxic products contained in granules inside the T cell and (b) the induction of apoptosis in the infected cell.**

8. **Some antigens, such as polysaccharides that have many repeating, identical epitopes on each molecule, are capable of triggering B cells without significant help from T cells. These so-called T-independent responses involve predominantly the production of IgM and do not include the development of immunologic memory.**

9. **Certain substances stimulate multiple clones of T and B cells to proliferate. These substances are referred to as mitogens. Superantigens activate all T cells that use a specific Vβ segment to form its TcR. Plant lectins such as Con A and phytohemagglutinin activate all T cells by binding to cell-surface glycoproteins. Similarly, lipopolysaccharide from bacterial cell walls activates all mouse B cells. Some antibodies specific for molecules on the T- and B-cell surface are also mitogenic.**

10. **Cytokines are nonantigen-specific mediators secreted by many different cell types. Cytokines act via cell surface receptor to affect the function of cells of the immune system as well as other systems in the body.**

REFERENCES

Cambier JC, Pleiman CM, Clark MR (1994): Signal transduction by the B cell antigen receptor and its coreceptors. Annu Rev Immunol 12:457.

Clark EA, Ledbetter JA (1994): How B and T cells talk to each other. Nature 367:425.

Durie FH, Foy TM, Masters SR, Laman JD, Noelle RJ (1994): The role of CD40 in the regulation of humoral and cell mediated immunity. Immunol Today 15:406.

Kishimoto T, Taga T, Akira S (1994): Cytokine signal transduction. Cell 76:253.

Knight SC, Stagg AJ (1993): Antigen presenting cell types. Current Opinion Immunol 5:374.

Marrack P, Kappler JW (1994): Subversion of the immune response by pathogens. Cell 76:323.

Mosmann TR, Coffman RL (1989): Th1 and Th2 cells: different patterns of lymphokine secretion lead to different functional properties. Annu Rev Immunol 7:145.

Paul WE (1993): Infectious diseases and the immune system. Sci Am 269:91.

Paul WE, Seder RA (1994): Lymphocyte responses and cytokines. Cell 76:241.

Weiss A, Littman DR (1994): Signal transduction by lymphocyte antigen receptors. Cell 76:263.

For each question, choose the ONE BEST answer or completion.

1. The role of the antigen-presenting cell in the immune response is all of the following *except:*
   A) the limited digestion of polypeptide antigens
   B) to allow association of MHC gene products and peptides
   C) supplying second signals required to activate T cells
   D) enzymatic degradation of T-cell receptors
   E) presentation of peptide–MHC complexes to T cells with the appropriate receptor

2. Which of the following statements about interleukin 2 (IL-2) is *incorrect*?
   A) it is produced primarily by activated macrophages
   B) it is produced by CD4$^+$ T cells
   C) it can induce the proliferation of CD4$^+$ T cells
   D) it binds to a specific receptor on CD4$^+$ T cells
   E) it activates CD8$^+$ T cells in the presence of antigen

3. Which of the following is *not* produced by Th1 CD4$^+$ T cells?
   A) IL-2 receptor
   B) IL-2
   C) cytokines that induce macrophage activation
   D) IL-4
   E) cytokines that activate CD8$^+$ T cells

4. Which of the following is *incorrect* concerning cytokines?
   A) one cytokine may act on many different target cells
   B) each cytokine binds to a specific cell-surface receptor
   C) all cytokines are produced by T cells
   D) within T cells, activation of cytokine genes occurs within hours
   E) cytokine receptor expression may be regulated by the cytokine itself

5. T cell-derived cytokines
   A) are the antigen-specific products of T-cell activation
   B) are stored in the resting T cell and released on activation
   C) are MHC-restricted in their effects
   D) influence the class of antibodies produced by B cells

6. Which would you expect to activate cytotoxic CD8$^+$ T cells?
   A) a killed viral preparation that has retained its antigenic properties but cannot replicate
   B) an attenuated (altered) viral preparation that can still replicate within the host's cells
   C) a small protein such as chicken γ-globulin
   D) all of the above
   E) none of the above

7. Infection with vaccinia virus results in the priming of virus-specific CD8$^+$ T cells. If these vaccinia virus-specific CD8$^+$ T cells are subsequently removed from the individ-

ual, which of the following cells will they kill in vitro?

A) vaccinia-infected cells expressing MHC class II molecules from any individual
B) influenza-infected cells expressing the same MHC class I molecules as the individual
C) uninfected cells expressing the same MHC class I molecules as the individual
D) vaccinia-infected cells expressing the same MHC class I molecules as the individual
E) vaccinia-infected cells expressing the same MHC class II molecules as the individual

8. Bacterial lipopolysaccharide (LPS), a T-independent antigen, stimulates antibody production in mice. Which of the following is *incorrect*?

A) the antibody produced will be predominantly IgM
B) memory B cells will not be induced
C) IL-4 and IL-5 are required for the production of antibody during the response
D) The polymeric nature of the antigen cross-links B-cell surface receptors and leads to activation

Clinical problem: Great effort is now being directed at developing vaccines for a variety of diseases. In one study, it was found that antibody to a particular epitope on a protein of the pathogen's surface membrane was protective. The structure of this epitope was determined to be a peptide 10 amino acids in length. This peptide was synthesized and used to immunize individuals exposed to the pathogen. Disappointingly, no protection was seen. Can you suggest any reasons for this failure?

ANSWERS TO REVIEW QUESTIONS

1. *D* The antigen-presenting cell does not enzymatically degrade the T-cell receptor. The other statements are all features of the antigen-presenting cell.

2. *A* IL-2 is produced almost exclusively by activated T cells.

3. *D* IL-4 is produced not by the Th1 subset of $CD4^+$ cells but by the Th2 subset.

4. *C* Activated T cells synthesize cytokines,

some of which are lymphocyte-specific, but many other cells of the immune system can produce cytokines.

5. *D* T cell-derived cytokines play a key role in the phenomenon of isotype switching. They are neither antigen-specific nor MHC-restricted: the IL-4, for example, synthesized by every individual is identical, irrespective of the antigenic stimulus.

6. *C* A pathogen that can infect and live with-

in the host's cells would activate CD8+ T cells. This would be unlikely to occur in the case of the same organism in a noninfectious state or for a "harmless" exogenous antigen, such as chicken gamma globulin.

7. **D** The principle of MHC restriction indicates that the TcR of CD8+ T cells will recognize and respond to target cells that express specific peptide bound to self MHC class I molecules. Thus, vaccinia-primed CD8+ T cells will recognize and hence kill only vaccinia-infected targets that express self MHC class I.

8. **C** T-independent antigens, because they do not generate T cell-derived cytokines, do not produce IL-4 or IL-5. Thus, no isotype switching or memory cell induction occurs in the response to T-independent antigens.

Clinical problem: Several possibilities may be considered, such as size and complexity of the peptide, which are required for immunogenicity. The more likely failure, however, was that the response to the pathogen's membrane protein was almost certainly a thymus-dependent response. Therefore, immunization with the epitope seen by the B cells would not work unless epitopes seen by helper T cells were also present.

Attempts at producing synthetic vaccines are now directed toward incorporating the B cell-specific epitopes in carriers containing adequate helper T epitopes that will induce both help and memory responses. This would provide a better possibility for protection following exposure to the pathogen.

CONTROL MECHANISMS IN THE IMMUNE RESPONSE*

INTRODUCTION

An understanding of the immune response as a complete physiologic system requires, in addition to an understanding of the "on" signals described in previous chapters, some understanding of the "off" signals. Only with such a complete understanding of the system is it possible to approach such questions as

1. Why does the response to any particular antigen not continue to increase in magnitude until it takes over the whole immune apparatus?

2. Why is the development of an autoimmune response against antigens of our own tissues an exceptional rather than a commonplace event?

In a system as complex as one that produces an immune response, multiple levels of control exist. Conceptually, there are two major aspects to regulation of the immune response: one occurs in the *developmental pathways of immunocompetence;* the other concerns the regulation of the *response of mature lym-*

*Contributed by Karen Yamaga, University of Hawaii.

phocytes to antigen. These are discussed in the present chapter. Breakdown of control mechanisms may lead to autoimmunity and autoimmune disease, subjects that are discussed in Chapter 17.

TOLERANCE

Tolerance is the ***state of unresponsiveness to a particular antigenic epitope***. It occurs when the interaction of antigen with an antigen-specific lymphocyte results in ***inactivation*** (turn off), rather than activation (turn on). ***Only cells with antigen-specific receptors, that is, lymphocytes, can be tolerized*** and this state of tolerance can be achieved any time in the ontogeny of the cell, provided it expresses a receptor for the antigen.

As a consequence of inactivation by antigen, the lymphocyte may be ***deleted*** or, alternatively, become ***anergic*** (i.e., nonresponsive). In deletion, exposure to antigen results in the physical removal or elimination of cells by the process of ***apoptosis*** (programmed cell death) that we have referred to in previous chapters. In an anergic state, the inactivated cell is still physically present but unable to respond to a further antigenic stimulus.

As we described in Chapter 11, antigen-specific activation is a complex multistep process. The end result of this process is proliferation and differentiation. Interfering with one of the many steps in cellular activation can result in the cell being able to complete some but not all of its program. As a result the cell may be rendered anergic. It is also worth noting that anergy and deletion are not mutually exclusive. Cells that are initially anergized by exposure to antigen may be deleted at a later time.

In this section we will discuss how both immature and mature lymphocytes can be made tolerant to antigen.

Induction of Tolerance in Immature T and B Lymphocytes

As we have already discussed in Chapters 6 and 9, the unique process of rearranging V genes, insertion of D and J segments, and random assortment of two chains (H and L or α and β) are responsible for the generation of a huge number of possible specificities for B- and T-cell receptors. Since this enormous number of different possible specificities (10^7–10^8 by some estimates) must inevitably have some binding sites specific for some of the many self antigens present in any individual, the first problem to be confronted is the avoidance of immune reaction against self.

To address this problem, throughout the life of an individual both immature T and B cells appear to undergo a process of *negative selection,* in which cells with potential reactivity to self molecules are *functionally inactivated.* For the developing T cell, this occurs in the thymus, at a stage when the cell expresses both the T-cell receptor, $\alpha\beta$, as well as CD4 and CD8 (see Chapter 9). For the developing B cell the steps in negative selection are less well defined but presumably occur in the bone marrow. Evidence suggests that negative selection of B and T cells can result in both *deletion* and *functional inactivation* of self-reactive precursor cells.

It is also important to note that *if immature B and T cells are exposed to foreign antigens the result is inactivation rather than activation.* When this occurs, the developing immune system may be fooled into believing that the foreign antigen is a self antigen and thus become tolerant to the foreign antigen. One of the earliest experiments that demonstrated that the immune system could be tricked came from the observations of Owen in 1945 that *dizygotic cattle twins,* which shared common vascular supplies in utero, developed into erythrocyte *chimeras;* that is, each calf possessed a mixture of its own erythrocytes plus those of the twin with which an intrauterine vascular anastomosis existed.

The study of this accident of nature was extended by the demonstration that such dizygotic cattle twins were mutually tolerant of skin grafts from one another, regardless of differences in sex and color. These observations provided the basis for experiments by Medawar and his colleagues that reproduced natural tolerance in the laboratory and led to a Nobel Prize.

Medawar and his colleagues injected *neonatal* mice of one strain (A) with viable spleen cells of another histoincompatible strain (CBA). When such mice grew to adulthood, they were tested and found to be specifically tolerant of skin grafts from the normally histoincompatible donor CBA strain (see Fig. 12.1), even though grafts from a third and different strain were rejected in a normal fashion. These studies indicated that in the neonatal mouse the injected CBA cells interacted with immature antigen-specific host cells (now known to be T cells) and specifically switched them off, resulting in long-lasting tolerance.

A most important observation was that the tolerant state of the injected animals of strain A could be abolished by transfer of lymphoid cells from normal adult donors of strain A. The abolition of tolerance indicated that the original induced tolerance occurred, during the neonatal stage.

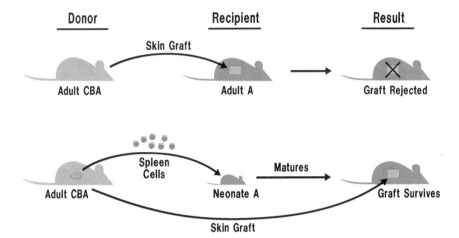

Figure 12.1

The induction of tolerance to an allograft in a neonatal mouse.

In spite of this graphic demonstration that the process of self/nonself discrimination occurs during the maturation of the immune system, clonal deletion of self-reactive lymphocytes is not perfect. If it were perfect, autoimmune reactions should never occur. Why do such reactions happen at all? Among the many mechanisms which have been proposed, we will present three that are not mutually exclusive.

1. Self-reactive T lymphocytes, especially those that are just below the threshold of critical affinity for antigen required for deletion, may escape the negative selection process and may find their way to the periphery.

2. Only those self antigens that find their way into the thymic microenvironment or are abundant will be able to delete T lymphocytes that recognize them. Those antigens absent from the thymus or present in low levels may not be recognized by developing lymphocytes and these T cells may avoid deletion or anergic events. Thus, these lymphocytes may be found in the periphery.

3. There is evidence that B-cell-negative selection may not be as stringent as T-cell-negative selection and that B-cell reactivity to self components is more common. However, as responses to self antigens generally require both B *and* T cells, the mere presence of autoreactive cells does not imply that they would become activated to participate in harmful immunological responses. In fact, stringent conditions are imposed on lymphocytes before they become activated to function. As was discussed in Chapter 11 and will be discussed later in this chapter, activation requires stimulation by costimulating molecules and cytokine signals.

MECHANISMS THAT INHIBIT T- AND B-CELL ACTIVATION

Inhibition of T-Cell Activation. Much recent work has begun to change our view of how specific acquired tolerance is achieved in mature populations of T and B cells. The production of *peripherally acquired tolerance* is now thought to be due to the *presentation of antigen to the T-cell receptor in an incomplete or ineffectual way.* As we have learned in Chapter 10, stimulation of T cells to active proliferation and secretion of T-cell products (e.g., IL-2) requires recognition by the T-cell receptor of the antigen in the context of the proper MHC class II molecule, followed by secondary costimulatory signals. The best studied costimulatory signal on an antigen-presenting cell results from the interaction of its B7 molecule with a CD28 receptor on the T cell (as described in Chapter 9). The recognition of antigen in the context of MHC by the TcR complex and of B7 by the CD28 receptor on naive T cells results in the active proliferation of T cells. If the costimulatory molecule is destroyed or absent, or the interaction of B7 and CD28 is blocked, T cells fail to respond and are rendered *anergic,* a state in which the cell loses its ability to respond to subsequent antigen challenge.

In vitro experiments have provided details to explain the mechanism of anergy by using certain cells that are able to initiate the first signal by presenting antigen on MHC class II molecules, but are unable to deliver the second costimulatory signal. The delivery of the first signal to the T-cell receptor in these cells leads ultimately to the induction of several transcription factors, one of which binds to the promoter region of the IL-2 gene allowing for its transcription in the T cell. However, if T-cell antigen recognition is not followed by the costimulatory signal, the activation process is aborted because the CD28–B7 interaction is needed to stabilize the IL-2 mRNA. The end result is anergy.

This in vitro model of inducing clonal anergy is now felt to be the operative mode for induction of unresponsiveness to antigens in the periphery that have not induced clonal deletion by appearing in the thymic cortical cells. Thus, antigens presented by cells of the pancreas, kidney, liver, and other organs, which have been induced by IFN-γ to express MHC class II molecules but do not provide the costimulatory signal, may be responsible for the induction of this clonal anergy. If, by virtue of infection or other activation processes, they also acquire the ability to provide the second signal (by B7 induction or other costimulatory molecules), they now become capable of triggering T cells and are susceptible to immunologic attack with resultant damage and disease. It is even more likely that an antigen-presenting cell with costimulatory activity may acquire a tissue-specific antigen and thus trigger T cells to autoreact.

Functionally, ***anergized T cells do not generally produce IL-2,*** although they may be able to produce certain other cytokines, such as IL-3. In some cases, anergic T cells can produce IL-2 but do not express an IL-2 receptor and thus are unable to respond to IL-2.

<u>Inhibition of B-Cell Activation.</u> As we saw in Chapter 11, B cells require multiple sequential signals to properly proliferate and differentiate into antibody-secreting cells. Most of this signaling after the Ig receptors are engaged comes from T-cell help in the form of cytokines. In the ***absence of such T-cell help, B cells also undergo negative signaling or downregulation*** induced by a Ca^{2+} flux leading to an anergic state. Thus, administration of antigen in ways that avoid the engagement of T cells (such as large doses, and soluble antigen, as we shall see later) leads to the partial activation of B cells by engagement of its specific Ig receptors and the development of unresponsiveness when the costimulatory signals are absent.

The state of anergy in both B and T cells does not necessarily involve cell death or even loss of receptors, but rather some physiologic change leading to an inability to subsequently activate the cell by specific antigen.

ACTIVE SUPPRESSION VIA T CELLS.   The production of ***suppressor T cells*** may play a major role in inhibiting anti-foreign antigen responses as well as providing a fail-safe mechanism against those anti-self reactive cells that have escaped the protective screen of clonal deletion and clonal anergy.

Some early studies showed that mice rendered tolerant to a particular antigen did not demonstrate a restoration of specific immunity after they were grafted with large numbers of normal T cells. This effect remained something of a mystery until Gershon showed that such animals possessed a class of antigen-specific T cells capable of actively suppressing the normal T cells. He further demonstrated that the adoptive transfer of the T cells from such a tolerant animal into a normal recipient prevented the development of immunity to that particular antigen. He called this process "infectious tolerance."

The phenomenon of active or infectious tolerance as a mechanism of specific unresponsiveness is the subject of intense scrutiny at present. There are well-documented experimental models in which this phenomenon can be demonstrated. Certain T cells appear to be capable of specifically suppressing the functional response of other lymphocytes to antigen. However, a unique phenotype for suppressor cells is not yet known and the exact nature of the receptors they use or the factors they release that induce suppression is still controversial. Among the many mechanisms that have been proposed only two will be described here.

One mechanism to explain suppression is that suppressor cells produce ***inhibitory cytokines*** that act on other lymphocytes. An example is IFN-γ, which may prevent IL-4-mediated switching of B cells. Also, T cells produce TGF-β, a powerful suppressant of T- and B-cell proliferation. Thus, it is possible that a population of T cells may temporarily function as a suppressor cell if they produce an appropriate cytokine, and there may not be a unique population of T cells whose sole function is to suppress immune responses.

Another mechanism is that CD8$^+$ cells may have cytotoxic activity toward either other T cells or B cells that express foreign peptides in association with MHC molecules. They may recognize and lyse activated cells using mechanisms common to all cytotoxic CD8$^+$ T cells.

IDIOTYPE NETWORK. An alternative view of immune regulation has been put forward by Jerne (a Nobel Prize winner), who postulated that the immune system was controlled by a network, in which the products of V-region genes (idiotypes), present on antibody, and antigen-specific receptors on T and B cells may be recognized as immunogenic in the host and, thus, activate B cells and/or helper or suppressor T cells, depending on the particular circumstances. These events would lead to complex control loops, which modulate the extent of the immune response. In this model, the loop can be entered and homeostasis perturbed at any point. Thus, introduction of antigen provides only one of the mechanisms by which the system can be driven. Idiotype- or anti-idiotype-bearing agents (cells or antibody) may also perturb the equilibrium. Although some of these phenomena have been demonstrated in experimental animals, the extent of their biological relevance is still unclear.

REGULATION OF THE RESPONSE IN THE INDIVIDUAL

In the previous section we discussed the regulation of the immune response, focusing on the specific effects of T and B lymphocytes. In this section we will discuss the regulation of the response as it affects the immune system in general. As we shall see, some of the factors are very specific and affect the response to only a specific antigen—not to others. In contrast, some factors affect the response in a nonantigen-specific manner; that is to say, the response to many or all antigens is diminished or completely turned off.

Age

As one would expect, age extremes have an effect on the immune responsiveness to almost all antigens. Very young individuals do not respond to many antigens. While the fetus may respond with IgM antibodies to some antigens, IgG responses in the fetus are rare because of its still undeveloped immunocompetence. Generalized immunocompetence develops only a few months after birth. It is therefore important to note as we shall see in Chapter 22 that there is a lower age limit for immunization of infants against several diseases.

The diminution of immunocompetence of very old individuals is less well documented. It is probably associated with the generalized decrease in the functions of many organs and systems, including the immune system. It should be noted however, that immunizations to several organisms are recommended for older people (Chapter 22).

Nutrition

Just as with age, the nutritional status affects many organs and functions including the immune response. The most dramatic effects are seen in protein-energy malnutrition cases. Reduced circulating T lymphocyte count and poor delayed skin reactions are early indications of protein-energy malnutrition. The complement system and phagocytic killing mechanisms are also impaired. Here again the effect is nonantigen-specific.

MHC Molecules

The role of MHC and of antigen presentation in the immune response has been discussed in detail in Chapters 10 and 11. To refresh our memory, every individual has MHC class I and MHC class II molecules that have a "groove" on which the peptides of the processed antigen are presented to the T cell. Those areas that bind with the antigenic peptides exhibit a wide degree of polymorphism. However, it is probable that the MHC molecules of a given individual will not have the correct or appropriate motif to bind and present a given peptide epitope. This is not very common in outbred individuals such as humans, but can easily be demonstrated in experiments with highly inbred animals such as mice.

The significance of the MHC in humans is demonstrated by those rare cases in which some individuals have no MHC expression on cells that are normally presenting antigen ("bare lymphocyte" syndrome). These individuals make an

IgM response to some antigens but do not make a T-cell response, nor do they make a response with other isotypes which require T-cell help. Up regulation of MHC class I and II molecules on APC by IFN-γ may restore responsiveness.

Effects of Cytokines

As we have seen in Chapter 11, T-cell activation and proliferation are dependent on signals from *cytokines.* Within the population of CD4$^+$ T cells are subsets that produce distinct cytokines with different functions. Thus, Th1 cells produce IFN-γ, a potent activator of macrophages, and TNF-β, a lymphotoxin. On the other hand, Th2 cells secrete IL-4, IL-6, and IL-10, all of which are involved in B-cell activation and differentiation. Therefore, Th1 cells are important in cell-mediated immunity that involves macrophage activation, whereas Th2 cells are involved in IgE antibody production. Furthermore, IL-4 (as well as IL-10 and IL-13) inhibits IFN-γ activation of macrophages and conversely, IFN-γ may prevent IL-4 mediated switching of B cells. Another cytokine, IL-12, which is produced primarily by monocyte–macrophages, is necessary for the initiation of Th1. Other examples can be given, but it is clear that the influence of cytokines on T cells, B cells, and macrophage offer a potent, short-acting, proximal level of controlling the immune responses.

Effects of Antigen

DOSAGE. Not every injection of an antigen results in an immune response. Generation of a response is a highly empirical process, depending on *dose, timing,* and *nature of the antigen* involved.

The importance of dosage was recognized by Mitchison in 1964, who found that immunologic tolerance in adult animals could be induced by opposite extremes of dosage. The initial studies showed that tolerance could be induced in adult animals by the use of relatively large doses of antigen, given repeatedly over long periods of time. Very small doses given similarly were also found to induce tolerance. Intermediate doses resulted in immunity.

The elegant experiments of Chiller and Weigle helped explain some of the parameters of immunological tolerance and defined differences in the control mechanisms between T and B cells. They demonstrated (1) that both *T and B lymphocytes are susceptible* to induction of tolerance, (2) that the susceptibilities of these two classes of lymphocytes differ considerably, with respect to both the *dose of antigen* against which tolerance is induced and the *time* required for induction of tolerance, (3) that the *duration* of tolerance is significantly *shorter in B cells* than in T cells, and finally (4) that the *immunologic status* of the whole animal reflects the status of the population of T cells (in the cases of thymus-dependent antigen).

By transfer of various cell mixtures into irradiated recipients (that are immunologically incompetent as a result of irradiation), it was shown that T cells were apparently rendered tolerant very rapidly after injection of antigen (within 24 hours) and that the tolerant state was maintained in T cells for around 100 days (see Fig. 12.2). The population of bone marrow B cells also becomes tolerant, but not until somewhat later (day 10–11) and recovery in this population occurred by day 49. Normal animals injected with the antigen manifested tolerance in parallel with the tolerance of the T-cell population. Therefore, an animal whose population of bone marrow B cells had recovered from tolerance by day 60 would, nevertheless, remain functionally unresponsiveness because of the continued absence of immunocompetent antigen-specific T cells.

The reasons for the different recovery times of T- and B-cell populations lie in the ontogenetic origins of these cells. It may be recalled that the thymus is most active after birth and tends to atrophy with maturity. Thus, little replacement of T cells occurs in adult animals, and tolerance of existing T cells would be long-lasting. By contrast, bone marrow functions throughout life and constantly provides new B cells to replace those made tolerant. Thus, when antigen is gone, new reactive B cells repopulate the host.

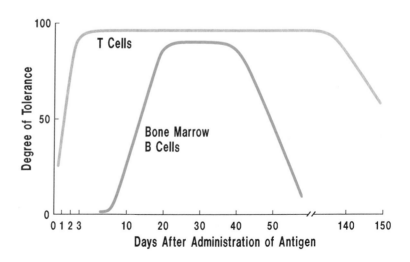

Figure 12.2

The kinetics of the induction, maintenance, and loss of B- and T-cell tolerance.

The essential conclusions from the experiments described above—that T cells become tolerant at lower doses of antigen and remain tolerant for longer periods than B cells—serve to explain the observations by Mitchison on tolerance induced by high and low doses of antigen by assuming that tolerance was induced only in T cells at low doses of antigen, while tolerance was induced in both T and B cells by high doses of antigen.

ANTIGEN SEQUESTRATION. Antigens of proven immunogenicity will not provoke an immune response if they fail to reach lymphoid tissues. One example of how this may occur is called ***antigen sequestration,*** which is operationally the simplest method to understand, but applied to only a select few antigens. The lens protein of the eye, certain spermatozoal antigens, and chondrocyte antigens of cartilage are sequestered behind anatomical barriers and are normally not "seen" by the immunologic system. However, under certain circumstances, such as trauma to the lens, they are seen to be highly immunogenic and elicit destructive autoimmune responses. Tissues that do not induce an immune response or that immune components cannot reach are termed ***immunologically privileged sites.***

NATURE OF ANTIGEN. The inherent ***immunogenicity*** of the substance being used for induction tolerance is critically related to the ease of induction of tolerance. For example, a very weak immunogen, such as bovine γ-globulin (BGG), requires a less stringent regimen for induction of tolerance to it in mice than a very strong immunogen, such as hen egg albumin or diphtheria toxoid. In general, the more chemically complex the antigen is, the more immunogenic it is. This is because complexity increases the number of epitopes and the chances for cell interaction necessary to trigger a response.

FORM OF THE ANTIGEN. The ***form*** of the antigen is also important. BGG in soluble form is not immunogenic and it also readily induces tolerance in mice; however, if it is given in an adjuvant (see Chapter 3) or in an aggregated form, BGG is immunogenic. If a normally antigenic material is injected in solution in its monomeric form, tolerance rather than immunity frequently results. This effect is exemplified by the following: if a suspension of BGG in saline, which is normally immunogenic in rabbits, is subjected to ultracentrifugation, then the supernatant that contains the monomeric BGG is no longer immunogenic, but is, in fact, ***tolerogenic,*** while the sediment, which consists of aggregated BGG, is highly immunogenic.

The most likely explanation of these findings is that forms of antigen that are not readily phagocytized by macrophages or not taken up by other antigen-presenting cells are more likely to induce tolerogenicity rather than immunogenicity. This explanation is supported by the fact that changing the physical state of such tolerogenic substances by heating, which causes aggregation of proteins, or by incorporating into adjuvants converts them to potent immunogens. Thus, generally, if antigen reaches this type of cell, immunity results; if the processing cell is bypassed, some form of tolerance is induced. Thus, destruction of APC or blocking their antigen-processing and antigen-presenting function by various agents, before antigen is given, leads to tolerance, and tolerance is easily induced in newborns with small or absent populations of APC.

METABOLISM OF THE ANTIGEN. *Nonmetabolizable substances* may be tolerogenic. Pneumococcal polysaccharides and synthetic D-polypeptides (made with the unnatural D rather than L isomers of amino acids) are resistant to enzymatic digestion. These substances are immunogenic when administered in very low quantities (1 μg), but slightly higher doses (10 μg) induce a long-lasting state of specific tolerance. One contributing factor in this case may be that the antigen is taken up by APC but is not broken down and is repeatedly released back into circulation, where it can bind to antibody, if present, and prevent its detection in serum.

Regulation by Antibody

The production of antibody results in a *feedback inhibition* of further production of antibody- and cell-mediated responses. For example, the appearance of IgG antibody results in a shutoff of synthesis of IgM antibody. The shutoff presumably is the result of several mechanisms that may be operating simultaneously. The first is the result of competition for antigen. The IgG receptors with increased affinity on B cells represent a more efficient system for capture of antigen than that of IgM receptors. Similarly, as the level of antibody rises, the concentration of antigen declines, and the net affinity of resulting antibody increased as competition for the remaining antigen favors those B cells with high-affinity receptors.

The second mechanisms by which antibodies regulate the immune response may be due to the formation of immune complexes composed of the eliciting antigen and antibody. These complexes may bind FcR (Fc receptors) on either B cells (via CD32, as described in Chapter 8) or subpopulations of T cells. This interaction may inhibit their responses by suppressing the generation of intracellular signals.

A third mechanism is that antibodies may perturb the idiotype–anti-idiotype network that may result in the down regulation of immune responses.

IMMUNOSUPPRESSION BY DRUGS OR RADIATION

Finally, we will briefly mention nonspecific methods of dramatically inhibiting immunologic responses through the use of immunosuppressive agents and irradiation. Some of these are also described in Chapter 20 dealing with transplantation immunology.

The most commonly used immunosuppressive drugs include *cytotoxic* agents (such as methotrexate and cyclophosphamide) that kill rapidly dividing cells and thus target lymphocytes (as well as hematopoietic cells of the bone marrow, gastrointestinal lining cells, and hair follicles). *Corticosteroids,* also widely used drugs, affect a wide range of cell types and are potent inhibitors of inflammatory responses. A major class of immunosuppressants acts specifically on T cells to prevent activation. These include *cyclosprine* and *FK506,* which block the action of nuclear transcription factors and inhibit the synthesis of IL-2 and other cytokines; also *rapamycin*, which interferes with protein kinases used in the signaling pathway of the IL-2/IL-2 receptor complex. Because these drugs are antigen-nonspecific, they also inhibit protective immunity as well as the unwanted response, there is a search for more selective forms of immunosuppression. One approach is to use antibodies to cell surface molecules that are coupled to toxin chain enabling them to kill specific lymphocytes effectively and selectively (see Chapter 21).

The hematopoietic and lymphoid systems are extremely sensitive to *radiation.* This susceptibility can be exploited as a treatment therapy for leukemias and lymphomas, but, obviously the dose rate of exposure is important. Whole-body irradiation may be lethal. With sublethal doses, regeneration of hematopoietic cells may be prompt and the lymphocytes in the blood may be restored within weeks.

SUMMARY

1. In the regulation of the immune response, multiple controls are used to ensure the correct functioning of the system.

2. As a consequence of differentiation in the thymus, T cells potentially reactive with self antigens are deleted or functionally inactivated. Self-reactive B cells are also deleted or inactivated during the early stages of development.

3. Acquired tolerance, or unresponsiveness, to foreign antigen may be induced in neonates by "fooling" the developing cells into recognizing the foreign antigen as self.

4. In adults, tolerance may be regulated at four different levels: (a) during the induction process, (b) by controlling the activation of T and B cells, (c) by suppressing ongoing immune response, and (d) by impairing the lymphoid system through radiation and drugs.

5. The induction process can be controlled by manipulating the dosage of the antigen (low- or high-zone tolerance), by altering its immunogenicity (soluble, nonmetabolizable), or by using routes that bypass APC.

6. T and B cells require multiple signals (costimulatory molecules, cytokines) to induce activation; preventing these signals may lead to an anergic state.

7. Immune responses may be actively suppressed by T suppressor cells, by perturbing the idiotype network, by antibody-mediated feedback inhibition or by drugs.

REFERENCES

Ashton-Rickardt PG, Tonegawa S (1994): A differential avidity model for T cell selection. Immunol Today 15:362.

Blackman M, Kappler J, Marrack P (1990): The role of the T cell receptor in positive and negative selection of developing T cells. Science 248:1335.

Goodnow CC, Adelstein S, Basten A (1990): The need for central and peripheral tolerance in the B cell repertoire. Science 248:1373.

Green RG, Webb DR (1993): Saying the "S" word in public. Immunol Today 124:523.

Nossal GJV (1994): Negative selection of lymphocytes. Cell 76:229.

Paul WE, Seder RA (1994): Lymphocyte responses and cytokines. Cell 76:241.

Powrie F, Coffman RL (1993): Cytokine regulation of T cell function: potential for therapeutic intervention. Immunol Today 14:270.

Robey E, Fowlkes BJ (1994): Selective events in T cell development. Ann Rev Immunol 12:675.

Seder RA, Paul WE (1994): Acquisition of lymphokine producing phenotype by CD4[+] T cell. Annu Rev Immunol 212:635.

Sprent J, Gao E, Webb SR (1990): T cell reactivity to MHC molecules: Immunity versus tolerance. Science 248:1357.

Choose the ONE BEST answer or completion.

1. Immunologic unresponsiveness, induced by immunosuppressive drugs, is different from immunological tolerance because
   A) only B cells are affected by the drugs
   B) only T cells are affected by the drugs
   C) liver enzymes are involved in the former and not in the latter
   D) drug-induced unresponsiveness is not antigen-specific but tolerance is
   E) drug-induced unresponsiveness is antigen-specific but tolerance is not

2. Immunologic tolerance
   A) involves only humoral immunity
   B) involves only cell-mediated immunity
   C) may involve only some antigenic determinants on a protein
   D) is induced with ease in adults
   E) is best achieved with particulate antigens

3. All of the following procedures would be likely to induce tolerance to a protein antigen *except*:
   A) intramuscular injection of the antigen in adjuvant
   B) intravenous injection of deaggregated protein
   C) injection of cyclophosphamide with the antigen
   D) injection of antigen into the fetus in utero

E) intravenous injection of small amounts of antigen

4. Regulatory elements in the Jerne idiotype network hypothesis include
   A) products of V-region genes
   B) anti-idiotypic suppressor T cells
   C) T-cell idiotypes
   D) all of the above
   E) none of the above

5. When a tolerogenic injection of a protein antigen is given experimentally, it can be shown that
   A) B-cell tolerance is more rapidly induced than T-cell tolerance
   B) B-cell tolerance is lost as new B cells come from the bone marrow
   C) B-cell tolerance can be induced only when low doses are used
   D) T-cell tolerance can be induced only when high doses are used
   E) T-cell tolerance is shorter lasting than B-cell tolerance

6. The induction of immunologic tolerance may be facilitated by
   A) the use of high doses of nonmetabolizable antigens
   B) haptens
   C) previous immunization of the individual
   D) the use of aggregated forms of the antigen
   E) none of the above

7. Peripherally acquired tolerance of mature T cells may occur because the following processes are negatively affected:
   A) the binding of antigen with MHC gene product
   B) the recognition of the TcR to the antigen–MHC complex
   C) the binding of costimulatory molecules on T cell to their ligands on APC
   D) activation of the IL-2 gene
   E) any of the above

8. All of the following are true regarding suppressor T cells *except*:
   A) adoptive transfer of antigen-specific T cells from a tolerant animal will prevent the development of immunity to that antigen
   B) suppressor T cells have a phenotype easily discernible from cytotoxic T cells
   C) suppressor T cells may produce inhibitory cytokines that block the function of other T and B cells
   D) one mechanism of suppression is that suppressor T cells lyse other T and B cells
   E) the exact nature of the receptors on suppressor T cells for recognizing antigen is not known

9. The following factors may affect the immunological response to antigens:
   A) extreme age
   B) poor nutrition
   C) cyclosporin
   D) the presence of preexisting antibody
   E) all of the above

ANSWERS TO REVIEW QUESTIONS

1. ***D*** Drugs eliminate B and T cells nonspecifically; only antigen-induced tolerance has the elements of specificity.

2. ***C*** Tolerance is achieved in specific clones of B or T cells and may involve only those clones specific for certain epitopes on an antigen and not others.

3. ***A*** Use of adjuvant is designed to achieve immunity and avoid tolerance. All other procedures could induce tolerance.

4. ***D*** All are regulatory or recognition elements in the network. Products of V-region genes would be the idiotypes of receptors on B and T cells.

5. ***B*** T-cell tolerance is more rapidly achieved, occurs with lower doses, and lasts longer than B-cell tolerance. As new B cells are produced by the bone marrow, tolerance in this compartment wanes. T-cell tolerance, by contrast, persists because the thymus of an adult no longer actively produces new T cells.

6. *A* Induction of tolerance is favored by large amounts of nonmetabolizable antigens; they make B cells tolerant by direct binding to receptors whereas aggregated forms of the antigen are readily phagocytized and make potent immunogens (*D*). Haptens have no ability to affect the response, unless they are coupled to carriers (*B*). Immune animals (*C*) are difficult to make tolerant, because they already have expanded clones of mature T and B cells.

7. *E* Inhibiting any of the above processes may lead to peripheral tolerance of T cells.

8. *B* Suppressor T cells do not have a distinctive phenotype at the present time. Furthermore, the nature of their antigen-binding receptors is not known and it is possible that it is the same for all CD8$^+$ T cells. Suppressor cells may lyse other T and B cells or may produce inhibitory cytokines to inhibit immune responses.

9. *E* Immune response is lower in the very young and very old. Preexisting antibody may exert a negative feedback mechanism. Poor nutrition decreases immune responses and cyclosporin blocks the transcription of IL-2.

COMPLEMENT

INTRODUCTION

In 1894 Pfeiffer discovered that cholera bacilli (*Vibrio cholerae*) were dissolved or lysed in vitro by the addition of guinea pig anticholera serum. Heating the serum at 56°C for 30 minutes abolished this activity, but did not abolish the activity of antibodies against the bacilli, since the heated serum could still transfer immunity passively from one guinea pig to another. Pfeiffer discovered that the addition of normal, fresh serum to the heat-treated antiserum restored its lytic activity. From these experiments, he concluded that antibodies to the bacilli, plus a heat-labile component present in immune as well as normal serum, were necessary for the lysis of *V. cholera* in vitro.

A few years later, Bordet (a Nobel Prize winner) confirmed that bacteriolysis by immune serum required a heat-labile component that he termed "Alexine." The term *complement,* applied some years later by Ehrlich (another Nobel Prize winner), displaced "Alexine" and is used to denote, collectively, those components in normal serum that, together with antigen-bound antibodies, exhibit a variety of biological properties, one of which is the ability to lyse cells or microorganisms. Complement consists of a group of serum proteins that act in concert and in an orderly sequence to exert their effect. These proteins are not immunoglobulins;

they are synthesized by liver hepatocytes or by tissue macrophages, epithelial cells of the gastrointestinal tract, and blood monocytes. Their concentrations in serum do not increase after immunization. Like antibodies, they appear to have arisen late in evolution and are found only in vertebrates. Bordet discovered that the action of complement, in the presence of the appropriate antiserum, results in the lysis of red blood cells. Based on this observation, Bordet developed the *complement fixation test,* described later in this chapter.

We now know that in addition to lysis, the activation of complement results in the generation of many powerful biologically active substances. This chapter describes the complement system and the properties of the complement components and their biological relevance.

THE COMPLEMENT SYSTEM

Nature has devised two pathways for the activation of complement, the so-called *classical pathway* and the *alternative pathway.* Although both pathways share some common components, they differ in the ways in which they are initiated. The classical pathway requires antigen–antibody complexes for initiation, while the alternative pathway does not. In the sections that follow, both pathways, their activation, and their products will be described.

The Classical Complement Pathway

The *classical complement system* involves the activation, in an orderly fashion, of nine major protein components designated C1 through C9. For several steps in the activation process, the product is an enzyme that catalyzes the subsequent step. This cascade provides amplification and activation of large amounts of complement by a relatively small initial signal. To safeguard against the system going awry, the series of reactions also provides several sites for regulation. The sequence of the classical complement pathway is given in Figure 13.1 and is discussed below.

ACTIVATION OF C1. The first component to become activated is the C1 complex, consisting of three proteins, C1q, C1r, and C1s, with molecular weights of approximately 400,000, 95,000, and 85,000 daltons, respectively. The C1 complex that contains a hexamer of C1q and dimers of C1r and C1s is held together by calcium ions.

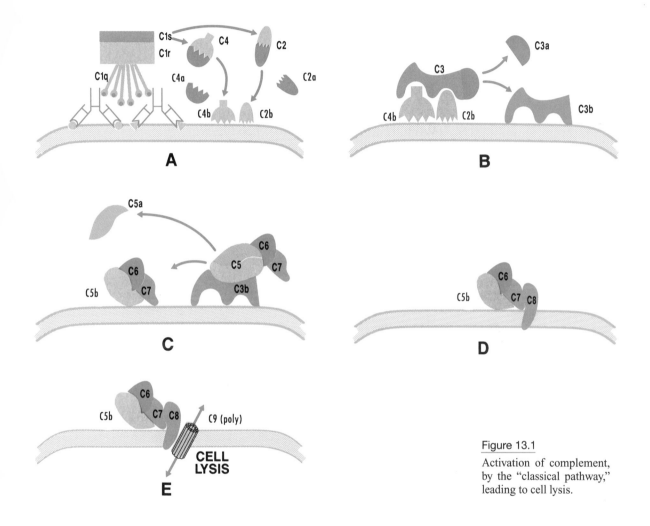

Figure 13.1

Activation of complement, by the "classical pathway," leading to cell lysis.

C1q is a polymer of six identical subunits. The activation of C1q requires the binding of C1q subunits to C1q-specific receptors on the Fc regions of at least two adjacent molecules of IgG. However, C1q can become activated by binding two or more Fc regions of a single pentameric IgM; thus, IgM is an efficient complement-activating antibody. The receptors for C1q become available following conformational changes that take place on at least two antibody molecules, each binding with two epitopes on a multivalent antigen. Since such cross-linking cannot occur with a hapten or monovalent antigen, the binding of antibodies with such molecules does not activate complement. *IgG₄*, *IgA*, and *IgE* do not have C1q receptors and thus cannot bind C1q; consequently, these isotypes are not able to activate the complement system. Activated C1q activates C1r which, in turn, activates C1s. Activated C1s has esterolytic and proteolytic properties which act on the next component of complement, namely, C4.

ACTIVATION OF C4. C4 is the second component of complement to be activated. It is called C4 (rather than C2) because historically it was the fourth component of complement discovered. C4 is a glycoprotein of molecular weight 180,000 daltons synthesized by macrophages. The action of activated C1s on C4 results in cleavage of C4 into C4a and a larger fragment C4b. C4b has several functions, one of which is to bind to the cell membrane adjacent to the antibody–antigen complex that has initiated the process. In addition, C4b attaches to the next complement component in the pathway, C2.

ACTIVATION OF C2. C2 is a glycoprotein with a molecular weight of approximately 115,000 daltons. It is cleaved by the action of C1s and C4b, but remains associated with activated C4b. This complex constitutes a new enzyme designated $C\overline{42}$ (a bar above the numbers designates an active complex of the components under the bar), also called *C3/5 convertase.* It acts on and activates C3 and C5.

ACTIVATION OF C3. Compound C3 is a β-globulin with a molecular weight of 180,000 daltons. It is secreted (as pro-C3) by macrophages. C3 becomes activated by C3 convertase ($C\overline{42}$), which splits C3 into a small fragment, C3a, and a larger fragment, C3b. It has been determined that a single, biomolecular complex of $C\overline{42}$ (i.e., C3 convertase) is able to activate hundreds of C3 molecules to yield hundreds of C3a and C3b fragments. Thus, the action of C3 convertase on C3 constitutes a very important *amplification* step in the system cascade, as it generates C3a and C3b fragments.

Both C3a and C3b have several important biological properties and functions, some of which we will describe later. However, one of the properties of C3b is its ability to attach to the cell membrane in the immediate vicinity of its site of activation. Thus, through the action of C3 convertase, many C3b molecules are split from C3 and become attached to the target-cell membrane. Many cell types such as red blood cells, polymorphonuclear cells, macrophages, and platelets as well as bacteria, yeasts, and certain viruses may serve as targets. C3b also combines with $C\overline{42}$ to form $C\overline{423}$, an enzyme that is also called C5 convertase because it activates C5. The small C3a fragment remains in the fluid phase and, as we shall see later, it has important biological properties.

THE MEMBRANE ATTACK COMPLEX. The assembly and activation of complement components C5–C9 constitute the cytolytic complex of the complement system; is collectively referred to as the ***membrane attack complex.***

ACTIVATION OF C5, C6, AND C7. Complement components C5, C6, and C7 are globular proteins of molecular weight 180,000, 130,000, and 120,000 daltons, respectively. By the action of C5 convertase ($\overline{C423}$), C5 is split into two fragments: a small fragment, C5a, which has several important biological properties (described later); and C5b, which binds stoichiometrically with C6 and C7 to form a complex $\overline{C5b67}$ designated simply as $\overline{C567}$ on the cell membrane. This complex, through conformational changes, inserts itself into the lipid bilayer of the cell membrane and focuses the activities of the next components, C8 and C9, onto and into the target cell membrane.

ACTIVATION OF C8 AND C9. Compounds C8 and C9 consist of proteins with molecular weights of approximately 160,000 and 80,000 daltons, respectively. The complex $\overline{C5}b678$ interacts with the cell membrane and forms small pores that may lead to lysis. However, the final "hit" that leads to lysis is caused by the polymerization of C9, a perforin-like molecule (see Chapter 11) around the $\overline{C5}b678$ complex. This polymerization results in the formation of transmembrane channels that are the major cause of lysis.

The passage of ions through these channels disturbs the osmotic equilibrium, and there is a rapid influx of water into the cell. As the cell swells, the membrane becomes permeable to macromolecules, which can then escape from the cell. The end result is lysis of the target cell.

The Alternative Complement Pathway

The classical pathway of complement activation involves components C1 through C9, and it is initiated by antibody complexed to multivalent antigens (or aggregated antibody, without antigen). One important aspect of this classical pathway is that the antibody focuses the activities of the components of complement on the antigen. Another important aspect is that the activation of C3 by C3 convertase (designated simply as $\overline{C142}$) results in the release of various physiologically active substances at the site of the reaction. Thus, the activation of C3 is an important event in the classical pathway of complement activation.

Compound C3 can also be activated by another route, termed the ***alternative pathway*** of complement activation. It arose in evolution earlier than the classical pathway, and it does not require antigen-antibody complexes for initiation. The alternative pathway of complement activation (shown in Fig. 13.2) may be triggered by various substances among which are ***lipopolysaccharides (LPS)*** or endotoxin from the cell walls of gram-negative bacteria, ***the cell walls of some bacteria, cell walls of some yeasts (zymosan), aggregated IgA,*** and a factor present in ***cobra venom.*** C3b exists in trace amounts in normal serum and can bind foreign surface antigens. It combines with a serum factor called ***factor B,*** forming a complex, C3bB. This complex is further activated by serum ***factor D,*** which cleaves factor B while it is attached to C3b to generate the enzyme complex C3bBb. C3bBb acts as a C3 convertase and, as in the classical pathway, releases C3a and C3b from C3. The C3b fragment complexes with factor B and becomes activated with factor D to yield more C3 convertase, thereby amplifying the amount of C3 convertase and the amount of C3 that becomes activated. This amplification is delicately balanced by the fact that the C3bB complex dissociates rapidly. However, this disso-

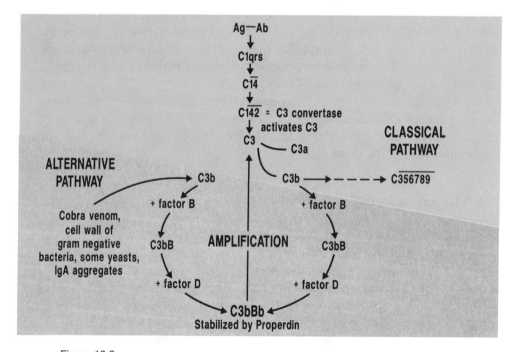

Figure 13.2

The relationship between the classical and the alternative pathways of complement activation.

ciation is regulated by a serum protein called ***properdin,*** which acts to stabilize the C3bBb complex. As mentioned above, C3b is present in trace amounts in normal serum. It probably originates from a low level of activity of factors B and D on C3, which causes the release of C3b. The released C3b is largely inactivated by yet two other factors: ***factor H*** and ***factor I*** (the C3b inactivator). It is believed that lipopolysaccharides of gram-negative bacteria and other substances that initiate the alternative pathway of complement activation somehow protect the small amounts of C3b from inactivation, so that the presence of these substances triggers the alternative pathway.

In addition to the activation of C3b, which ultimately leads to the activation of the membrane attack complex (C5–C9), C3b promotes ***immune adherence,*** especially between bacteria and macrophages, an activity that enhances phagocytosis. C3b also activates C3, an event that is followed by the activation of the remaining components of the complement cascade. C3b also helps to solubilize large immune complexes, leading to their clearance from the circulation and their ultimate destruction by the liver.

The two pathways of complement are interconnected; in fact, the amplification process involved in the alternative pathway of activation is also operative in the classical pathway. Thus, the alternative pathway amplifies both antibody-dependent and antibody-independent cleavage of C3.

BIOLOGICAL ACTIVITY OF COMPLEMENT COMPONENTS

In addition to its function of producing cell lysis, the activation of complement yields fragments of complement components that possess various important biological activities. Some of the important activities are summarized below.

Anaphylatoxins (C3a, C5a)

An ***anaphylatoxin*** is a substance (usually of low molecular weight) that induces the degranulation of mast cells and/or basophils, causing, among other things, release of histamine. Histamine has several important physiological functions (e.g., it increases capillary permeability and causes contraction of smooth muscle) that are associated with ***anaphylaxis*** and other allergic reactions (see Chapter 14).

The anaphylatoxins that are elaborated during the activation of complement are C3a and C5a. Recently C4a was also shown to possess weak anaphylatoxin activity. The increase in capillary-permeability caused by histamine results in ***lo-***

cal edema (accumulation of fluid) in the tissue. The influx of edema fluid, which contains more antibodies and more components of complement, causes additional release of anaphylatoxins, thus amplifying the reaction.

Chemotaxins (C5a)

Chemotaxins are substances that attract phagocytic cells and cause their migration from an area of lesser concentration to an area of higher concentration *(chemotaxis).* The chemotaxin produced during complement activation is C5a, which is the most potent chemoattractant for neutrophils.

Immune Adherence (C3b)

Immune adherence is a phenomenon in which a particular antigen, coated with antibodies and in the presence of complement, adheres to various surfaces. In vivo, these surfaces include the walls of blood vessels. Its adherence to the walls of blood vessels makes the particular antigen easy prey for circulating phagocytic cells. The complement component C3b is responsible for immune adherence.

Opsonization (C3b)

Opsonization refers to the coating of particulate antigen by antibody and/or by complement components that render the particle more attractive to phagocytic cells and allow them to be phagocytized more readily. The attachment is facilitated by the presence, on the surface of the phagocytic cells, of receptors for the Fc portion of the antibody and for the C3b component of complement. Thus, not only are antibodies, notably IgG, referred to as *opsonins* but also the C3b component of complement is called an opsonin.

COMPLEMENT RECEPTORS (CRs)

Receptors to many of the products released during complement activation are found on the surface of many cells. These include not only surfaces on cells of the body but also surfaces of various microorganisms. Receptors for activated C1q are present on neutrophils, monocytes, and B cells. Interaction with these receptors activates the cells for a variety of functions, such as increased phagocytosis by phagocytic cells. Receptors to the anaphylatoxins, released during complement activation (C3a, C4a, and C5a), are present on mast cells, basophils, and several other cell types. Interaction of C3a, C4a, or C5a with their corresponding receptors on mast cells or basophils activates the cells to release histamine and other vasoactive compounds, causing smooth-muscle contraction and increased vascular permeability, inducing a host of physiological effects, as we shall see in Chapter 14.

Various receptors for activation and degradation products of C3b have been identified on all human peripheral blood cells except platelets. These receptors have been classified into four major types: CR1, CR2, CR3, and CR4. They have been identified as cell-surface molecules CD35, CD21, CD11b/18, and CD11c/18 for CR1, CR2, CR3, and CR4, respectively, where "CD" stands for cluster determinants on the cell surface and the number gives their identification. Interaction of C3b products with the appropriate receptors results in cell activation and many biological activities, ranging from immune adherence, B-cell activation, and phagocytosis.

So, in addition to the complement cascade, whether through the classical or alternative pathway, the activation of complement and its components and their interactions with the various receptors amplify and maximize the effects of complement, with the ultimate objective of destroying and eliminating the invader. The invader can be an infectious microorganism or, as we shall see later, a foreign particle or cell, which may be injurious or even harmless.

REGULATION OF COMPLEMENT ACTIVATION

The serum proteins that are components of the classical or the alternative activation routes of complement are synthesized in the liver, by macrophages and blood monocytes, and by intestinal epithelial cells. They are released into the serum in their inactive forms and become activated during the events of the complement cascade.

On one hand, complement activation necessitates the formation of stable molecular complexes in a cascading sequence for short periods. On the other hand, this activation generates physiologically powerful molecules. Consequently, the activation of complement requires careful control and regulation by a variety of mechanisms, in order to prevent adverse effects. Indeed, many inactivators of the various components of complement are known. These act on several key components of the classical as well as the alternative activation pathway. Notably, *C1 esterase inhibitor (C1INH)* forms a complex with C1r and C1s, causing their dissociation from C1q and thus inhibiting the initiation of the classical activation pathway. Similarly, a factor called *decay accelerating factor (DAF)* prevents the assembly and causes dissociation of C3 convertase. Some other inhibitors are C3b inhibitor, anaphylatoxin inactivator, and C4b inhibitor.

There are rare genetic disorders that result in deficiencies in the proteins that regulate the complement pathways. One such disorder is associated with a deficiency of C1 esterase inhibitor (*C1INH*). This deficiency results in uncontrolled activation of C4 and C2 by C1, and allows production of more and more fragments that are, in turn, activated by *plasmin* to yield vasoactive peptides. Thus, a small stimulus that activates C1 may trigger a large response that cannot be interrupted.

C1INH deficiency is transmitted in an autosomal dominant manner. Individuals with this disorder have *hereditary angioedema.* They suffer from local edema in various organs, such as skin, the gastrointestinal tract, and the upper respiratory tract, induced by the vasoactive peptides. The edema may become life-threatening when it occurs in the larynx and obstructs air passage.

COMPLEMENT DEFICIENCY

Genetic deficiencies in complement components have been reported for almost all of the major complement components of the system. Heterozygous individuals, with a single defective allele for any complement component, have about half the normal level of that component in their serum. Individuals with a homozygous defect in a given complement component are rare, but they do exist. As would be expected, many of the latter individuals suffer from recurrent infections, most notably gonococcal and meningococcal infections. The consequences of a deficiency in a particular component of complement may vary, depending on the deficient component. Thus, for example, deficiency in C2 does not appear to be particularly harmful to some individuals' ability to fight infection, probably because the mechanism for activation of the alternative complement pathway is not affected. In contrast, individuals deficient in C3 usually suffer from recurrent infections with pyogenic and gram-negative bacteria, probably because of the absence of chemotactic, opsonizing, and bactericidal activities from their serum complement. In Chapter 18 we discuss in more detail several disorders that result from complement deficiency.

THE COMPLEMENT FIXATION TEST

The ***complement fixation test*** was used extensively in the past for the detection of hepatitis B surface antigen, anti-DNA antibodies, and the Wassermann test for syphilis, but now less labor-extensive, less expensive, and more sensitive analyses are used in clinical medicine.

The complement fixation test is based on the competition, for complement, between various antigen–antibody complexes and the lytic system consisting of red blood cell-specific antibodies and red blood cells (RBCs), which, together with complement, bring about the lysis of RBC.

The complement fixation test is shown in Table 13.1. The test consists of an ***indicator system*** composed of predetermined amounts of sheep red blood cells (SRBCs), rabbit antibodies to SRBC (also termed ***hemolysin***), and complement (C′), which is generally supplied as guinea pig serum. The amounts of each reagent are predetermined in such a way that the introduction of complement, given at a slight deficiency, to SRBC/anti-SRBC complexes (often termed "sensitized" SRBC) results in almost complete (e.g., 95%) lysis. The degree of lysis can be determined spectrophotometrically by measuring the intensity of the red color of hemoglobin released into the solution.

Since the concentration of complement is limiting, any loss or consumption of complement would be reflected by a decrease in the extent of lysis. Such a loss could occur during preincubation of that fixed amount of complement with an antigen–antibody system (not related to SRBC and anti-SRBC) that would result in the attachment of complement to the antibody in this antigen–antibody complex. This attachment or ***fixation*** of complement results in the activation of the ***complement cascade*** and the consumption of complement components by the antigen–antibody complexes. Subsequent introduction of sensitized SRBC into the mixture does not result in lysis of the SRBC, because complement has been fixed or "used" by the first antigen–antibody system. The greater

TABLE 13.1   The Complement Fixation Test

Test system	C′ (complement)		Sheep RBC (SRBC)		Anti-sheep RBC (hemolysin)	Hemolysis release of hemoglobin)
Antigen X	+	C′	+	SRBC	+	Anti-SRBC	Hemolysis
Antibody to X	+	C′	+	SRBC	+	Anti-SRBC	Hemolysis
X-anti-X complex	+	C′	+	SRBC	+	Anti-SRBC	No hemolysis

the concentration of the antigen–antibody complexes, the more complement would be fixed by this system, and the more limited would be the lysis of the SRBC.

SUMMARY

1. Complement consists of a group of serum proteins that activate each other in an orderly fashion to generate biologically active molecules, such as enzymes, opsonins, anaphylatoxins, and chemotoxins.

2. Complement can be activated through two pathways: (a) the classical pathway that is initiated by antigen–antibody complexes and (b) the alternative pathway, in which complement components become activated by the cell walls of some bacteria and yeasts, in combination with several serum factors.

3. The activation through the classical pathway requires C1q for initiation; the alternative pathway requires C3b, serum factors B and D, and properdin.

4. The activity of complement and its components is tightly regulated by various inhibitors.

5. The level of complement does not increase after immunization.

REFERENCES

Arland GJ, Colomb MC, Gagnon J (1988): A functional model of the human C1 complex. Immunol Today 8:106.

Boackle RJ (1986): The complement system. In Virella G, Goust JM, Fudenberg HH, Patrick CC (eds): Introduction to Medical Immunology. New York: Marcel Dekker.

Fearon DT, Austen KF (1980): The alternative pathway of complement—a system for host resistance to microbial infection. New Engl J Med 303:259.

Frank MM (1994): Complement and kinin. In Stites DP, Terr AI, Parslow TG (eds): Basic and Clinical Immunology, 8th ed. Norwalk, CT: Appleton & Lange.

Kuby J (1992): Immunology. New York: Freeman.

Liszewski MK, Atkinson JP (1993): The complement system. In Paul WE (ed): Fundamental Immunology, 3rd ed. New York: Raven Press.

Lublin DM, Atkinson JP (1989): Decay accelerating factor: biochemistry, molecular biology and function. Annu Rev Immunol 7:35.

Muller-Eberhard HJ, Colten HR (1986): The complement system. Prog Immunol 6:267.

Pascual M, French LE (1995): Complement in human diseases: looking toward the 21st century. Immunol Today 16:58.

Reid KBM, Day AJ (1989): Structure function relationship of the complement components. Immunol Today 10:177.

Ross GD (ed) (1986): Immunobiology of the Complement System. An Introduction for Research and Clinical Medicine. London: Academic Press.

REVIEW QUESTIONS

> For each question, choose the ONE BEST answer or completion.

1. A patient is admitted with multiple bacterial infections and is found to have a complete absence of C3. Which complement-mediated function would remain intact in such a patient:
   A) lysis of bacteria
   B) opsonization of bacteria
   C) generation of anaphylatoxins
   D) generation of neutrophil chemotactic factors
   E) none of the above

2. Which of the following screening tests would be most useful for confirming a presumptive diagnosis of a congenital absence of a complement component?
   A) quantitation of serum opsonic activity
   B) quantitation of serum hemolytic activity
   C) quantitation of C3 content of serum
   D) quantitation of C1 content of serum
   E) electrophoretic analysis of patient's serum

3. Complement is required for
   A) lysis of erythrocytes by lecithinase
   B) lysis of erythrocytes by specific antibodies
   C) phagocytosis
   D) bacteriolysis by specific antibodies
   E) only A and C are correct
   F) only B and D are correct

4. Complement activation by an immune complex may result in
   A) precipitation
   B) release of anaphylatoxins
   C) release of macrophage-inhibiting factor
   D) opsonization
   E) only A and C are correct
   F) only B and D are correct

5. Active fragments of C5 can lead to the following *except*:
   A) contraction of smooth muscle
   B) vasodilation
   C) attraction of leukocytes
   D) attachment of lymphocytes to macrophages
   E) all of the above
   F) none of the above

6. The alternative pathway of complement activation is characterized by the functions listed below *except*:

A) activation of complement components beyond C3 in the cascade
B) participation of properdin
C) generation of anaphylatoxin
D) utilization of C4

7. Immunoglobulins that activate the first component of complement (C1q) via the Fc portion include
A) IgG
B) IgA
C) IgM
D) IgE
E) only A and B are correct
F) only A and C are correct
G) only B and C are correct
H) only C and D are correct

8. The following activate(s) the alternative pathway of complement:
A) endotoxin
B) monomeric IgG
C) yeast cell wall

D) C1
E) only A and C are correct
F) only B and D are correct
G) only A and B are correct

9. Which component(s) of complement could be missing and still leave the remainder of the complement system capable of activation by the alternative pathway?
A) C1, C2, and C3
B) C3 only
C) C2, C3, and C4
D) C1, C2, and C4
E) C1, C3, and C4

10. An antigen–antibody immune complex in a C3-deficient individual will still result in
A) anaphylatoxin production
B) depression of factor B
C) production of chemotactic factors
D) activation of C2
E) activation of C5

ANSWERS TO REVIEW QUESTIONS

1. **E** All these functions are mediated by complement components that come after C3 and in its absence cannot be activated.

2. **B** The hemolytic assay would reveal a defect in any one of the C components since all are required to effect hemolysis. The tests for specific components are likely to work only if you happen to pick the right one. They are not useful for screening. Electrophoretic analysis is good for the major serum components (albumin and globulin) but unlikely to give information on many of the complement components.

3. **F** Complement is required for the lysis of erythrocytes by anti-erythrocyte antibody (IgG or IgM) (**B**), and (**A**) for lysis of bacteria by specific anti-bacteria IgM or

IgG (**D**). Complement is not required for phagocytosis or lysis of erythrocytes by lecithinase. (However, the C3b opsonins, which are generated during complement activation, enhance phagocytosis of the opsonized particle.)

4. **F** C3a and C5a are activated during complement activation. Both are anaphylatoxins (**B**) and their presence leads to the degranulation of mast cells. C3b, which is generated during complement activation, is an opsonin (**D**), it coats particles and enhances phagocytosis by phagocytic cells that have receptors for C3b.

5. **D** C5a is an anaphylatoxin, which induces degranulation of mast cells, resulting in the release of histamine, which causes vasodilation and contraction of smooth muscles. C5a is also a chemotaxin, attracting leukocytes to the area of its release (where the antigen is reacting with antibodies and activates the complement system). It does not promote attachments of lymphocytes to macrophages.

6. **D** The alternative pathway of complement activation connects with the classical pathway at the activation of C3. Thus, it does not require C1, C4, or C2. Properdin is essential for the activation

through the alternative pathway, since it stabilizes the complex (C3bBb) formed between C3b and activated serum factor B, which acts as a C3 convertase and activates C3. During the activation of the alternative pathway both C3a and C5a are generated; both are anaphylatoxins and cause degranulation of mast cells.

7. **F** Only IgG (**A**) and IgM (**C**) have receptors for C1q.

8. **E** Endotoxin (lipopolysaccharide) from cell walls of gram-negative bacteria (**A**) and cell walls of yeasts (**C**) can activate the alternative pathway of complement.

9. **D** C3 is required for the alternative pathway of complement activation, while C1, C2, or C4 are not required.

10. **D** The immune complex will activate C2 (and C4) but will not activate C3 or any other components. Since the alternative pathway of complement activation also requires C3, this pathway will not be activated. Anaphylatoxins and chemotactic factor generation require C3, while the synthesis of factor B is not related to C3.

HYPERSENSITIVITY REACTIONS: ANTIBODY-MEDIATED, TYPE I—ANAPHYLACTIC REACTIONS

INTRODUCTION

Under some circumstances, *immunity,* rather than providing protection, produces damaging and sometimes fatal results. Such deleterious reactions are known collectively as *hypersensitivity* or *allergic* reactions; antigens that commonly cause hypersensitivity or allergic reactions are referred to as *allergens.* It should be remembered that hypersensitivity reactions differ from protective immune reactions only in that they are exaggerated or inappropriate and damaging to the host. The cellular and molecular mechanisms of the two types of reaction are virtually identical.

Hypersensitivity reactions were divided into four classes, designated types I–IV by Gell and Coombs:

Type I: Anaphylactic reactions are mediated by IgE antibodies, which bind through the Fc portion to receptors on *mast cells* and *basophils.* When cross-linked by antigens, the IgE antibodies trigger the mast cells and basophils to release pharmacologically active agents that are responsible for the characteristic symptoms of anaphylaxis. Reactions are rapid, occurring within minutes after challenge, that is, reexposure to antigen.

Type II: Cytolytic or cytotoxic reactions occur when *IgM* or *IgG* antibodies bind to antigen on the surface of cells and activate the complement cascade, which culminates in destruction of the cells.

Type III: Immune complex reactions occur when complexes of antigen and IgM or IgG antibody accumulate in the circulation or in tissue and activate the complement cascade. Granulocytes are attracted to the site of activation, and damage results from the release of lytic enzymes from their granules. Reactions occur within hours of challenge with antigen.

Type IV: Cell-mediated immunity (CMI) reaction—also called *delayed-type hypersensitivity (DTH)* or the *tuberculin reaction*—is mediated by T cells rather than by antibody. On activation, the T cells release lymphokines that cause accumulation and activation of macrophages, which, in turn, cause local damage. This type of reaction has a delayed onset and occurs 1–2 days after challenge with antigen.

This chapter deals with type I hypersensitivity, which involves anaphylactic reactions; types II and III are discussed in Chapter 15; cell-mediated immunity (type IV) is discussed in Chapter 16.

GENERAL CHARACTERISTICS OF TYPE I HYPERSENSITIVITY

The term *anaphylaxis* was coined by Portier and Richet (the latter is a Nobel Prize winner), who studied the effects of the toxin from a Mediterranean Sea anemone on dogs. Several weeks after an initial administration of the toxin, a second dose was given to determine whether the dogs had developed immunity to it. Some of the dogs, rather than showing increased resistance to the effects of the toxin, experienced excessive salivation, defecation, difficulty in respiration, paralysis of the hind limbs, and death within minutes of receiving the dose. Portier and Richet named this phenomenon *anaphylaxis,* from the Greek *ana,* which means "away from," and *phylaxis,* which means "protection." The term is the antithesis of the phenomenon of *prophylaxis* ("toward protection"). Subsequent studies revealed that anaphylaxis is the result of hypersensitivity rather than decreased resistance to the toxin. The discovery of anaphylaxis provided the first example of the ability of the immune system to cause harm.

The sequence of events involved in the development of anaphylactic sensitivity can be divided into several phases: (1) the *sensitization phase,* during which IgE antibody is produced in response to an antigenic stimulus and binds to specific receptors on mast cells and basophils; (2) the *activation phase,* during which reexposure to antigen triggers the mast cells and basophils to respond by release of the contents of their granules; and (3) the *effector phase,* during which a complex response (anaphylaxis) occurs as a result of the effects of the many pharmacologically active agents released by the mast cells and basophils.

SENSITIZATION PHASE

The antibody responsible for type I hypersensitivity is IgE, formerly called *reagin* or *reaginic antibody.* All normal individuals can make IgE antibody specific for a variety of antigens when the antigen is introduced parenterally in the appropriate manner. Approximately 50% of the population generates an IgE response to airborne antigens (also referred to as *allergens*) that are encountered only on mucosal surfaces, such as the lining of the nose and lungs and the conjunctiva of the eyes. However, 10% of the general population develops clinical symptoms (hay fever) after repeated exposure to a plethora of these airborne allergens such as plant pollens, mold spores, and animal dander. Allergists frequently use the term *atopy* (which means uncommon) to refer to this syndrome and the term *atopic* to describe affected patients. Since all members of a given population in a given locale have roughly the same quantitative contact with any particular allergen, such as ragweed pollen, it is unclear why a clinically significant response is made by only a small proportion of that population. It has been suggested that the response is under the control of MHC genes (see Chapter 10) (since familial tendencies are seen) and that differences in mucosal permeability may restrict the effects of antigens lodging on the surface.

IgE antibody production is T-cell-dependent and, in experimental animals, neonatal thymectomy abolishes the capacity to produce it. *Interleukin-4 (IL-4)* produced by CD4$^+$ Th2 cells is an important requirement for IgE production (see Chapters 10 and 15) since neutralizing antibodies against IL-4 can suppress IgE responses. It has also been suggested that the low level of IgE antibody in nonallergic individuals is maintained by suppressor T cells (see Chapter 12) and by IFNγ, which decreases IgE production. Thus a balance is maintained between those factors that upregulate and downregulate IgE responses. Natural events such as viral infection may disturb this balance and stimulate IgE-producing B cells. Therefore, allergic sensitization may result from failure of a control mechanism.

In any event, once adequate exposure to the allergen has been achieved by repeated mucosal contact, ingestion, or parenteral injection, and IgE antibody has been produced, an individual is considered to be **sensitized.** IgE antibody is made in small amounts (its concentration in the blood is the lowest of all immunoglobulins) and very rapidly becomes attached to mast cells and basophils as it circulates past them.

Mast cells, the main effector cells responsible for type I responses, are a ubiquitous family of cells generally found around blood vessels in the connective tissue, in the lining of the gut, and in the lungs. They are large **mononuclear cells,** heavily granulated and deeply stained by basic dyes such as toluidine blue (see Fig. 14.1). They are derived from progenitor cells that migrate to the tissue, where they differentiate into mature mast cells. In some species, a circulating, polynuclear granulated cell, called a **basophil,** also takes part in type I responses and

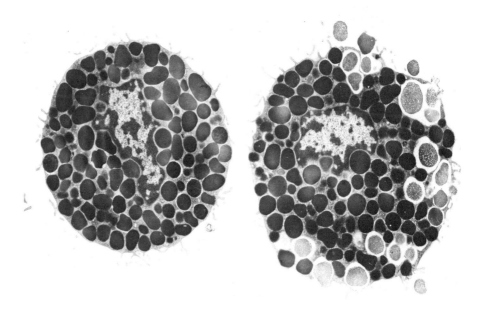

Figure 14.1

Electron micrograph of a normal mast cell illustrating the large monocyte-like nucleus and the electron-dense granules. On the right, a mast cell has been triggered and is beginning to release the contents of its granules, as seen by their decrease in opacity and the formation of vacuoles connecting with the exterior. (Photos courtesy of Dr. T. Theoharides, Tufts Medical School.)

functions in much the same way as the tissue-based mast cells. Unlike the mast cells they mature in the bone marrow and are present in the circulation in their differentiated form. One of the most important features that mast cells and basophils have in common is that both have specific receptors on their cell membranes that bind the Fc portion of IgE molecules with very high affinity. Once bound, the IgE molecules persist at the cell surface for weeks, and that cell will remain "sensitized" as long as enough antibody remains attached, and will trigger the activation of the cell when it comes into contact with antigen.

Sensitization may also be achieved passively by transfer of serum that contains IgE antibody to a specific antigen. A procedure of historical interest only known as the ***Prausnitz–Küstner (P–K)*** test used to be performed as a test for the antibodies responsible for anaphylactic reactions. In the P–K test serum from an allergic individual was injected into the skin of a normal person. After a lag period of 1–2 days, during which the locally injected antibody diffused toward neighboring mast cells and became bound to them, the site of injection was said to be sensitized, and would respond with an urticarial (hives) reaction when injected with that antigen to which the donor was allergic. Such a reaction in passively sensitized animals is called ***passive cutaneous anaphylaxis (PCA).***

ACTIVATION PHASE

The anaphylactic reaction itself may be triggered by injection of the specific antigen into the skin of a sensitized individual. This is commonly referred to as the ***challenge.*** Such challenge, when performed by intradermal injection into the skin, may result in local ***cutaneous anaphylaxis;*** when the challenging allergen is distributed throughout the body (such as following intravenous injection), the challenge may trigger ***systemic anaphylaxis.***

The response to intradermal challenge, called ***"wheal and flare,"*** is characterized by ***erythema*** (redness due to dilation of blood vessels) and ***edema*** (swelling produced by release of serum into tissue) (see Fig. 16.4A,B in Chapter 16). The anaphylactic reaction is the most rapid of all hypersensitivity reactions and reaches its peak within 10–15 minutes; then it fades without leaving any residual damage.

The size of the local skin reaction observed when an allergic patient is tested or challenged by intradermal injection of a battery of potential antigens (allergens) is roughly indicative of the degree of sensitivity to that particular substance. In addition, if the clinical history of symptoms correlates well with the time of contact with the antigen, then the cutaneous anaphylactic response may be taken as evidence that the symptoms (e.g., sneezing, itchy eyes) are attributable to the allergens of that particular plant pollen or animal dander that engendered the skin response. Other more quantitative tests are used as well (see below).

The activation phase of type I hypersensitivity reaction begins with the triggering of the mast cell to release its granules, and their pharmacologically active contents. It requires that at least two of the receptors for the Fc portion of the IgE molecules be bridged together in a stable configuration. In the simplest and immunologically most relevant manner, this linkage is accomplished by a multivalent antigen that can bind a different molecule of IgE to each of several epitopes on its surface, thus cross-linking them and effectively triggering the cell to respond (see Fig. 14.2). This linking of receptors may also be accomplished in other experimentally useful ways, such as by addition of an antibody that is specific for IgE molecules, or for the IgE receptor molecules on the surface of mast cells, or even by use of dimers or aggregates of IgE (see Fig. 14.2).

It should be pointed out that mast cells may be activated through mechanisms other than IgE. The anaphylatoxins C3a and C5a, products of complement activation (see Chapter 13), as well as various drugs such as codeine, morphine, and iodinated radiocontrast dyes, produce anaphylactoid reactions. Physical factors such as heat, cold, or pressure can also activate mast cells, as seen, for exam-

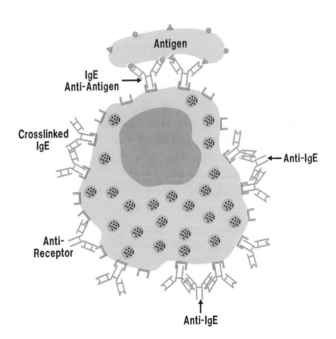

Figure 14.2

Various modes of cross-linking receptors leading to mast cell activation and degranulation.

ple, in cold-induced urticaria (an anaphylactic rash induced in certain individuals by chilling an area of skin).

The triggering of a mast cell by the bridging of its receptors initiates a rapid and complex series of events culminating in the degranulation of the mast cell and the release of pharmacologically potent molecules. Because of the ease with which its outcome can be measured, the mast cell has served as a model for the study of activation of cells in general. Among the rapid events known to occur are receptor aggregation, and changes in membrane fluidity, which result from methylation of phospholipids, leading to an influx of Ca^{2+} ions. The intracellular levels of *cyclic adenosine monophosphate (cAMP)* and cyclic *guanosine monophosphate (cGMP)* are known to affect subsequent events and are important in the regulation of those events. In general, an increase in intracellular cAMP at this stage will slow, or even stop, the process of degranulation. Thus, activation of *adenylate cyclase,* the enzyme that converts adenosine triphosphate (ATP) to cAMP, provides an important mechanism for controlling anaphylactic events.

As a very rapid consequence of this series of events, the mast-cell granules are moved by microfilaments to the cell surface, where their membranes fuse with the cell membrane and all the contents are released to the exterior (see Fig. 14.1). Depending on the extent of cross-linking on the cell surface, any cell can release some or all of its granules. Furthermore, this explosive release of granules is physiologic and does not imply lysis or death of the cell. In fact, the degranulated cells regenerate and, once the contents of the granules have been synthesized, the cells are ready to resume their function.

EFFECTOR PHASE

The symptoms of anaphylaxis are entirely attributable to the pharmacologically active materials released by the activated mast cells. It is helpful to consider these mediators in two major categories (Fig. 14.3). One category consists of basic *preformed mediators,* which are stored in the granules by electrostatic attraction to a matrix protein and are released as a result of the influx of ions, primarily Na^+. Recently it has been recognized that substances derived from the granule matrix itself produce inflammatory reactions and are involved in so-called late-phase reactions. The other category consists of *substances synthesized de novo,* in part from membrane lipids, and released during the anaphylactic response. Many potent substances are released during degranulation, however, only the most important members of each category are considered here.

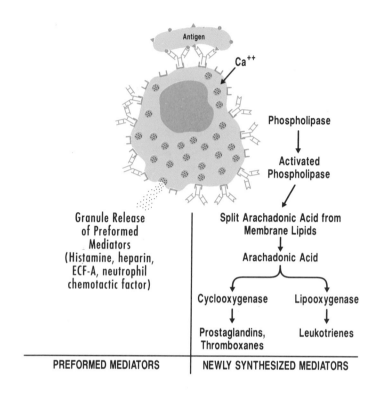

Figure 14.3

Mediators during activation
of mast cells.

Preformed Mediators

HISTAMINE. Histamine is formed in the cell by decarboxylation of the
amino acid histidine, and it is stored bound by electrostatic interaction to an acid
matrix protein called **heparin.** When released, histamine binds rapidly to a variety
of cells via two major types of receptor, **H1 and H2,** which have different distribution in tissue and that mediate different effects. When histamine binds to H1 receptors on smooth muscles it causes constriction; when it binds to H1 receptors
on endothelial cells it causes separation at their junctions, resulting in **vascular
permeability.** H2 receptors are those involved in mucus secretion and increased
vascular permeability, as well as in the release of acid from stomach mucosa. All
these effects are responsible for some of the major signs in systemic anaphylaxis:
difficulty in breathing **(asthma)** or asphyxiation due to **constriction of smooth
muscle** around the bronchi in the lung, and a **drop in blood pressure** that results
from extravasation of fluid into tissue spaces as the **permeability of blood vessels
increases.** H1 receptors are blocked by **antihistamines,** such as benadryl, by direct competition, and when these drugs are given soon enough, they can counter-

act the effects of histamine. Blockage of H2 receptors requires other drugs, such as cimetidine. However, some time after the introduction of antihistamines, it was noted that they were ineffective in controlling constriction of smooth muscles that was slower in onset and more persistent than that produced by histamine. This observation led to the discovery of SRS-A, the slow-reacting substance of anaphylaxis (see below), now known to consist of a group of *leukotrienes.*

SEROTONIN. Serotonin is present in the mast cells of only certain species, such as rodents. Its effects are similar to those of histamine, in that it causes *constriction of smooth muscle* and *increases vascular permeability.*

EOSINOPHILIC CHEMOTACTIC FACTOR OF ANAPHYLAXIS (ECF-A). Eosinophilic chemotactic factors are a set of low-molecular-weight *peptides* that produce a chemotactic gradient capable of attracting *eosinophils* to the site of release of these peptides. In anaphylactic reactions eosinophils appear to serve as a belated indicator of the presence of IgE-mediated reactions, especially the late-phase reaction of type I hypersensitivity discussed later; they may also release arylsulfatase and histaminase, which destroy several mediators of the hypersensitivity reaction, thus serving as one of the mechanisms to limit the reaction. Eosinophils have an additional function in parasitic worm infections, which is discussed later in this chapter.

NEUTROPHIL CHEMOTACTIC FACTORS (NCFs). Activated mast cells release several substances that are chemotactic for neutrophils, another set of polymorphonuclear granulocytes. Again, as we shall see later, granulocytes are important in the late phase of type I (IgE-mediated) hypersensitivity.

HEPARIN. Heparin is an *acidic proteoglycan* that constitutes the matrix of the granule, and to which basic mediators, such as histamine and serotonin, are bound. Its acidic nature accounts for the metachromatic (high-staining) properties of the mast cell when basic dyes such as toluidine blue are applied to it. Release of heparin causes *inhibition of coagulation,* which may be of some use in the subsequent recovery of the mast cell or further introduction of antigen into the reaction area; however, it is not directly involved in the symptoms of anaphylaxis.

Newly Synthesized Mediators

LEUKOTRIENES. When a preparation of smooth muscle, such as a guinea pig uterine horn, is treated with histamine, rapid contraction occurs. The contractions are the basis of a sensitive bioassay for histamine, the ***Schultz–Dale reaction.*** When the histamine is washed out, rapid relaxation occurs. Addition of an antihistamine to the assay prior to the addition of histamine inhibits the contraction effect of histamine. If the supernatant solution from a preparation of activated mast cells is also included in the assay, the immediate contraction effect of histamine is blocked by the antihistamine and does not occur; however, a slower prolonged contraction results, and it cannot be easily reversed by washing.

This observation led to the discovery of the ***slow-reacting substance of anaphylaxis (SRS-A),*** which is so potent and is present in such low concentration that its chemical structure defied analysis for many years. It is now known to consist of a set of peptides that are coupled to a metabolite of arachidonic acid and are called ***leukotrienes.*** The leukotrienes have been named LTB4, LTC4, and LTD4; in minute amounts, they cause ***prolonged constriction of smooth muscle.*** They are considered to be the cause of much antihistamine-resistant asthma in humans.

THROMBOXANES AND PROSTAGLANDINS. Leukotrienes are only a small part of the complex series of products produced from ***arachidonic acid*** released from cell membrane lipids by phospholipases during mast cell triggering. Arachadonic acid is a polyunsaturated, long-chain hydrocarbon that can be oxygenated in two separate pathways (Fig. 14.3): by lipoxygenase to give the above-mentioned leukotrienes and by cyclooxygenase to give prostaglandins and thromboxanes. Many of these latter compounds are vasoactive, causing bronchoconstriction, and are chemotactic for a variety of white cells, such as neutrophils, eosinophils, basophils, and monocytes.

PLATELET-ACTIVATING FACTOR. Platelet-activating factor (PAF) induces platelets to aggregate and release their contents of mediators, which include histamine and, in some species, serotonin. Activation of platelets may also induce release of metabolites of arachidonic acid, thus augmenting effects generated by mast cells. PAF itself is one of the most potent causes of bronchoconstriction and vasodilation known, producing shock-like symptoms rapidly in very small doses.

LATE-PHASE REACTION

In addition to the anaphylactic reaction described above, the many substances released during mast-cell activation and degranulation are responsible for the initiation of a profound inflammatory response with infiltration and accumulation of eosinophils, neutrophils, basophils, lymphocytes and macrophages. Most important, and constituting a large percent of the cells, are eosinophils and neutrophils that become activated and exacerbate the type I IgE-mediated hypersensitivity. This response often follows the IgE-mediated anaphylactic reaction within 4–8 hours and may persist for several days. This is referred to as the ***late-phase reaction*** and is shown diagrammatically in Figure 14.4. The mast cell, degranulated by cross-binding of IgE on its surface by antigen, releases ***eosinophil chemotactic factor (ECF-A)*** that recruit ***eosinophils*** to the reaction area. Their passage, as well as the passage of other leukocytes from the circulation to the tissue, is facilitated by the increased vascular permeability caused by histamine and other mediators. Various cytokines, notably ***granulocyte macrophage colony-stimulating factor (GM-CSF),*** IL-3, and IL-5, play an important role in eosinophil growth and differentiation.

Eosinophils bind via their Fc receptors to the Fc portion of IgE and IgG present on the antibody bound to antigen. They become activated and degranulate, releasing leukotrienes that cause muscle contraction. They also release platelet-activating factor (PAF) and major basic protein (MBP). MBP has the ability to destroy various parasites (such as schistosomes) by affecting their mobility and damaging their surface. Also, MBP is toxic to mammalian epithelium of the respiratory tract. Finally, the eosinophilic degranulation releases eosinophilic cationic protein (ECP), a potent neurotoxin and helminthotoxin. All these biologically active substances, while directed towards foreign invaders, cause tissue damage.

In addition to these eosinophil-mediated events, mast-cell degranulation releases neutrophil chemotactic factor (NCF), which attracts neutrophils to the area. The neutrophils come into close contact with antibody-coated antigen via Fc receptors on the neutrophils and become activated to phagocitize. In addition, they release their powerful lysosomal enzymes, which cause great tissue damage. Like degranulation products of eosinophils, degranulation products of neutrophils also include leukotrienes and platelet activating factor (PAF). Lymphocytes (both T and B) as well as macrophages enter the area, further sensitizing or immunizing the host against the offending antigen or microorganism. This dramatic series of events triggered and mediated by IgE is involved in the elimination of parasites, as described later in this chapter. Unfortunately, the same events take place in certain individuals when the antigen is a harmless substance such as pollen or animal hair and dander, resulting in tissue damage.

CLINICAL ASPECTS OF TYPE I HYPERSENSITIVITY

To summarize all the events that follow the release of the mediators of the anaphylactic response, we can describe a typical sequence of events. Contact with

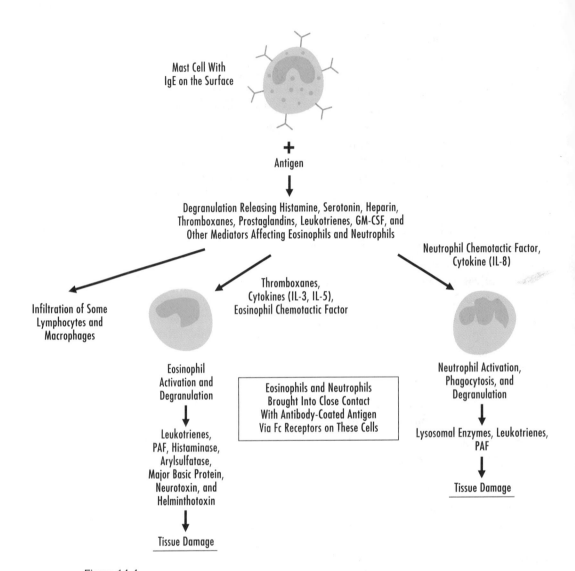

Figure 14.4

A diagrammatic representation of late-phase reaction of type I IgE-mediated hypersensitivity with some of the involved mediators.

antigen causes cross-linking of IgE receptors on mast cells. The cross-linking induces each mast cell to release its contents of mediators. Probably the first mediator to act would be histamine (or serotonin in some species). If release of histamine occurred locally as a result of intradermal injection of antigen (such as mosquito saliva injected during a mosquito bite), this would induce a typical "wheal and flare" reaction consisting of blood vessel dilation (flare) and increase in permeability (wheal). If release of histamine occurred systemically, as a result of the widespread dispersion of antigen, then much more severe consequences would ensue. This could include difficulty in breathing (asthma) because of constriction of bronchiolar muscles, uterine cramps, or involuntary urination and defecation. In addition, widespread vascular permeability could produce a massive loss of fluid into tissue spaces (hives and edema) and a drastic fall in blood pressure (shock).

The symptoms of anaphylaxis seen in systemic reactions vary widely with the species observed, although the basic mechanisms are the same. Guinea pigs, for example, die from asphyxiation produced by histamine-induced constriction of bronchioles, whereas dogs suffer from a pooling of the blood in the intestine and liver, vomiting, and diarrhea. Humans are confronted with three different possibilities of a lethal outcome: (1) asphyxiation from laryngeal edema, (2) suffocation from bronchiolar contraction, or (3) loss of adequate blood pressure from overwhelming peripheral edema.

A second set of pharmacologically active agents comes into play next as a result of de novo synthesis from arachidonic acid. Arachidonic acid is metabolized in one of two ways: the cyclooxygenase pathway leading to prostaglandins and thromboxanes or the lipoxygenase pathway leading to leukotrienes. The former are known to be involved in inflammation and vasoconstriction, while the leukotrienes, as we have seen, were called SRS-A because of their ability to produce prolonged contraction of smooth muscle and increased vascular permeability.

"Classic" anaphylactic reactions develop in minutes and abate within a half to one hour, but these are often followed by inflammatory sequelae called "late-phase" reactions. Clinically, they evolve from the immediate "wheal and flare"-type response into an area of redness, burning, itching, and warmth some 6–8 hours after contact with antigen. As already pointed out, where these occur they serve to prolong and extend the consequences of the immediate response mediators. The effectors of this phase of response are many, as we have discussed earlier and shown in Figure 14.4.

It is widely recognized that many allergic reactions are due to food allergens.

Various foods or their metabolic derivatives sensitize the gastrointestinal tract, leading to the production of IgE antibodies. Subsequent exposure to these allergens may result in mast-cell degranulation and the release of mediators that cause changes in gut permeability, with the possible dissemination of antigen–antibody complexes into distal areas of the body such as the skin or lungs, initiating urticaria or asthmatic disorders.

Thus, as we can see, continued study of the IgE-mediated anaphylactic response has revealed several layers of complexity, each with profound clinical implications, produced by the multiple active products formed and released when mast cells are triggered.

Detection

In a clinical setting, the degree of sensitivity to a particular allergen is usually determined by the patient's complaints and by the extent of skin test reactions. To avoid serious consequences from intradermal challenge in patients who may be extremely sensitive to certain allergens, a skin-prick test that introduces minute amounts of antigen is first given. Generally the extent of the skin test reaction (wheal and flare) observed within 30 minutes of challenge correlates roughly with the degree of sensitivity. We should, however, not forget the possibility of a late-phase reaction, which may occur in some individuals within several hours following the challenge and that sometimes may last 24 hours.

A more quantitative assay that correlates, albeit not 100%, with clinical symptoms, is available in the laboratory. Known as the ***radioallergosorbent test (RAST),*** this procedure involves covalent coupling of the allergen to an insoluble matrix, such as paper disks or beads. The antigen-coated matrix is then dipped into a sample of the patient's serum and allowed to bind any antibody that is specific for the allergen. After the disk is washed, a radiolabeled antibody specific for IgE is added. The amount of radioactivity bound is a measure of the amount of specific IgE antibody in the serum sample (see Fig. 14.5).

Intervention

ENVIRONMENTAL INTERVENTION. In some cases, the easiest treatment for allergy is avoidance, an advice followed infrequently. If some pollens are the cause of the reaction, it may be possible for the patient to go to pollen-free

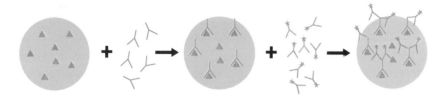

Antigen covalently   Human IgE   Isotopically
linked to paper disk   against the   labeled antibodies
                     antigen   to human IgE

Figure 14.5

The radioallergosorbent test (RAST).

areas during the season when the offending plant is pollinating. Masks and air filters also have a useful role to play, but usually avoidance is difficult for the general atopic population.

PHARMACOLOGIC INTERVENTION. Modern pharmaceutical chemistry has provided a host of drugs that are more or less effective at various stages in the evolution of the anaphylactic reaction. In brief, these drugs include (1) *cromolyn sodium,* which stabilizes membranes, prevents Ca^{2+} influx, and decreases or prevents mast cell degranulation when administered before antigen exposure [also, theophylline (and several other substances), which causes increase in cAMP and thus inhibits mast-cell degranulation, is given orally or by inhalation to asthmatic patients, hopefully prior to exposure to antigen]; (2) *corticosteroids,* especially when topically applied, which block the metabolic pathways involving arachidonic acid and have general anti-inflammatory effects, thus preventing late phase reactions; (3) *antihistamines,* which compete with histamine for receptor sites, thereby decreasing or preventing immediate symptoms such as sneezing, itching, and runny nose; and (4) *epinephrine,* which most effectively treats the life-threatening systemic effects of anaphylaxis. It directly reverses the effects of histamine by relaxing smooth muscle and decreasing vascular permeability.

IMMUNOLOGIC INTERVENTION. For many years, allergists have practiced a form of therapy, called injection therapy or *hyposensitization,* whereby they inject patients, over an extended period, with increasing doses of the antigen to which they are sensitive. The improvement in symptoms noted in some patients has been ascribed to several different factors. The most popular rationale is based on the observation that such injections serve to increase the synthesis of IgG antibody specific for the allergen. Such antibody in the circulation presumably binds to and removes the allergen before it has a chance to reach and react with the IgE antibody on the surface of mast cells. Thus, the term ***blocking antibody*** has become associated with this IgG, and there is a rough correlation between titers of this IgG antibody generated and clinical improvement.

Other findings during hyposensitization include an initial increase in levels of IgE antibody, followed by a prolonged decrease on continued therapy. This decrease has been linked to a decrease in intensity of symptoms and is attributed either to induction of ***tolerance,*** to a ***switch from Th2 to Th1*** T cells or to the induction of ***suppressor T cells.*** After repeated subclinical doses of the antigen, there is also a progressive decrease in the sensitivity of mast cells and basophils to triggering by antigen. It is likely that the explanation for the apparent benefits of this immunologic therapy encompasses more than one of these demonstrable effects. Whatever the reason, this form of therapy is generally more successful in dealing with allergens that enter the circulation directly, such as bee-sting venom, than for those allergens contacted via mucosal surfaces, such as pollen, where IgG antibody is unlikely to be effective.

Hyposensitization therapy should be distinguished from ***desensitization.*** Occasionally, patients must be treated promptly with substances to which they are allergic, for example, when horse antivenom serum for treatment of a rattlesnake bite is given to someone who is sensitive to the horse serum antigens. The sensitive patient must then be given increasingly large doses of the horse antivenom over a short period of time (hours), with each dose below the level that will precipitate a serious systemic reaction. During this period, sufficient horse antigens are given to trigger enough sublethal discharges from mast cells that a therapeutic dose of antitoxin can now be given without danger of inducing fatal anaphylaxis. The risk of severe reactions may also be reduced by prior administration of antihistamines and steroids. Such preliminary treatment causes a more or less temporary period of unreactivity during which, presumably, the available supply of IgE-sensitized mast cells is used up. In time, recovery of mast cells and new synthesis of IgE antibody lead to a restoration of the original sensitivity.

MODIFIED ALLERGENS. Experiments in animals have demonstrated that administration of a ***chemically altered allergen*** (e.g., ragweed pollen denatured by urea or coupled to polyethylene glycol) will suppress a primary or established IgE response. The mechanism may involve the induction of ***suppressor T cells*** that are both antigen-specific and isotype-specific. The modified allergens do not combine with preexisting IgE antibodies and, therefore, do not trigger anaphylactic responses. Use of such modified allergens *(allergoids)* seems to offer a promising approach to treatment of allergy. A more rational approach would involve determining the specific epitopes on the allergen to which the helper T cells are directed and to induce tolerance specifically to these epitopes.

THE PROTECTIVE ROLE OF IgE

The protective effects of anaphylactic reactivity may be seen in the situation where the causative antigen of the anaphylactic response is derived from one of many parasitic worms such as helminths. The immune response to these worms favors the induction of IgE for reasons which are still not clear. As a consequence of antigens from the worm cross-linking IgE on the surface of mast cells, histamine and other mediators associated with the anaphylactic response are released. The effects of increased permeability due to histamine release serve to

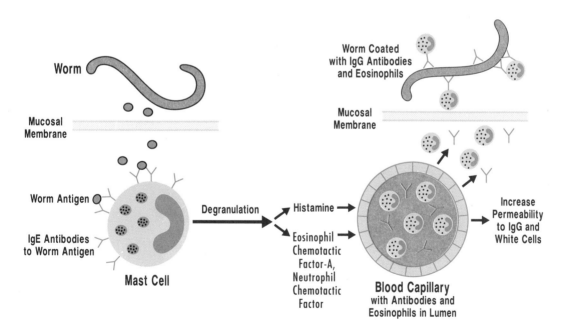

Figure 14.6A

A diagrammatic representation of the destruction of a worm by eosinophils that have been liberated and activated following IgE- and antigen-mediated mast cell degranulation.

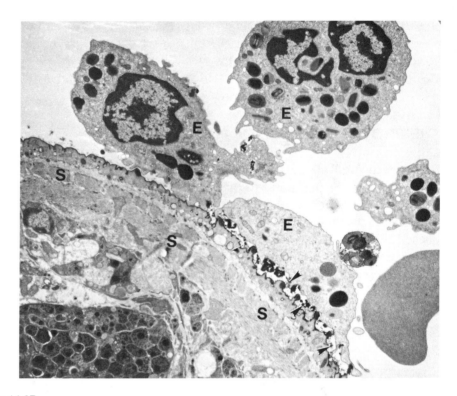

Figure 14.6B

Electron micrograph (×6,000) of eosinophils (E) adhering to an antibody-coated schistosomulum (S). The cell on the left has not yet degranulated, but the one on the right has discharged electron-dense material (arrows), which can be seen between the cell and the worm. (Photo courtesy of Dr. J. Caulfield, Harvard Medical School.)

bring serum components, which include IgG antibody, to the site of worm infestation. The IgG antibody binds to the surface of the worm and attracts the eosinophils, which have migrated to the area as a result of the chemotactic effects of the ***eosinophilic chemotactic factor (ECF-A).*** The eosinophils then bind to the IgG-coated worm, by virtue of their membrane receptors for Fc, and release the contents of their granules (Fig. 14.6A,B). The major constituent of the contents of these granules is a ***major basic protein,*** referred to previously, which coats the surface of the worm and leads, in some unknown way, to the death of the worm and its eventual expulsion. Thus, all components of the type I reaction combine to perform this protective function. This beneficial effect of the anaphylactic response in many animals suggests that responses involving IgE may have evolved to play a role in dealing with worm parasitism and not just to be a nuisance in human allergies.

SUMMARY

Type I anaphylactic reactions are mediated by IgE antibodies, which bind to specific receptors on the surface of mast cells and basophils. When these receptors are cross-linked by contact with specific antigen, the cell is triggered to respond by releasing its granules and their contents, as well as synthesizing other products from its membrane.

The combined pharmacologic effects of these mediators produce the immediate symptoms typical of this response: increased vascular permeability, constriction of smooth muscles, and influx of eosinophils.

A "late-phase" reaction consisting of redness and itching may appear later as a result of the inflammatory response to granule–matrix constituents of the mast cell.

Despite the dangerous systematic reactions produced by this mode of immune response, its value probably lies in its ability to provide immunity to parasitic infections.

REFERENCES

Bevan MA, Metzger H (1993): Signal transduction by Fc receptors: The Fc RI case. Immunol Today 14:222.

Galli SJ, Austin KF (eds) (1989): Mast Cell and Basophil Differentiation and Function in Health and Disease. New York, Raven Press.

Hamawy MM, Mergenhagen SE, Siraganian RS (1994): Adhesion molecules as regulators of mast cell and basophil function. Immunol Today 15:62.

Ishizaka K (1988): IgE binding factors and regulation of the IgE antibody response. Annu Rev Immunol 6:513.

Kuby J (1992): Immunology, New York: Freeman.

Lichenstein LM (1993): Allergy and the immune system. Sci Am (Sept):126.

Mygid N (1986): Essential Allergy. Oxford: Blackwell Scientific Publications.

Plant M, Zimmerman EM (1993): Allergy and mechanisms of hypersensitivity. In Paul WE (ed): Fundamental Immunology, 3rd ed. New York: Raven Press.

Terr AI (1994): Mechanisms of hypersensitivity. In Stites DP, Terr AI, Parslow TG (eds): Basic and Clinical Immunology, 8th ed. Norwalk, CT: Appleton & Lange.

Terr AI (1994): The atopic diseases. In Stites DP, Terr AI, Parslow TG (eds): Basic and Clinical Immunology, 8th ed. Norwalk, CT: Appleton & Lange.

Terr AI (1994): Anaphylaxis and urticaria. In Stites DP, Terr AI, Parslow TG (eds): Basic and Clinical Immunology, 8th ed. Norwalk, CT: Appleton & Lange.

REVIEW QUESTIONS

For each question, choose the ONE BEST answer or completion.

1. Injection therapy (hyposensitization)
   A) is safe if used initially with high concentrations of antigen
   B) is more effective for symptoms of hay fever than for wasp sting
   C) directly affects stability of membranes
   D) is a form of active immunity
   E) induces large amounts of endogenous antihistamines

2. Epinephrine
   A) causes bronchodilation
   B) is effective even after anaphylactic symptoms commence
   C) relaxes smooth muscle
   D) decreases vascular permeability
   E) all of the above

3. An IgE myeloma protein
   A) can competitively inhibit binding of normal IgE to mast cells
   B) is the most commonly found form of myeloma protein
   C) will inhibit binding of antigen to IgE antibody
   D) will spontaneously induce anaphylaxis
   E) will increase a patient's immediate skin test response to an antigen

4. The following mechanism(s) may be involved in the clinical efficacy of injection therapy:

A) enhanced production of IgG, which binds allergen before it reaches mast cells
B) enhanced production of suppressor T cells
C) decreased sensitivity of mast cells and basophils to degranulation by allergen
D) decreased production of IgE antibody
E) all of the above

5. Fatal anaphylaxis in humans and dogs
   A) has identical symptoms
   B) involves mast cells in humans only
   C) is very rapid
   D) has similar target organs
   E) occurs only in genetically susceptible individuals

6. Immediate hypersensitivity skin reactions
   A) usually occur within 15 minutes
   B) exhibit a raised wheal due to infiltration by mononuclear cells
   C) exhibit a red flare due to vasodilation
   D) can be elicited by monovalent haptens
   E) only A and C are correct
   F) only B and D are correct
   G) all are correct

7. Mast cells
   A) are found circulating in the blood
   B) release their granules by lysing
   C) are basophilic after complete degranulation
   D) are very similar to basophils
   E) all are correct

8. Antihistamines
   A) bind to receptors for histamine, thereby preventing the histamine from exerting a pharmacologic effect

B) are more effective given before, rather than after, the onset of allergic symptoms

C) do not influence the activity of leukotrienes

D) do not affect binding of IgE to mast cells

E) all are correct

9. In the RAST assay for ragweed pollen

A) the patient's serum is first mixed with a radiolabeled anti-IgE

B) only IgE anti-ragweed antibodies are detected

C) the patient's serum competitively inhibits binding of the anti-IgE

D) monovalent IgE is used

E) complement is utilized

10. Antigen interaction with IgE antibody is associated with

A) Prausnitz–Küstner reaction

B) Schultz–Dale reaction

C) rhinitis due to ragweed pollen

D) eosinophilia

E) all of the above

11. Anaphylactic reactions

A) evolve in minutes and abate within 30 minutes

B) may be followed by inflammatory sequelae hours later

C) are the consequences of released pharmacologic agents

D) may involve components of mast-cell granule matrix

E) all of the above

Case study: While playing tennis on a warm day a young man felt a wasp on his arm and brushed it off, but still received a mild sting, which he ignored. Ten minutes later he felt dizzy and began to itch under his arms and on his scalp. When he broke out in hives and felt a tightness in his chest, he headed for the hospital. On the way he felt cold and clammy and collapsed on the seat of the taxi. In the emergency room his pulse was barely detectable. What happened, and why?

ANSWERS TO REVIEW QUESTIONS

1. **D** At least one of the proposed rationales for use of injection therapy involves the production of IgG-blocking antibody induced by active immunization. Thus, *A*, *B*, and *E* are false, and there is no basis for *C*.

2. **E** All are effects of epinephrine and make it useful for treatment of acute anaphylactic symptoms.

3. **A** IgE is the least common myeloma protein because of the smaller number of

precursor B cells for this type of antibody. Production of large amounts of IgE globulin will compete for binding sites on mast cells, preventing specific IgE from binding. Therefore, *C* and *D* are false; the converse of *E* is true.

4. *E* All are considered to be involved to varying degrees in injection therapy.

5. *C* Anaphylaxis is very rapid in all species but differs in symptomatology. Anaphylactic sensitivity can be induced in virtually all individuals, but only a proportion becomes sensitized through normal airborne contact.

6. *E* The wheal is due to fluid, not cells, and multivalent antigens are required to cross-link IgE molecules. Thus only *A* and *C* are true statements.

7. *D* Mast cells release granules physiologically and not by lysing, they are basophilic before but not after they de-

granulate, and they are not found circulating freely. Mast cells are similar to circulating basophils.

8. *E* All are correct statements.

9. *B* The RAST assay measures IgE antibody that is allowed to bind to allergen coupled to an insoluble matrix. It detects IgE antiragweed antibodies. It does not utilize monovalent IgE, and complement is not utilized in the test.

10. *E* All involve IgE-mediated responses: (*A*) in the skin, (*B*) in an experimental system in vitro, (*C*) in an atopic nose, and (*D*) in response to a chronic antigenic challenge (to worm parasites, for example).

11. *E* All are true. *A* and *C* are true of the classic "wheal and flare" type response, while *B* and *D* describe features of the "late-phase" response, which is a complication of some anaphylactic reactions.

Case study: This is a classic case of systemic anaphylaxis. In the emergency room epinephrine was promptly administered and the symptoms due to vascular permeability (hives, low blood pressure) and smooth muscle constriction (difficulty in breathing) were reversed. When he revived sufficiently, he revealed that he had been stung by similar-looking insects in the past, the last time 3 months ago, but without any noticeable effects. These stings were apparently the priming injections building up sufficient levels of IgE antibody to sensitize his mast cells. Thus the last sting, despite the fact that little venom was injected, was sufficient to precipitate a systemic reaction. A careful skin test involving intradermal injection of very dilute wasp venom should show an immediate "wheal and flare" response, confirming the existence of sensitivity. The young man should be advised to (1) avoid wasps, (2) carry an emergency vial of injectable epinephrine, and (3) undergo injection therapy aimed at hyposensitization to the wasp venom antigen.

HYPERSENSITIVITY REACTIONS: ANTIBODY-MEDIATED, TYPE II—CYTOTOXIC REACTIONS AND TYPE III—IMMUNE COMPLEX REACTIONS

TYPE II—CYTOTOXIC REACTIONS

Introduction

In type II hypersensitivity, binding of the specific antibody directly to an antigen on the surface of a cell produces damage to that cell through a variety of mechanisms. These mechanisms involve either the complete complement sequence and eventual lysis of the cell or opsonic effects mediated by receptors for Fc or C3b. These lead to phagocytosis and destruction of the cell by macrophages and neutrophils which have on their surface receptors for Fc or C3b. Some clinically important examples of type II reactions are given below.

Transfusion Reactions

The simplest form of cytotoxic reaction is seen after transfusion of ABO incompatible blood (see Chapter 19). As an example, people with type O blood have in their circulation, for reasons that are still not completely clear, IgM anti-A and anti-B antibodies which react with the A and B blood-group substances. If such a person were to be transfused with a unit of type A red cells, the immediate consequences could be disastrous. Since there is a considerable amount of IgM anti-A antibody in this person's circulation, all the transfused type A red cells will bind some antibody. Because of the efficiency of IgM antibody in activating complement (a single IgM molecule is sufficient to activate many complement molecules; see Chapter 13), and because of the absence of repair mechanisms, red cells will be lysed intravascularly by the destructive action of complement on their membranes. Not only does this nullify the desirable effects of the transfusion; the individual is also faced with the risk of kidney damage from blockage by large quantities of red cell membrane, plus the possible toxic effects from the release of the heme complex.

Rh Incompatibility Reaction

A somewhat similar mechanism is exemplified by the ***rhesus (Rh) incompatibility reaction*** seen in infants born of parents with Rh-incompatible blood groups (see Chapter 19). In the simplest case, an Rh$^+$ child born to an Rh$^-$ mother releases some of its red cells into the mother's circulation during birth. If the mother is thereby sufficiently immunized to produce anti-Rh antibody of the IgG isotype, subsequent Rh$^+$ fetuses will be at risk, since, as we saw in Chapter 5, only IgG antibody is capable of crossing the placenta. Thus, in second or subsequent pregnancies, when the anti-Rh IgG antibodies have crossed the placenta, they bind to the Rh antigen on the red cells of the fetus. Because the density of Rh antigen on the surface of red blood cells is low, these antibodies usually fail to agglutinate or lyse the cells directly. However, the antibody-coated cells are readily destroyed by the opsonic effect of the Fc portions of the IgG, which interact with the receptors for Fc on the phagocytic cells of the reticuloendothelial system. The result is progressive destruction of the fetal or newborn red cells, with the pathological consequences that come from decreased transport of oxygen and result in jaundice from the products of the breakdown of hemoglobin.

Autoimmune Reactions

As a consequence of certain infectious diseases, or for other, still unknown reasons, some people produce an antibody reactive against their own red cells. This antibody, on binding to the red cells, shortens their life span or destroy them altogether by mechanisms that involve hemolysis or phagocytosis via receptors for Fc and C3b. This may lead to progressive anemia if the production of new red cells cannot keep pace with destruction. Occasionally, the antibody only binds effectively at lower temperatures *(cold agglutinin)*, in which case lowering of body temperature, particularly the lower temperature of the arms and legs, leads to effective antibody binding and destruction of the red cells.

Another example of cell destruction by autoantibodies is *idiopathic thrombocytopenia purpura*. In this condition antibodies directed to platelets result in platelet destruction by complement or phagocytic cells with Fc or C3b receptors. Decrease in platelet numbers may lead to bleeding *(purpura)*.

Drug-Induced Reactions

In some people, certain drugs act as haptens and combine with cells or with other circulating blood constituents and induce antibody formation. When antibody combines with cells coated with the drug, cytotoxic damage results. The type of pathologic injury depends on the type of cell that binds the drug. Thus, for example, Sedormid (a sedative) binds to platelets and the resulting antibody directed against it causes lysis of the platelets and resulting *thrombocytopenia* (low blood platelet count). This disorder, in turn, can give rise to *purpura*, which is the main problem in drug-induced thrombocytopenia purpura. Withdrawal of the offending drug leads to a cessation of symptoms. Other drugs, such as chloramphenicol (an antibiotic), may bind to white cells; phenacetin (an analgesic) and chlorpromazine (a tranquilizer) may bind to red cells. The consequences of an immune response to these drugs can lead to an *agranulocytosis* (decrease in granulocytes) in the case of white cells and a *hemolytic anemia* in the case of red cells. Damage to the target cell in these examples may be mediated by either of the two mechanisms described above: by cytolysis via the complement pathway or by destruction of cells by phagocytosis mediated by receptors for Fc or C3b.

It should be pointed out that whereas the preceding discussion emphasizes type II reaction induced by drugs, type I, II, III, and IV reactions may be induced because of hypersensitivity to drugs. Some reactions are induced by a drug acting as a hapten conjugated to some body components; other reactions (type IV) can be induced by the drug acting as a contact sensitizer (see Chapter 16).

Antireceptor Antibody Disease

A number of clinical disorders are known that involve the production of antibodies against various cell receptor molecules on cells, leading, in some cases, to the loss of function of those cells by cytotoxic effects or, in other cases, to the activation of the cell by the antibody. Myasthenia gravis, for example, is associated with antibody to the acetylcholine receptors on motor endplates of muscles and leads to muscle weakness of all striated muscle groups. Graves' disease, on the other hand, involves antibodies to the thyroid-stimulating hormone (TSH) receptor of thyroid cells and gives rise to hyperthyroidism through the activation of the thyroid cells by engagement of the TSH receptor. These disorders are discussed in more detail in Chapter 17, which deals with the subject of autoimmunity.

TYPE III—IMMUNE COMPLEX REACTIONS

Introduction

In 1903, a French scientist named Arthus immunized rabbits with horse serum by repeated intradermal injection. After several weeks, he noted that each succeeding injection produced an increasingly severe reaction at the site of inoculation. At first a mild *erythema* (redness) and *edema* (accumulation of fluid) were noticed within 2–4 hours of injection. These reactions subsided without consequence by the following day, but subsequent injections produced larger edematous responses, and by the fifth or sixth inoculations the lesions became hemorrhagic with *necrosis* and were slow to heal. This phenomenon, known as the *Arthus reaction*, is the prototype of all type III immune complex reactions or reactions mediated by aggregates of antibody and antigen.

A second type of immune complex reaction is called *serum sickness*. This term derives from observations made at the turn of the century by von Pirquet and Schick of the consequences of the treatment of certain infectious diseases, such as diphtheria and tetanus, with antisera made in horses. It was well known that the pathologic consequences of infection by both the *Corynebacterium* and the

Clostridium organisms were due to the secretion of exotoxins that are extremely damaging to host cells. The bacteria themselves are relatively noninvasive and of little consequence. Hence, the strategy that evolved to treat these diseases was to neutralize the toxins rapidly, before quantities large enough to kill the host became fixed in tissues. Since active immunization required several weeks before useful levels of antibody were produced, it was necessary to protect the individual through passive immunization by injecting large amounts of a preformed antitoxin antibody as soon as the disease was diagnosed, in order to prevent death by toxin. Horses, which were readily available, easily immunized, and capable of yielding large quantities of useful antisera, were the animals of choice for the production of antitoxin. Today, we know that the administration of large quantities of heterologous serum, from another species, causes the recipient to synthesize antibodies to the foreign Ig, leading to the formation of antigen–antibody complexes that result in the clinical symptoms associated with serum sickness.

The Arthus reaction and serum sickness represent two classical examples of type III hypersensitivity, also referred to as immune complex reactions.

The Arthus Reaction

Antigen injected intradermally in an immune animal diffuses toward blood vessels that contain the circulating antibody. When antigen and antibody meet, at the appropriate concentrations, in or near vessel walls (venules), they form *insoluble antigen–antibody complexes* and accumulate (see Fig. 15.1), much as they would

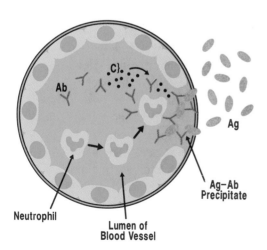

Figure 15.1.

A diagrammatic representation of the Arthus reaction.

on a gel-diffusion (Ouchterlony) plate (see Chapter 7). When the aggregates become large enough, the adjacent Fc regions of the IgG molecules bind the first component of complement and begin the *activation of the complement cascade*, as we have discussed in Chapter 13. The formation of *C3a and C5a (anaphylotoxins)* causes an increased local permeability of blood vessels, with leakage of fluid from the vessels (edema). Other components are chemotactic and attract *neutrophils*, and these neutrophils, together with *platelets*, begin to pile up at the site of the reaction. Eventually, stasis of blood flow and complete blockage of the blood vessel occurs. The activated neutrophils phagocytize the immune complexes and, together with the clumped platelets, release a complex array of *proteases, collagenases*, and *vasoactive substances*. The end result is rupture of the vessel wall and *hemorrhage*, accompanied by *necrosis* of local tissue (see Fig. 16.4C,D in Chapter 16).

The experimental proof of this course of events involves the demonstration, by the use of fluorescent antibodies, that antigen, antibody, and various complement components can all be detected at the site of damage to the vessel wall. The requirement for complement and granulocytes together was shown in experiments in which animals depleted of complement (*by cobra venom factor*) or of neutrophils (by specific antipolymorphonuclear cell serum) formed aggregates of antigen and antibody, but did not produce the characteristic Arthus reactions.

Although it is the prototype for type III hypersensitivity reactions, the Arthus reaction is clinically the least commonly seen. Nevertheless, it best illustrates the underlying mechanism for immune aggregate reactions.

Serum Sickness

The strategy of passive immunization for treatment of diseases whose effects were due to production of toxins worked very well and was widely used until universal active immunization of children became standard practice. However, some recipients of this therapy with horse antisera, while spared the bacteriologic disease and the effect of the toxin, developed undesirable reactions. About 1–2 weeks after receiving the horse serum they developed fever and itchy, edematous rashes over parts of their bodies, painful swollen joints, and enlarged lymph nodes. Occasionally their urine was found to contain red cells and albumin, a sign of inflammation in the glomerular apparatus of the kidney. In time, all these symptoms subsided with little residual damage, but a repeat injection of horse serum could induce much more severe symptoms and even death. While this sequence of events, as we shall see, can be induced by many other types of antigens, it still bears the name *"serum sickness."* This form of hypersensitivity is again becoming an important consideration in patients being treated for malignancy, graft rejection, or autoimmune disease with monoclonal antibodies made in mice or rats. The mechanism of the type of reaction typified by serum sickness is best understood by reference to the animal model that was instrumental in its clarification. In this model, a rabbit is injected with a large amount of a foreign protein, such as bovine serum albumin (BSA). After equilibration in the body fluid spaces, the protein begins to disappear at a rate characteristic of normal biodegradative processes (Fig. 15.2). After about 8–10 days, there is a sudden change in the rate of disappearance, and the residual free protein is completely cleared from the circulation. This event, termed ***immune elimination***, is soon followed by the appearance of free circulating antibodies to BSA. It is during the period that corresponds with the onset of rapid disappearance of antigen and ends with the rise in the level of free antibody that the symptoms of serum sickness appear. At the same time, there is a drop in the normal level of complement activity in the serum. These changes were explained by the discovery, in the circulating blood, of soluble complexes of the antigen BSA and antibodies to BSA. With the onset of production of antibody, the first complexes formed are those that involve a relatively small amount of antibody and an excess of antigen. Reference to the precipitin curve (see Chapter 7) will show that such complexes are small (of the order of Ag_2Ab or Ag_3Ab_2) and soluble.

Circulating immune complexes may normally be removed by phagocytic cells of the reticuloendothelial system. In addition, red blood cells that have C3b

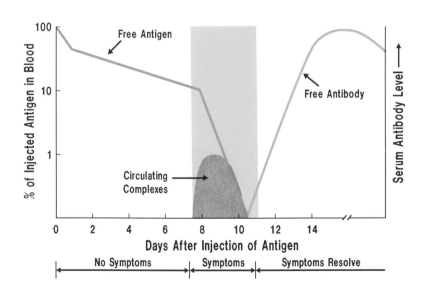

Figure 15.2.

The relationship between circulating antigen–antibody complexes and serum sickness.

receptors may bind complexes that have fixed complement and transport them to the liver, where the complexes are removed by Kupffer cells. Under some circumstances, circulating complexes are not removed by the reticuloendothelial system and may deposit in such tissues as kidney, joints, or skin. The size of the complex is important; large complexes are removed by the liver, whereas small complexes may not be deposited at all. Intermediate-size complexes are most likely to localize and produce tissue damage. The sites of deposition of the complexes in tissues is generally dependent on a change in vascular permeability, which permits the complexes to escape from blood vessels into tissue spaces. This permeability may be IgE-mediated with release of vasoactive amines (histamine) from mast cells, basophils, or platelets, or the result of anaphylatoxins (C3a, C5a).

An important observation in the rabbit model of serum sickness was that if several rabbits were similarly injected with a large dose of BSA, they subsequently tended to fall into three groups. The first group made no antibody and cleared the antigen at a steady slow rate with no symptoms of serum sickness. The second group produced copious amounts of antibody, cleared the antigen very rapidly, and had only transient and minimal symptoms. Apparently, large amounts of antibody produce large complexes, which are removed by the macrophages of the reticuloendothelial system and produce few clinical symptoms. It was in the third group—the group that made only small amounts of antibody—that symptoms of serum sickness were most prolonged and most severe. In this group, a chronic disease resulted from the continual production of soluble complexes generated from excess antigen and low levels of antibody. The continuous pileup of such complexes on membranes leads to the appearance of so-called *lumpy-bumpy deposits* that are visualized by fluorescence microscopy of lesions on glomerular basement membrane lesions (see Fig. 16.4I in Chapter 16). Once deposited, the complexes behave much as those in the Arthus reaction. Adjacent Fc regions of the IgG molecules bind C1q and initiate the *complement* cascade. The chemotactically induced influx of *granulocytes* into the lesion is the critical event that leads to the loss of integrity of the basement membrane. As a result of the actions of the degradative enzymes released from the *lysosomal granules* of the *neutrophils*, the basement membrane is disrupted and leaks serum and red cells into the urine. The attendant *necrosis*, if sufficiently widespread, can jeopardize the entire kidney function.

Similar events may occur in blood vessels of the skin, heart, and lung, as well as in joint synovial spaces. While there tends to be preferential localization of lesions in certain clinical conditions (e.g., in skin, rather than in glomerular basement membrane or joints), the reasons for this preferential localization are not completely understood.

A mechanism for generating complexes at a specific site has been described recently. This mechanism involves the nonspecific infiltration of a tissue site by antigen before synthesis of antibody commences. When circulating antibody appears, it binds to the tissue-fixed antigen, thus generating complexes in situ rather than in the circulation. This mechanism may be particularly relevant for certain antigens, such as DNA, which is known to bind preferentially to the collagen of basement membranes. In all other details, however, the consequences are identical whether the complexes are formed locally or in the circulation.

Infection-Associated Immune Complex Disease

In a variety of infections and for as yet unknown reasons, some individuals produce an antibody that cross-reacts with some constituent of normal tissue. Thus, in *Goodpasture's syndrome*, for example, *pulmonary hemorrhage* and *glomerulonephritis* have been shown to be due to an antibody that binds directly to *basement membrane* in the lung and kidney, activates complement, and causes membrane damage as a consequence of accumulation of neutrophils and release of degradative enzymes. Goodpasture's syndrome is sometimes considered to be a type II hypersensitivity reaction since it involves an antibody-mediated cytotoxic effect on normal cells. The distinction between this infection-associated antibody-mediated disease and the immune aggregate disease of serum sickness is that microscopic examination of the lesions reveals a linear, *ribbon-like deposit* along the basement membrane (see Fig. 16.4J in Chapter 16), as would be expected if an even carpet of antibody were bound to surface antigens. In contrast, in serum sickness the pileup of preformed aggregates on the basement membrane leads to "lumpy-bumpy" deposits.

Rheumatic fever, a disease that can follow a throat infection with group A streptococci, involves inflammation and damage to heart, joints, and kidneys. A variety of antigens in the cell walls and membranes of streptococci have been shown to be cross-reactive with antigens present in human heart muscle, cartilage, and glomerular basement membrane. It is presumed that antibody to the streptococcal antigens binds to these components of normal tissue and induces inflammatory reactions via a pathway similar to that described above. In *rheumatoid arthritis*, discussed in Chapter 17, there is evidence for the production of *rheumatoid factor*, an IgM autoantibody, that binds to the Fc portion of normal IgG. These immunoglobulin complexes participate in causing inflammation of joints and the damage characteristic of this disease.

In a number of *infectious diseases* (malaria, some viral infections, leprosy) there may be times during the course of the infection when large amounts of antigen and antibody exist simultaneously and cause the formation of immune aggregates that are deposited in a bewildering variety of locations. Thus, the complex of symptoms in any of these diseases may include a component attributable to a type III hypersensitivity reaction.

Occupational Diseases (Hypersensitivity Pneumonitis)

Farmer's lung is a prototypic form of the type III reactions classified as *"occupational diseases."* In sensitive individuals, exposure to moldy hay leads, within 6–8 hours, to severe respiratory distress or *pneumonitis*. It has been shown that affected individuals have made large amounts of IgG antibody specific for the spores of thermophilic actinomycetes that grow on spoiled hay. Inhalation of the bacterial spores leads to a reaction in the lungs that resembles the Arthus reaction seen in skin, namely, the formation of antigen–antibody aggregates and consequent inflammation.

There are many similar pulmonary type III reactions that bear names related to the occupation or causative agent, such as *pigeon breeder's disease, cheese washer's disease, bagassosis* (*bagasse* refers to sugarcane fiber), *maple bark stripper's disease, paprika worker's disease*, and the increasingly rare *thatched roof worker's lung*. Dirty work environments, involving massive exposure to potentially antigenic material, obviously lend themselves to the development of this form of occupational disease.

SUMMARY

1. *Type II hypersensitivity reactions* involve damage to target cells and are mediated by antibody through two major pathways. In the first pathway, antibody (usually *IgM*, but also *IgG*) activates the entire *complement* sequence and causes *cell lysis*. In the second pathway, antibody (usually *IgG*) serves to engage receptors for *Fc on phagocytic* cells, and C3b engages receptors on phagocytic cells with C3b receptors, causing destruction of the antibody—and/or C3b-coated target. These reactions usually involve circulating blood cells, such as red cells, white cells, and platelets, and the consequences are those that would be expected from destruction of the particular type of cell.

2. *Type III immune complex reactions* involve the formation of antigen–antibody complexes that can activate the complement cascade. Release of certain products of complement (*C3a* and *C5a*) causes a local increase in vessel permeability and permits the release of serum (*edema*) and the chemotactic attraction of *neutrophils*. The neutrophils, in the process of ingesting

the immune complexes, release degradative *lysosomal enzymes* that produce the tissue damage characteristic of these reactions. If the site of reaction is a vessel wall, the outcome is *hemorrhage* and *necrosis;* if the site is a glomerular basement membrane, loss of integrity and release of protein and red cells into the urine results; and if the site is a joint meniscus, destruction of synovial membranes and cartilage occurs. Multiple forms of this response exist, depending on the type and location of antigen and the way in which it is brought together with antibody. In all cases, however, the outcome depends on complement and granulocytes as mediators of tissue injury.

REFERENCES

Cotran RS, Kumar V, Robbins SL (1989): The Kidney in Pathologic Basis of Disease. Philadelphia: Saunders.

Dixon FJ, Cochrane CC, Theofilopoulus AN (1988): Immune complex injury. In Samter M, Talmage DW, Frank MM, Austen KF, Claman HN (eds): Immunological Diseases, 4th ed. Boston: Little, Brown.

Fye KH, Sack KE (1994): Rheumatic diseases. In Stites DP, Terr AI, Parslow TG (eds): Basic and Clinical Immunology, 8th ed. Norwalk, CT: Appleton & Lange.

Lawley TJ, Frank MM (1980): Immune complexes and immune complex diseases. In Parker CW (ed): Clinical Immunology, Vol I. Philadelphia: Saunders.

Terr AI (1994): Immune Complex Disease. In Stites DP, Terr AI, Parslow TG (eds.): Basic and Clinical Immunology, 8th ed. Norwalk, CT: Appleton & Lange.

Theofilopoulos AN, Dixon FJ (1979): The biology and detection of immune complexes. Adv Immunol 28:89.

REVIEW QUESTIONS

For each question, choose the ONE BEST answer or completion

1. Which of the following clinical diseases is most likely to involve a reaction to a hapten in its etiology?
   A) Goodpasture's syndrome
   B) hemolytic anemia after treatment with penicillin
   C) rheumatoid arthritis
   D) farmer's lung
   E) Arthus reaction

2. An IgA antibody to a red cell antigen is unlikely to cause autoimmune hemolytic anemia because

A) it would be made only in the gastrointestinal tract

B) its Fc region would not bind receptors for Fc on phagocytic cells

C) it can fix complement only as far as C1, C4, C2

D) it has too low an affinity

E) it requires secretory component to work

3. The glomerular lesions in immune complex disease can be visualized microscopically with a fluorescent antibody against

A) IgG heavy chains

B) κ light chains

C) C1

D) C3

E) all of the above

4. The lesions in immune complex-induced glomerulonephritis

A) are dependent on erythrocytes and complement

B) result in increased production of urine

C) require both complement and neutrophils

D) are dependent on the presence of macrophages

E) require all nine components of complement

5. Serum sickness occurs only

A) when anti-basement membrane antibodies are present

B) in cases of extreme excess of antibody

C) when IgE antibody is produced

D) when soluble immune complexes are formed

E) in the absence of neutrophils

6. Immune complexes are involved in the pathogenesis of

A) post-streptococcal glomerulonephritis

B) pigeon breeder's disease

C) serum sickness

D) an edematous hemorrhagic reaction in the skin of a beekeeper, 2 hours after he was stung for the 20th time

E) all of the above

7. The Arthus reaction and farmer's lung *differ* because

A) only the former is due to antigen–antibody complexes

B) the mode of contact with the antigen is different

C) only the former requires complement

D) only the latter can occur in farmers

E) the reactions in farmer's lung are much more rapid

8. The final damage to vessels in immune complex-mediated arthritis is due to

A) lymphokines from T cells

B) histamine and SRS-A

C) the C5, C6, C7, C8, C9 attack complex

D) lysosomal enzymes of polymorphonuclear leukocytes

E) cytotoxic T cells

9. Serum sickness is characterized by

A) deposition of immune complexes in blood vessel walls when there is a moderate excess of antigen

B) phagocytosis of complexes by granulocytes

C) consumption of complement

D) appearance of symptoms before free antibody can be detected in the circulation

E) all of the above

10. The Arthus reaction involves

A) lymphocytic infiltrate around veins

B) formation of antigen–antibody precipitates on vessel walls

C) cross-linking of IgE antibody

D) complement activation

E) only A and C are correct

F) only B and D are correct

11. Circulating immune complexes are an etiologic factor in the following diseases:
    A) skin lesions of systemic lupus erythematosus
    B) farmer's lung
    C) glomerulonephritis, after treatment with horse anti-tetanus antiserum
    D) Goodpasture's syndrome
    E) only A and C are correct
    F) only B and D are correct

12. A patient is suspected of having farmer's lung. A provocation test involving the inhalation of an extract of moldy hay is performed. A sharp drop in respiratory function is noted within 10 minutes and returns to normal in 2 hours, only to fall again in another 2 hours. The most likely explanation is
    A) the patient has existing T-cell-mediated hypersensitivity
    B) this is a normal pattern for farmer's lung
    C) the patient developed a secondary response after the inhalation of antigen
    D) the symptoms of farmer's lung are complicated by an IgE-mediated reactivity to the same antigen
    E) all of the above

Case study: A technician in a snake venom-producing farm got careless one day and was bitten by a rare lethal Egyptian cobra. He was rushed to the emergency ward and a call went out immediately for antivenom serum. Fortunately some was located and within 5 hours he was given 15 ml intravenously. The next day he received another 10 ml, the last available. Within days he was well on the way to recovery and left the hospital a week later. He returned 10 days after leaving the hospital complaining of joint pain, fever, and recurrent itchy hives on his trunk, arms, and legs. What do you suspect is happening, and how would you confirm it?

ANSWERS TO REVIEW QUESTIONS

1. *B* Penicillin can function as a hapten, binding to red cells and inducing a hemolytic anemia. *A*, *C*, and *D* are examples of immune aggregate (type III) reactions requiring complement and neutrophils for pathologic effects.

2. *B* Since phagocytic cells have Fc receptors for IgG, bound IgA would not cause engulfment and damage. Thus, *A, C, D*, and *E* are false.

3. *E* The lesions in immune complex disease are dependent on the presence of antigen, antibody, and complement. Hence, all can be demonstrated by immunofluorescence

at a lesion: *A* and *B*, because they are parts of IgG; *C* and *D*, because they are the early components of complement activated by the immune aggregated.

4. *C* Damage by immune complexes requires complement components to attract neutrophils, which are the agents responsible for subsequent tissue damage. Lysis by the final sequence of C6, C7, C8, and C9 is not required.

5. *D* Anti-basement membrane antibodies may produce damage but can be distinguished from serum sickness lesions by their ribbon-like appearance compared to the "lumpy-bumpy" appearance of serum sickness lesions. Excess of antibody would clear antigen rapidly with few lesions. IgE antibody is responsible for anaphylactic reactions and neutrophils are required for the lesions typical of serum sickness.

6. *E* All are examples of type III hypersensitivity reactions: *A*, by production of antibody, which reacts with normal kidney antigen; *B*, by inhalation of antigens from pigeon droppings; *C*, serum sickness is a classical example of an immune complex disease; and *D* is a description of an Arthus reaction in someone who has been immunized by repeated injection of bee venom.

7. *B* Both the Arthus reaction and farmer's lung are examples of immune aggregate reactions that require complement and neutrophils. The former involves antigen injected into the skin; the latter involves inhaled antigen.

8. *D* Neither T cells nor mast cells are responsible for the final tissue damage in immune complex disease. Therefore *A*, *B*, and *E* are eliminated. The final lytic complex of complement is similarly not involved, since complement activation up to C5 is sufficient to bring in the polymorphonuclear leukocytes, whose lysosomal enzymes cause the tissue damage.

9. *E* All are characteristics of serum sickness.

10. *F* Choice *A* is characteristic of cell-mediated immunity (type IV) reactions and *C* of anaphylaxis (type I) reactions. Thus, *B* and *D* are correct statements.

11. *E* Farmer's lung involves formation of local rather than bloodborne antigen–antibody aggregates, and Goodpasture's syndrome is caused by antibody binding to antigen in situ. Only *B* and *C* have circulating soluble complexes.

12. *D* The type III response in farmer's lung and similar occupational diseases has an onset of symptoms usually several hours after exposure. The appearance of breathing difficulties within minutes would create a strong suspicion that a type I anaphylactic response is also present. Presumably the patient made both IgE and IgG antibodies to the actinomycete antigens. A positive "wheal and flare" reaction on skin testing would provide further confirmation.

Case study: Most antivenoms of exotic species such as snake, spider, and scorpion would be made in horses. The horse antiserum neutralized the toxin and saved the patient's life. However, being a foreign protein, it induced an immune response with resultant formation of antigen–antibody complexes and the symptoms of type III hypersensitivity, serum sickness. The localization of these complexes in joints and the activation of complement to give anaphylatoxins were responsible for the joint pain, hives, and itching he experienced. It is possible that he could subsequently develop symptoms of glomerulonephritis as well. Treatment would consist of corticosteroid administration for its general anti-inflammatory effects. Confirmatory studies of your diagnosis might include looking for depressed levels of serum C3 and C4 as a result of activation in tissue by the antigen–antibody aggregates. In the convalescent stage one might also find antibody to horse Ig as a final definitive proof of your diagnosis.

HYPERSENSITIVITY REACTIONS: T-CELL-MEDIATED, TYPE IV—DELAYED-TYPE HYPERSENSITIVITY

INTRODUCTION

In contrast to antibody-mediated immunity, ***cell-mediated immunity (CMI)*** or delayed-type hypersensitivity (DTH) involves immune responses initiated primarily by antigen-specific T cells. When activated by contact with an antigen-presented by antigen-presenting cells, the T cells release soluble mediators, cytokines, some of which attract and activate other mononuclear cells that are not antigen-specific such as monocytes and macrophages. This activation is an example of a cascade: the activation of very few, antigen-specific T cells leads to a reaction in which the large majority of the mononuclear cells that are present and responsible for the eventual outcome of the reactions is nonantigen-specific. The antigen eliciting this type of response may be foreign tissue (as in allograft reactions), an intracellular parasite (e.g., viruses, mycobacteria, or fungi), a soluble protein, or one of many chemicals capable of penetrating skin and coupling to body proteins that serve as carriers.

In contrast to antibody-mediated hypersensitivity that can be transferred from an immunized or sensitized individual to a nonimmune individual via serum, cell-mediated immunity cannot be transferred with serum but can be ***transferred only with T cells.***

The nomenclature for this type of hypersensitivity response has varied over the years, according to historic usage. Originally the response was termed the ***tuberculin reaction***, from the observation by Koch, in 1890, that people infected with *Mycobacterium tuberculosis* gave a positive skin test when injected intradermally with a concentrated lysate of a mycobacterial culture [old tuberculin (OT)]. Subsequently, the delayed nature of the onset of these responses (days, in contrast to minutes or hours for antibody-mediated responses), has led to their collective designation as ***delayed-type hypersensitivity (DTH) reactions.*** With the discovery that all these reactions are the consequences of an initial response by T cells, they are now classified as T-cell-mediated or, more simply, cell-mediated immunity (CMI). According to the Gell–Coombs classification of hypersensitivity reactions, DTH or CMI reactions are classified as type IV reactions. This chapter deals with the nature and underlying mechanisms of these reactions.

GENERAL CHARACTERISTICS

Gross Appearance and Histology of the Reaction

An intradermal injection of antigen in a sensitized animal or person does not lead to an apparent response until approximately 18–24 hours after challenge. This time course characteristically distinguishes DTH from antibody-mediated reactions, which appear much more quickly (see Chapters 14 and 15). After about 18–24 hours, evidence of ***erythema*** (redness) and ***induration*** (raised thickening) appear, reaching maximal levels 24–48 hours after the challenge (see Fig. 16.4E). The induration can easily be distinguished from edema (fluid) by absence of pitting when pressure is applied. These reactions, even when severe, rarely lead to necrotic damage and resolve slowly.

A biopsy taken early in the reaction reveals primarily mononuclear cells of the monocyte/macrophage series with a few scattered lymphocytes. Characteristically, the mononuclear infiltrates appear as a perivascular cuff before extensively invading the site of deposition of antigen (see Fig. 16.3F). Neutrophils are not a prominent feature of the initial reaction. Later biopsies show a more complex pattern, with the arrival of B cells and the formation of *granuloma* in persistent lesions. The hardness or induration is attributable to the deposition of fibrin in the lesion.

Mechanism of DTH

The mechanisms involved in the sensitization to DTH and the elucidation of the reaction following antigenic challenge are now quite well understood, although some of the finer details are being filled in or are periodically changed. As in the other types of hypersensitivity reactions, DTH hypersensitivity consists of two main stages, namely, the sensitization stage and the challenge stage, which leads to the reaction. These are shown diagrammatically in Figure 16.1.

SENSITIZATION OR INDUCTION STAGE. This stage lasts 1–2 weeks. Contact of T cell with antigen on APC results in the activation of the T cell as described in Chapter 11. In DTH, the important key T cell is the Th1 CD4$^+$. The Th1 cell is also referred to as T_{DTH}. The cytokines produced by these cells, notably IL-2 and IFN-γ, are chemotactic for and activate macrophages. Another cytokine produced by the Th1 CD4$^+$ cell is IL-12. IL-12 suppresses the Th2 subpopulation of T cells that appear to be important in B-cell expansion and activation. Moreover, IL-12 promotes the expansion of Th1 subpopulation, driving the response to produce more Th1-synthesized cytokines which activate macrophages. Thus, IL-12 plays an important role in cell-mediated DTH. (It should be mentioned that during the induction phase, a small number of CD8$^+$ T cells—cytotoxic T cells or Tc cells also appear during T-cell expansion. These cells and their functions were described in Chapter 11.)

Activation of the T cells may be recognized in several ways: the T cells enlarge, become blastoid, and divide. While these events can be seen by direct visualization, such observations are difficult and tedious. Consequently, direct visualization has been replaced by a widely used assay that measures proliferation of cells (described below).

Cells stimulated to divide synthesize DNA. If they are supplied with a pulse of ^{3}H-labeled thymidine, they will incorporate that radiolabeled material into the newly synthesized DNA, and the cells themselves will become labeled. It is then a simple matter to expose the cells to antigen and after a certain period of time

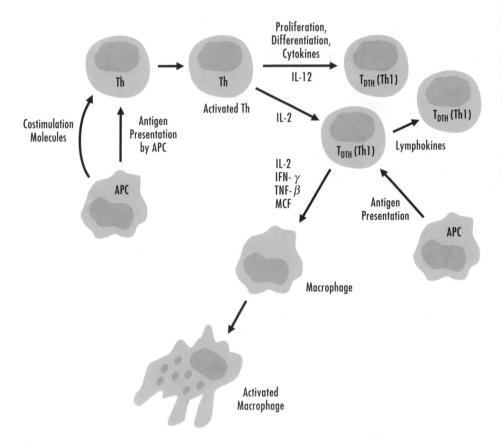

Figure 16.1.

Activation of T cells leading to the release of lymphokines, the expression of Th1 (T_DTH) cells, and activation of macrophages (APC = antigen-presenting cell).

count the incorporated radioactivity in a given aliquot of cells. Since incorporation is proportional to DNA synthesis, we can determine the extent to which the cells have proliferated in response to antigen and compare it to proliferation with no exposure to antigen. This ***proliferative assay*** is an in vitro correlate of CMI.

ELICITATION OF THE DTH REACTION. A second exposure to antigen—antigenic challenge—causes the delayed type reaction. The antigen, presented by APC, interacts with the expanded Th1 or T_DTH cells, resulting in the release of cytokines that have a variety of biological effects. These include the attraction of macrophages to the reaction site, the ***activation of the macrophages***, and the release of additional cytokines with important biological functions. It takes approximately 18–24 or even 48 hours from time of antigenic challenge to recruit and activate all these cells. Cytokines released by all the participating cells are the underlying cause of the delayed hypersensitivity reaction. Importantly, only a relatively few antigen-specific T cells are required to trigger the reaction. These constitute 1–5% of the total cellular, mostly monocytic component of the DTH reaction. The recruitment and activation of non-antigen specific cells by antigen specific cells demonstrate the interaction between acquired and innate immunity discussed in Chapter 2.

Release of Cytokines. The DTH reaction involves the release of numerous cytokines that exert their activity upon lymphocytes, macrophages, and several other cell types. As mentioned earlier, the picture is quite complicated. In order to avoid confusion, those cytokines deemed the most important are: ***interleukin 2 (IL-2), macrophage chemotactic factor (MCF), interferon γ (IFN-γ)*** (see Fig. 16.2), and ***tumor necrosis factor β (TNF-β). IL-2*** is important for ***proliferation and activation of T cells*** in the reaction area. ***MCF attracts monocytes*** into the area, ***IFN-γ activates mononuclear cells***, and ***TNF-β is cytotoxic.*** Activated macrophages, which constitute the majority of cells at the reaction site, have a highly enhanced ability to ingest and kill various microorganisms, the ultimate purpose of cell-mediated immunity. As is the case with hypersensitivity type II and III discussed earlier, the beneficial aspects of cell-mediated immunity become deleterious in delayed, type IV hypersensitivity or allergy.

Consequences of DTH

It should be apparent from the preceding discussion that many of the effector functions in CMI are performed by ***activated macrophages.*** In the most favorable circumstances, CMI results in destruction of the organism that elicited the response in the first place. This destruction is believed to result predominantly from ***ingestion*** of the organism by macrophages, their activation by IFN-γ, followed by ***degradation*** by ***lysosomal enzymes***, as well as by the by-products of the burst of ***respiratory activity***, such as ***peroxide*** and ***superoxide*** radicals. Foreign tissues, tumor tissue, and soluble or conjugated antigens are dealt with in a similar manner.

In circumstances where the antigen is readily disposed of, the lesion re-

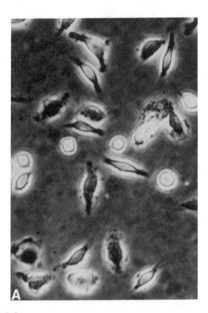 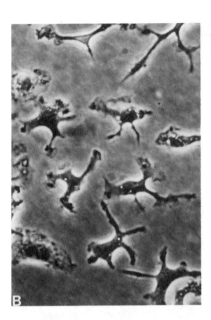

Figure 16.2.

The effect of IFN-γ on peritoneal macrophages: (A) normal macrophages in culture as they are just beginning to adhere; (B) macrophages that after activation with IFN-γ have adhered, spread out with the development of numerous pseudopodia, and grown larger. More lysosomal granules are also visible. (Photos courtesy of Dr. M. Stadecker, Tufts University Medical School.)

solves slowly, with little tissue damage. In some circumstances, however, the antigen is protected and very persistent; for example, schistosomal eggs and lipid-encapsulated mycobacteria are resistant to enzymatic degradation. In these cases, the response can be prolonged and destructive to the host. Continuous accumulation of macrophages leads to clusters of *epithelioid cells*, which fuse to form giant cells in *granulomas.* These granulomas, in turn, can be destructive because of their displacement of normal tissue and can result in *caseous (cheesy) necrosis.* The disease process may then be attributable not so much to the effects of the invading organisms as to the persistent attempts of the host to isolate and contain the parasite by the mechanisms of CMI. In diseases such as smallpox, measles, and herpes, the characteristic exanthems (skin rashes) seen are partly attributable to the responses of CMI to the virus, with additional destruction attributable to the attack by cytotoxic T cells on the virally infected epithelial cells.

Variants of DTH

Several known variants of classical DTH or tuberculin reactions have the same basic mechanisms, but have additional features, which are described in the sections that follow.

CONTACT SENSITIVITY. *Contact sensitivity* is a form of DTH in which the target organ is the skin, and the inflammatory response is produced as the result of contact with sensitizing substances on the surface of the skin. The prototype for this form of response is *poison ivy dermatitis* (Fig. 16.3G,H). The offending substance is *urushiol*, an oil secreted by the leaves of the poison-ivy vine and other related plants. Urushiol is a mixture of catechols (dihydroxyphenols) with long hydrocarbon side chains. These features allow it to penetrate the skin by virtue of its lipophilicity (which gives it the ability to dissolve in skin oils) and its ability to couple covalently (by formation of quinones) to some carrier molecules on cell surfaces. Other contact sensitizers are generally also *lipid-soluble haptens.* They have a variety of chemical forms, but all have in common the ability to *penetrate skin* and form *hapten-carrier conjugates.* Experimentally, chemicals such as 2,4-dinitrochlorobenzene (DNCB) are used to induce contact sensitivity. Since virtually every normal individual is capable of developing hypersensitivity to a test dose of this compound, it is frequently used to assess a patient's potential for T-cell reactivity. Various metals, such as nickel and chromium, which are present in jewelry and clasps of undergarments, are also capable of inducing contact sensitivity, presumably by way of *chelation* (ionic interaction) by skin proteins.

The induction of contact sensitivity is thought to proceed via presentation of the offending allergen by *Langerhans cells* (antigen-presenting cells in the skin). It is not yet resolved whether the sensitizer couples directly to components on the cell surface of the Langerhans cell or whether it couples first to proteins in serum or tissue that are then taken up by the Langerhans cells. The initial contact results in expansion of the clones of T cells capable of recognizing the specific contact sensitizer. Subsequent contact with the sensitizer triggers a sequence of events analogous to those described for CMI. In many cases, enough of the sensitizing substance remains at the site of the initial contact so that in approximately one week, when sufficient T-cell expansion takes place, the antigen that persists serves as a challenge and a reaction in this area will flare up without further antigenic challenge. An additional pathologic component of contact sensitivity reactions in humans is the separation of epidermal cells, *spongiosis*, and *blister* formation (Fig. 16.3H).

The commonly performed procedure for testing for the presence of contact sensitivity is the ***patch test*** in which a solution of the suspected antigen is spread on the skin and covered by an occlusive dressing. The appearance 2–3 days later of an area of induration and erythema indicates sensitivity.

ALLOGRAFT REJECTION. As we shall discuss in more detail in Chapter 20, if an individual receives grafts of cells, tissues, or organs taken from an ***allogeneic*** donor (a genetically different individual of the same species), it will initially be accepted and become vascularized. However, if the genetic difference is at any of the histocompatibility genes, especially genes in the MHC, a rejection process ensues whose duration and intensity is related to the degree of incompatibility between donor and recipient. The rejection reaction, in general, follows the course described for CMI. After vascularization, there is an initial invasion of the graft by a mixed population of antigen-specific lymphocytes and nonspecific monocytes through the blood vessel walls. This inflammatory reaction soon leads to destruction of the vessels; this deprivation of nutrients is quickly followed by necrosis and breakdown of the grafted tissue.

Figure 16.3A.

Type I (anaphylactic) hypersensitivity skin reaction—gross appearance, showing "wheal and flare" (urticaria). (Courtesy of Dr. M. Stadecker, Tufts University Medical School.)

Figure 16.3B.

Type I (anaphylactic) hypersensitivity skin reaction—histology, showing dermal edema with occasional eosinophils. (Courtesy of Dr. M. Stadecker, Tufts University Medical School.)

Figure 16.3C.

Type III hypersensitivity Arthus reaction—gross appearance, showing hemorrhagic appearance (purpura).

Figure 16.3D.

Type III hypersensitivity Arthus reaction—histology, showing neutrophil infiltrate, occluded arteriole, and hemorrhage. (Courtesy of Dr. M. Stadecker, Tufts University Medical School.)

Figure 16.3E.

Type IV delayed-type hypersensitivity reaction (tuberculin reaction)—gross appearance, showing induration and erythema 48 hours after tuberculin test. (Courtesy of Dr. Gottlieb, Tulane University Medical School.)

Figure 16.3F.

Type IV delayed-type hypersensitivity reaction—histologic picture showing dermal mononuclear cell infiltrate and perivascular cuffing. (Courtesy of Dr. M. Stadecker, Tufts University Medical School.)

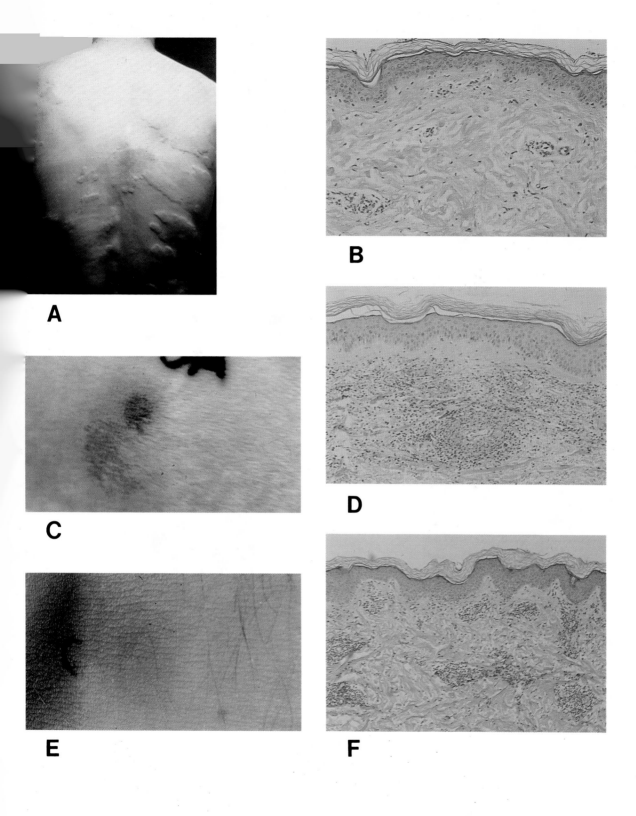

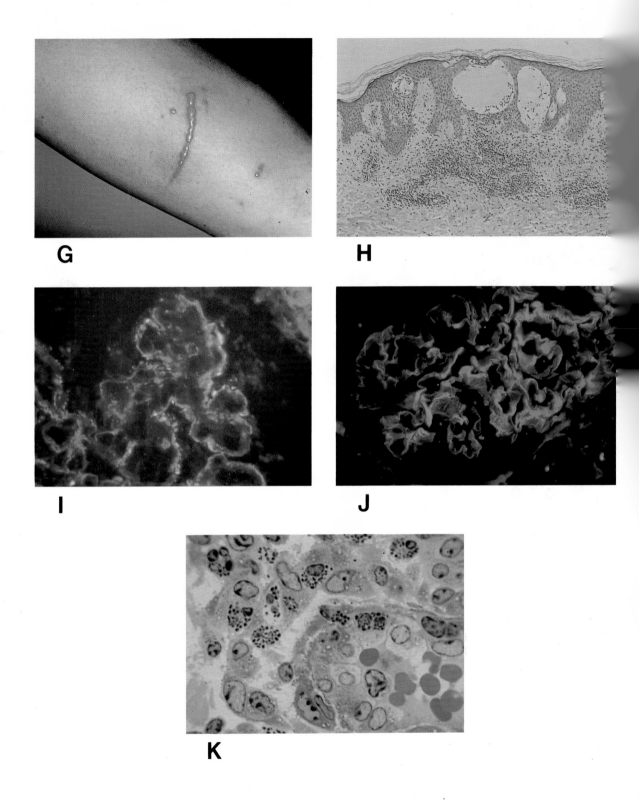

G

H

I

J

K

CUTANEOUS BASOPHIL HYPERSENSITIVITY (CBH). An unusual form of delayed reaction has been observed in humans following repeated intradermal injections of antigen. The response is delayed in onset (usually by about 24 hours) but consists entirely of erythema, without the induration typical of classic delayed-hypersensitivity reactions. When this condition was studied experimentally, it was found that the erythema was attended by a cellular infiltrate, but that the predominant cell type was the *basophil* (Fig. 16.3K). Studies in guinea pigs showed that the response was primarily mediated by T cells and was subject to the same MHC restrictions as classic T-cell-mediated responses. When classic delayed hypersensitivity was present, however, infiltrates of basophils were not seen. Thus, CBH seemed to be a variant of T-cell-mediated responses, but its exact mechanism was unknown. The picture was complicated still further when it was shown that passive transfer of serum could, under some circumstances, evoke a basophil response.

The function of CBH remained a mystery until it was shown that guinea pigs bitten by certain ticks had severe CBH reactions at the site of attachment of the tick. The infiltration of basophils and, presumably, the release of pharmacologically active materials from their granules resulted in death of the tick and its eventual detachment. Thus, CBH may have an important role in certain forms of im-

---

Figure 16.3G.

Type IV contact sensitivity reaction—gross appearance of reaction to poison ivy. (Courtesy of Dr. M. Stadecker, Tufts University Medical School.)

Figure 16.3H.

Type IV contact sensitivity reaction—histologic appearance showing intraepidermal blister formation and mononuclear cell infiltrate in the dermis. (Courtesy of Dr. M. Stadecker, Tufts University Medical School.)

Figure 16.3I.

Immune aggregate glomeruli lesions revealed by fluorescent antibody to human Ig: "lumpy-bumpy" immune aggregate deposit in glomerular basement membrane. (Courtesy of Dr. A. Ucci, Tufts University Medical School.)

Figure 16.3J.

"Ribbon-like" deposit of antibody along the basement membrane revealed by fluorescent antibodies to human Ig. (Courtesy of Dr. A. Ucci, Tufts University Medical School.)

Figure 16.3K.

Cutaneous basophil reaction showing basophils and some mononuclear cells 24 hours after skin test. (Courtesy of Dr. M. Stadecker, Tufts University Medical School.)

munity to parasites. More recently, basophil infiltrates have also been found in cases of contact dermatitis with allergens such as poison ivy, in cases of rejection of renal grafts, and in some forms of conjunctivitis. These observations indicate that basophils may also play a role in some types of delayed hypersensitivity disease.

TREATMENT OF CMI

CMI constitutes a cellular response similar to inflammation (see Chapter 2). It resolves after a period of time (days to weeks) following removal of the antigen. However, in severe cases or when exposure to antigen persists, corticosteroids, applied either topically or systemicly, constitute a very effective treatment.

SUMMARY

1. **All CMI (DTH) responses are T-cell-mediated and may be passively transferred with an appropriate quantity of such cells.**

2. **Unlike immediate-type hypersensitivity, type IV or delayed-type hypersensitivity reactions appear 18–24 hours after antigenic challenge of a sensitized individual.**

3. **CMI responses are initiated by the reaction of T cells with antigen that is presented in association with MHC class II molecules on antigen-presenting cells.**

4. **The triggering event leads to proliferation of the T cells and the release of several lymphokines, which cause the nonspecific accumulation and activation of monocytes and macrophages. It is the presence and activity of these macrophages that are the major histologic feature of CMI and that account for the protective outcome of CMI (by ingestion and destruction or by released enzymes.**

5. **CMI is a crucial mode of immunologic reactivity for protection against intracellular parasites, such as viruses, many bacteria, and fungi. However, the nature of the reaction and its mediators also cause delayed-type hypersensitivity reactions.**

6. In addition to DTH or tuberculin-type reactions, contact sensitivity and allograft rejection represent variants of the basic mechanism of CMI.

REFERENCES

Adams RM (1989): Occupational Skin Diseases, 2nd ed. Orlando, FL: Grune & Stratton.

Celada A, Nathan C (1994): Macrophage activation revisited. Immunol Today 15:100.

Gallin JI (1993): Inflammation. In Paul WE (ed): Fundamental Immunology, 3rd ed. New York: Raven Press.

Kapsenberg ML, Wierenga EA, Bos JD, Jensen HM (1991): Functional subsets of allergen-reactive human CD4$^+$ T cells. Immunol Today 12:392.

Mallory SB (1987): Allergic contact dermalitis. Immunol Allergy Clin N Am. 7:407.

Oppenheim JJ, Ruscetti FW, Faltynek C (1994): Cytokines. In Stites DP, Terr AI, Parslow TG (eds): Basic and Clinical Immunology, 8th ed. Norwalk, CT: Appleton & Lange.

Sauder DN (1986): Allergic contact dermatitis. In Theiss BD, Dobson AL (eds): Pathogenesis of Skin Disease. New York: Churchill Livingstone. Symposium on Cell-Mediated Immunity in Human Disease (1986): Hum Pathol 17:2, 17:3.

Terr AI (1991): Cell-mediated immunity. In Stites DP, Terr AI (eds): Basic and Clinical Immunology, 7th ed. Norwalk, CT: Appleton & Lange.

Terr AI (1994): Cell-mediated hypersensitivity disease. In Stites DP, Terr AI, Parslow TG (eds): Basic and Clinical Immunology, 8th ed. Norwalk: CT: Appleton & Lange.

Turk JL (1980): Delayed Hypersensitivity, 3rd ed. Amsterdam: Elsevier.

REVIEW QUESTIONS

> For each question, choose the ONE BEST answer or completion

1. Which of the following does not involve CMI?
   A) contact sensitivity to lipstick
   B) rejection of a liver graft
   C) serum sickness
   D) tuberculin reaction
   E) immunity to chicken pox

2. A positive DTH skin reaction involves the interaction of
   A) antigen, complement, and lymphokines
   B) antigen, antigen-sensitive lymphocytes, and macrophages
   C) antigen–antibody complexes, complement, and neutrophils
   D) IgE antibody, antigen, and mast cells
   E) antigen, macrophages, and complement

3. Cell-mediated immune responses are

A) enhanced by depletion of complement
B) suppressed by cortisone
C) enhanced by depletion of T cells
D) suppressed by antihistamine
E) enhanced by depletion of macrophages

4. Delayed skin reactions to an intradermal injection of antigen may be markedly decreased by
   A) exposure to a high dose of X irradiation
   B) treatment with antihistamines
   C) treatment with an antineutrophil serum
   D) removal of the spleen
   E) decreasing levels of complement

5. Patients with DiGeorge syndrome (congenital absence of a thymus) who survive beyond infancy would be capable of
   A) rejecting a bone marrow transplant
   B) mounting a DTH response to dinitrochlorobenzene
   C) resisting intracellular parasites
   D) forming antibody to T-dependent antigens
   E) all of the above
   F) none of the above

6. Which of the following statements is (are) characteristic of contact sensitivity?
   A) The best therapy is administration of the antigen

B) Patch testing with the allergen is useless for diagnosis
C) Sensitization can be passively transferred with serum from an allergic individual
D) Some chemicals acting as haptens induce sensitivity by covalently binding to host proteins acting as carriers
E) Corticosteroids constitute the treatment of choice
F) B and D are correct
G) D and E are correct

7. Interferon γ
   A) is synthesized by macrophages
   B) is released as a consequence of antigen- or mitogen-induced activation of T lymphocytes
   C) specifically binds to the antigen that induces its release
   D) induces macrophages to ingest and destroy bacteria in a nonspecific fashion
   E) only A and C are correct
   F) only B and D are correct

8. T-cell-mediated immune responses can result in
   A) formation of granulomas
   B) induration at the reaction site
   C) rejection of a heart transplant
   D) eczema of the skin in the area of prolonged contact with a rubberized undergarment
   E) all of the above

Case study: As a member of an anthropologic research team, you have occasion to visit a primitive tribe in the remote reaches of the Amazon jungle. During your visit the natives conduct a ceremony celebrating the rites of passage for young males. This consists, among other things, of covering their bodies with elaborate patterns of stripes and circles using a variety of colors extracted from local plants. On your return 3 weeks later you are asked to look at a young male who has developed alarmingly itchy and weepy red areas of skin that run in sharply demarcated stripes across his back and on one arm. Remembering your introductory course in immunology, you make an educated guess as to the cause. How, under such primitive conditions, could you confirm your diagnosis?

ANSWERS TO REVIEW QUESTIONS

1. *C* Serum sickness is an example of those reactions mediated by an antibody–antigen complex that involves components of the complement system and neutrophils. All others involve CMI to a significant extent.

2. *B* CMI reactions result from the triggering of T cells by antigen with recruitment of macrophages. Neither antibody, complement, nor mast cells plays a role in this process, although they do play a role in immediate hypersensitivity responses.

3. *B* Cortisone has a general anti-inflammatory effect and is also lytic for some T cells. Complement plays no role, and antihistamines have little effect on this type of response. Depletion of T cells or macrophages would suppress, not enhance, this type of response since the response is dependent on these cells.

4. *A* High doses of X irradiation will destroy T cells, which are responsible for initiating the response. Histamine, neutrophils, spleen, and complement do not play a role, and any treatment that affects them would not affect a DTH response.

5. *F* Patients with DiGeorge syndrome have a congenital thymic aplasia and lack all T-cell functions. Since *A, B,* and *C* are all aspects of a CMI response, they would be absent. Additionally, formation of antibody against T-dependent antigens is dependent on T helper cells and would not occur in these patients.

6. *G* Patch testing consists of application of the offending allergen under an occlusive dressing, and a positive DTH response after 24–48 hours is considered evidence of sensitivity; thus *B* is wrong. The allergens involved are those capable of penetrating skin and binding to host carrier proteins; thus *D* is correct. Oral ingestion of antigen, which, in certain experimental situations, was shown to induce suppression after subsequent induction of contact sensitivity, has not yet been shown to be an effective therapeutic maneuver in humans; thus *A* is wrong. However, corticosteroids constitute the treatment of choice for CMI; thus *E* is also correct. Since *D* and *E* are correct, the answer to question 6 is *G*. Passive transfer of CMI responses is accomplished with T cells, not with serum, thus *C* is wrong.

7. *F* Interferon γ is released during activation of T cells and induces macrophages to phagocytize and destroy nonspecifically any particles, organisms, or debris in the area.

8. *E* All of these effects are manifestations of CMI. Induration usually takes place at the reaction site. Formation of granulomas is characteristic of a chronic DTH reaction. Rejection of the heart is an example of an allograft response. Some of the chemicals used to cure rubber can induce contact sensitivity after prolonged exposure of the skin to them.

Case study: The appearance of the skin lesion and its sharp demarcations and weepy, itchy nature all suggest contact sensitivity. One of the dyes used to paint the body is most likely the sensitizer and, since it persisted on the skin, was also able to provoke a T-cell-mediated reaction after the initial expansion of the specific clones. In the absence of sophisticated testing equipment, a simple patch test using samples of the various dyes applied to healthy areas of skin should show a localized contact reaction 24–48 hours later at the site to which the causative dye was applied. (In the laboratory one might also look for an in vitro proliferative response of the patient's peripheral blood lymphocytes to added dye. A biopsy of the lesion should reveal an intense infiltrate of mononuclear cells.)

AUTOIMMUNITY*

INTRODUCTION

Tolerance to "self" is an evolutionary device that, as long as it remains intact, is necessary for normal growth, development, and existence. When something occurs to destroy the integrity of self-tolerance (and there are various exogenous as well as endogenous influences that can precipitate such an event), an immune response to self, *autoimmunity*, may develop. Such autoimmunity may be organ-specific, localized, or systemic.

The consequences of autoimmunity may vary from minimal to catastrophic, depending on the extent to which the integrity of self-tolerance has been affected. Thus, a distinction should be made between autoimmune response and autoimmune disease, in which autoimmunity evokes pathologic consequences with the possible involvement of antibody, complement, immune complexes, and cell-mediated immunity.

Many experimental models have been developed to study autoimmune phenomena, and, in general, these models rely on active immunization with known antigens. However, the inducing agents for most of the well-recognized naturally occurring autoimmune diseases are still not clear.

*Contributed by Karen Yamaga, University of Hawaii.

An important aspect of the susceptibility to autoimmune diseases is its correlation with HLA. This association has been discussed in Chapter 10.

In the present chapter, some of the more common and important of the numerous autoimmune diseases, together with the mechanisms most probably responsible for them, are given in order to present the reader with a framework to view autoimmunity and autoimmune diseases.

AUTOIMMUNITY AND DISEASE

Several major issues need to be addressed before we discuss specific autoimmune diseases. One concerns the definition of autoimmune diseases. A growing number of diseases are suspected of having an autoimmune basis, but the evidence for them may not be straightforward. Recognition of self components may not lead to pathologic consequences. How, then, does one distinguish between autoimmune response and autoimmune disease?

A second issue involves the etiology of the disease. Most infectious diseases can be ascribed to a single agent; some genetic diseases are due to a defect in a single gene. In contrast, it is much more difficult to ascribe the agent or agents responsible for autoimmune diseases. The most notable quality of autoimmune disease is that the cause is multifactorial, involving both genetic and environmental influences. Finally, some autoimmune phenomenon may occur secondary to a disease and may significantly contribute to the pathology but should not be considered as a primary autoimmune disease.

CRITERIA FOR AUTOIMMUNE DISEASE

Recently guidelines have been established for autoimmune disease using four types of evidence.

Direct Proof

The best guideline is ***direct proof*** by transferring autoantibody or self-reactive lymphocytes and reproducing the disease. For ethical reasons, this criterion has been achieved in only a few circumstances in humans, where ***pathogenic antibody is transplacentally transmitted from mother to fetus.*** This condition has been documented in neonatal myasthenia gravis, Graves' disease, and polychon-dritis. T-cell transfer is seldom feasible because MHC molecules of different in-dividuals must be matched. ***Severe combined immune-deficient (SCID)*** mice which, because of an absence of an immune system, are often used as a living "tissue culture flask" for human cells, may provide an approach to establishing the pathogen potential of T cell population. In fact, peripheral blood lymphocytes from patients with systemic lupus erythematosus transferred into these immuno-logically depleted mice have already been shown to induce immune complex le-sions in the kidney of the mice, mimicking human lupus nephritis.

Indirect Evidence

Because of the difficulty in providing direct proof for an autoimmune mecha-nism, ***indirect evidence*** must be used. One strategy is to identify the target anti-gen in humans, isolate the homologous antigen in an animal model, and repro-duce the disease in the experimental animal by administering the offending antigen. Among the examples in which this approach has succeeded are the in-duction of thyroiditis with thyroglobulin, myasthenia gravis with acetylcholine re-ceptor, uveitis with uveal S antigen, and orchitis with sperm.

   Problems arise, however, for those human diseases in which a suitable exper-imental animal model has not been found, when multifactorial events must occur before the disease arises, when several autoantigens are involved or when the pathogenetic antigen is not known.

   Another line of indirect evidence that has been used is to study genetically determined animal models. Thus, New Zealand black mice (NZB) spontaneously develop autoimmune hemolytic anemia while New Zealand white mice (NZW) do not. (NZB × NZW)F_1 strain has been used as a model for human systemic lu-pus erythmatosis (SLE).

Isolation of Self-Reactive Antibodies or T Cells

The third type of indirect evidence is based on isolating self-reactive antibodies or T cells from the target organs. For example, anti-erythrocyte antibodies can be eluted from erythrocytes of autoimmune hemolytic anemia patients, anti-DNA antibodies can be isolated from lupus nephritis patients, and cytotoxic T cells have been found in the thyroid of Graves' disease patients. However, the patholog-ic significance of these antibodies or T cells has not been easy to establish.

Circumstantial Evidence

The final criterion relies on ***circumstantial evidence***. This criterion is based on clinical clues that include familial tendency, lymphocyte infiltration, MHC association and, most importantly, clinical improvement with immunosuppressive agents.

ETIOLOGY OF AUTOIMMUNE DISEASE

As we have already said, unlike infectious diseases in which the cause can be described to a single organism, autoimmune diseases are multifactorial. This means that a constellation of events must occur before manifestation of the disease becomes apparent. This combination of events probably requires both genetic and environmental factors.

Genetic Factors in Autoimmune Disease

The most common evidence for the existence of a ***genetic predisposition*** to autoimmune disease is in the described increased incidence of the disease in monozygotic twins, dizygotic twins, and family members. However, while familial tendencies occur, the pattern of inheritance is generally complex and indicates involvement of several genes, that is, inheritance is ***polygenic***. Only recently has the existence of other genes been localized, and very little is known about the function of these genes. For example, as mentioned above, the $(NZB \times NZW)F_1$ mice develop a disease very similar to human SLE. The NZB mice develop autoimmune hemolytic anemia and glomerulonephritis, while the NZW strain mice have no clinical symptoms. However, when NZB and NZW mice are crossed, the F_1 offspring had a much earlier and more severe form of SLE-like glomerulonephritis than the NZB parent. The NZW mice must therefore contribute some gene(s) that affects the time of onset and severity of the disease. Recently, in a SLE susceptible strain of mice very similar to the NZB × NZW mice, genes on three different chromosomes were found to contribute to lupus glomerulonephritis and anti-double-stranded (ds) DNA antibody, traits commonly found in SLE patients. Similarly, at least 14 genes contribute to type 1 diabetes found in the non-obese diabetic mouse. It will be extremely important to identify similar human genes and determine their function in order to understand the complete etiology of the disease.

One gene family that is associated with autoimmune disease and has been extensively studied is the HLA complex, the human MHC. Considering the importance of HLA molecules in shaping the T-cell receptor (TcR) repertoire and their role in recognition by the TcR, this association is not surprising. This association will be discussed later in this chapter with regard to specific autoimmune disease.

Environmental Factors

Aside from a genetic predisposition, environmental factors play a role in many autoimmune diseases by triggering the manifestation of the disease. A few autoantigens are protected from the immune system, such that even if some individuals possess autoreactive T and B cells, they will not be activated to cause autoimmunity, that is, there is a *sequestration* of potential antigens from the lymphoid system. The lens and uveal proteins of the eye, the chondrocyte antigens in cartilage, and the antigens of spermatozoa are considered to be examples of sequestered antigens. However, when they are introduced to the immune system—by some physical accident or due to infection—an autoimmune response may result. However, sequestration cannot explain why so many other self antigens, such as thyroglobulin, IgG, and DNA, which circulate freely, are involved in autoimmune disease.

In view of all the potentially self-reactive lymphocytes with access to self antigens, the fact that autoimmune disease is the exception rather than the rule has led to the theory that mechanisms exist to hold autoreactive cells in check. Some of these control mechanisms have been described in Chapter 12. Several examples of control mechanisms, and how they may be upset to cause autoimmune disease, are described below.

ABSENCE OF HELPER T CELLS. Since, as we have seen in Chapter 12, low doses of antigen can produce tolerance in T cells without provoking an immune response, it is possible that some self antigens that circulate at low concentration (thyroglobulin is an excellent example) render specific T cells tolerant but have no similar effect on B cells. Thus B cells, capable of binding thyroglobulin, may exist in normal individuals but they are not triggered to make autoantibody because help by appropriate T cells is not available (see Fig. 17.1A).

Several mechanisms have been suggested to bypass the absence of $CD4^+$ T cells (helper T cells) in the development of autoimmunity. These include provision of a new or altered carrier determinant capable of activating helper T cells. Experimentally, such a bypass can be achieved by chemical alteration of the anti-

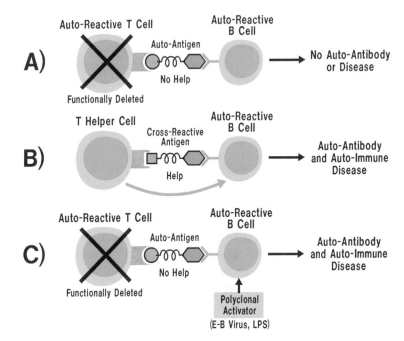

Figure 17.1.

Possible mechanisms of induction of autoimmunity.

gen, or by incorporating it into complete Freund's adjuvant or by using a cross-reactive antigen from a related species (see Fig. 17.1B). Another possible mechanism involves **polyclonal activation**, which could nonspecifically trigger many B-
cell clones (including the autoreactive ones) to produce antibody (see Fig. 17.1C).

Such conditions are believed to be mimicked to some extent by viral **infections** or by administration of **drugs** that may have the capacity to alter the carrier
molecule and elicit help from T cells. **Many bacterial infections,** such as streptococci infections, **elicit antibody that cross-reacts with normal tissue** (heart in the
case of streptococcal infection), **thus producing autoimmune disease.** Finally,
many bacteria, as well as Epstein–Barr viruses, are known to be powerful adjuvants and to induce polyclonal activation with a potential for eliciting an autoimmune response.

CONTROL BY SUPPRESSOR T CELLS. One way by which normal ani-
mals may control their immune responses is by induction of **suppressor cells** and,
in fact, some experimental autoimmune processes have been implicated to elicit

shutoff mechanisms that involve suppressor T cells (see Chapter 12). This effect may explain why the experimentally induced phenomena tend to be acute and self-limiting. When activity of suppressor T cells in experimental animals is impaired by a low dose irradiation or by treatment with cyclophosphamide, autoimmune diseases appear more rapidly and are more severe.

In addition to the experimental situations mentioned above, evidence of ***impaired immunoregulation*** has been found in several cases of human autoimmune disease, primarily as a deficiency in the functioning of T cells. In some cases, antibodies against suppressor T cells appear, so that the deficiency of these cells may represent a secondary phenomenon.

ABSENCE OF MHC CLASS II MOLECULES ON POTENTIAL TARGET CELLS. Since CD4$^+$ T cells (helper T cells) respond to antigen only when presented in association with MHC class II antigens, it is possible that certain autoantigens on cells that possess only class I antigens are not presented and therefore do not elicit autoimmune responses.

It has been shown experimentally that a number of normal cells, such as the endothelial cells in blood vessels and thyroid epithelial cells, may be induced by exposure to IFN-γ or other cytokines from activated T cells to express ***MHC class II antigens*** on their surface. These activated normal cells now become capable, in the absence of other antigen-presenting cells (APC), of presenting their surface antigens (such as thyroglobulin) to appropriate T cells, thus inducing autoimmune responses. Conceivably, therefore, viral infections of various tissues may lead, through the mechanism described above, to induction of MHC class II antigens in relevant cells, thus triggering a response to some self antigen they express.

The study of autoimmune diseases has the potential for a double reward: more successful treatment of many serious autoimmune diseases and elucidation of the normal control and regulation of the immune response, of which autoimmune disease may represent an aberration.

EXAMPLES OF AUTOIMMUNE DISEASE

The number of autoimmune diseases is growing as circumstantial evidence gives way to more direct proof of immunologic basis for a number of idiopathic diseases. We will discuss these autoimmune diseases according to their immunopathology and give a few examples of diseases that have been reasonably well characterized. A more exhaustive list can be found in references given at the end of the chapter.

Antibody-Mediated Autoimmune Disease

AUTOIMMUNE HEMOLYTIC ANEMIA. The disorder is autoimmune in nature if the antibodies react with self red blood cells. Sometimes these disorders are grouped under the more general category, immunohemolytic anemia. This includes diseases in which antibodies are generated as a result of induction by unmatched erythrocyte antigens in transfusion or in erythroblastosis fetalis.

One of the causes of a reduction in the number of red cells in the circulation is their destruction or removal by antibody directed against an antigen on the surface of the red cell. The destruction of the red cells can be attributed either to activation of the complement cascade and eventual lysis of the red cell (the resultant release of hemoglobin may lead to its appearance in the urine, i.e., hemoglobinuria) or to opsonization facilitated by antibody and the C3b components of complement. In the latter case, the red cells are bound to, and engulfed by, macrophages whose receptors for Fc and C3b attach to the antibody-coated red cells.

It is customary to divide the antibodies responsible for autoimmune hemolytic anemia into two groups, on the basis of their physical properties. The first group consists of the "warm" autoantibodies, so called since they react optimally with the red cells at 37°C. The warm autoantibodies belong primarily to the IgG class and some react with the Rh antigens on the surface of the red cells. Because activation of the complement cascade requires the close alignment of at least two molecules of IgG, the relatively sparse distribution of Rh antigens on the surface of the erythrocyte does not favor lysis via the complement pathway. On the other hand, IgG antibodies to these antigens are effective in the induction of immune adherence and phagocytosis. Thus individuals with autoimmune hemolytic anemia can be identified by a Coombs test, which is designed to detect bound IgG on the surface of red cells. The reasons for the formation of the antibody causing the hemolytic anemia are unknown.

A second kind of antibody, the *cold agglutinins,* attaches to red cells only when the temperature is below 37°C, and dissociates from the cells when the temperature rises above 37°C. Cold agglutinins belong primarily to the IgM class and are specific for the I or i antigens present in glycophorin, a major constituent of the surface of red cells. Since the cold agglutinins belong to the IgM class, they are highly efficient at activating the complement cascade and causing lysis of the erythrocytes to which they attach. Nevertheless, hemolysis is not severe in patients with autoimmune hemolytic anemia due to cold agglutinins, so long as body temperature is maintained at 37°C. When arms, legs, or skin are exposed to cold and the temperature of the circulating blood is allowed to drop, severe attacks of hemolysis may occur. Sometimes, cold agglutinins appear after infection by *Mycoplasma pneumoniae* or viruses, but the reason for their appearance is unknown.

Although the cause of autoantibody formation is often not known, some clues are offered by drug-induced anemia. A drug like penicillin, for example, may bind to some protein on the surface of red cells and induce formation of antibody, in much the same way as any hapten-carrier complex. The resulting antibody reacts with the drug (hapten) on the surface of the cell, causing lysis or phagocytosis. In such cases, however, the disease is self-limiting and disappears when use of the drug is discontinued. Another example is a disorder that occurs in a small minority of patients using α-methyldopa, an antihypertensive drug. It leads to a disorder that is almost identical to that characterized by worm autoantibodies.

MYASTHENIA GRAVIS. Myasthenia gravis is another autoimmune disease in which antibodies to a well-defined target antigen are implicated. In this disease, the targets are the acetylcholine receptors at neuromuscular junctions. Reaction of the receptor with antibody blocks the reception of a nerve impulse normally carried across the junction by acetylcholine molecules. This blockade results in severe muscle weakness, manifested by difficulty in chewing, swallowing, and breathing, and it eventually leads to death from respiratory failure. The disease can be experimentally induced in animals by immunization with acetylcholine receptors purified from torpedo fish or electric eel, which demonstrate significant cross-reactivity with mammalian receptors. The experimental disease, resulting from the formation of antibodies against the foreign receptors, which then bind to the mammalian receptors, mimics almost exactly the natural form of the disease and may be passively transferred with antibody. Some babies of myasthenic mothers have transient muscle weakness, presumably because these babies received sufficient amounts of pathogenic IgG by transplacental passage.

The development of myasthenia gravis may somehow be linked to the thymus, since many patients have concurrent ***thymoma***, or ***hypertrophy of the thymus***, and removal of the thymus sometimes leads to regression of the disease. Molecules cross-reacting with the acetylcholine receptor have been found on various cells in the thymus such as thymocytes and epithelial cells, but whether these molecules are the primary stimulus for the development of the disease is unknown. With regard to genetic predisposition, myasthenia gravis is associated with HLA-DR3 of the human MHC.

GRAVES' DISEASE. Although Graves' disease is a multisystem disease, one of its manifestations is a ***hyperactive thyroid gland (hyperthyroidism).*** This aspect of the disease serves as an example in which *antibodies directed against a hormone receptor may activate the receptor* rather than interfere with its activity. For reasons not yet understood, in Graves' disease, patients develop autoantibodies against thyroid cell surface receptors for thyroid-stimulating hormone (TSH). The interaction of these antibodies with the receptor activates the cell in a manner similar to the activation by TSH. The long-lasting stimulation by these antibodies causes hyperthyroidism due to the continuous stimulation of the thyroid gland.

The indirect evidence between an autoimmune pathogenesis and Graves' disease include familial predisposition, genetic association with HLA-DR3, presence of antibodies to TSH receptors, good correlation between the titer of antibody to TSH receptors, and the severity of hyperthyroidism. However, the best evidence is the transmission of thyroid stimulating antibodies from a thyrotoxic mother across the placenta, causing transient neonatal hyperthyroidism until the maternal IgG is catabolized.

Immune Complex–Mediated Autoimmune Disease

SYSTEMIC LUPUS ERYTHEMATOSUS. Systemic lupus erythematosus (SLE) presumably gets its name (literally "red wolf") from a reddish rash on the cheeks, which is a frequent early symptom. However, the distribution of the rash resembles the wings of a butterfly rather than the face of a wolf. The designation "wolf-like" is, thus, far-fetched, but the term "systemic" is quite appropriate since the disease attacks many organs of the body and causes fever, joint pain, and damage to the central nervous system, heart, and kidneys. The kidney lesions are most clearly understood and are the most probable cause of death from SLE.

Despite the mystery concerning the origin of this disease, a fair amount is known about the immunologic mechanisms responsible for the pathology that is observed. For unknown reasons, patients with SLE produce *antibody against several nuclear components of the body [antinuclear antibodies (ANA)], notably against native double-stranded DNA.* Occasionally antibodies are also produced against denatured, single-stranded DNA and against nucleohistones. Clinically, the presence of anti double-stranded DNA correlates best with the pathology of renal involvement in SLE (see below). The ANAs are of particular interest since no known method of immunization with DNA has yet succeeded in inducing such antibodies experimentally.

Whatever their origin, these antibodies are believed to form circulating soluble complexes with DNA derived from the breakdown of normal tissue, such as skin. The abnormal sensitivity of SLE patients to ultraviolet irradiation, which causes prompt exacerbation of symptoms, lends some credence to this idea. The soluble complexes, as in any immune-aggregate disease, are filtered out of the blood in the kidneys and get trapped against the basement membranes of the glomeruli. Other complexes may be similarly trapped in arteriolar walls and joint synovial spaces to form the characteristic "lumpy-bumpy" deposits. These complexes activate the complement cascade and attract granulocytes; the subsequent inflammatory reaction is characterized as glomerulonephritis. The resulting damage to the kidneys leads to leakage of protein *(proteinuria)* and sometimes hemorrhage *(hematuria),* with symptoms waxing and waning as the rate of formation of immune complexes rises and falls. More recently, an alternative model has been proposed in which antigen alone (double-stranded DNA) becomes trapped in the glomerular basement membrane, through electrostatic interactions with a constituent of the membrane. When the antibody appears, it binds to the antigen in the membrane and activates the same sequence of inflammatory events. This sequence of events could explain the failure, in some instances, to detect any circulating DNA–antibody complexes. Furthermore, it should be realized that, as in any chronic inflammatory response, it is entirely possible that inflammatory $CD4^+$ cells may be attracted to the site and contribute to the pathological lesions.

Although, as already mentioned, the antigen that initiates production of these antibodies is unknown, some recent findings suggest a plausible explanation that offers an attractive approach to therapy. Animals immunized with certain strains of encapsulated bacteria, such as *Klebsiella*, make **antibodies that cross-react very strongly with DNA**. A common antigenic epitope appears to be the phosphorylated backbone of many of the cross-reacting polysaccharides and DNA. Thus, it is conceivable that SLE is the result of an immune response made by only a few genetically disposed individuals to some common environmental organism. Other environmental influences include the ultraviolet light that exacerbates the disease, the influence of hormones (SLE is 10 times more frequent in women than in men during reproductive years, and exacerbation occurs during pregnancy), and the induction of SLE-like symptoms by drugs (such as penicillamine). Evidence for the genetic predisposition include the increased risk of developing SLE among family members, the higher rate of concordance (25%) in monozygotic twins when compared with dizygotic twins (<3%), linkage with HLA-DR3, and the presence of an inherited deficiency of an early complement component in 6% of SLE patients.

T-Cell-Mediated Autoimmune Diseases

MULTIPLE SCLEROSIS. Multiple sclerosis involves *demyelinization of central nervous system tissue* and leads either to a relapsing–remitting or a chronic progressive paralytic course. It is considered to be a T-cell-mediated autoimmune disease. The lesions resemble the cellular infiltrates associated with Th1 cells reminiscent of delayed-type hyperactivity. It is not clear whether the autoimmune response is due to failure of clonal deletion, from sensitization by neuroantigens or following a virus infection with molecular mimicry to a neuroepitope. The evidence that MS is an autoimmune disease is indirect and has relied on an experimentally induced model in rodents, namely, *experimental allergic encephalomyelitis (EAE)*. Following immunization of animals with myelin protein in complete Freund's adjuvant, the animals develop many of the characteristics of multiple sclerosis. CD4$^+$ T-cell clones specific for myelin basic protein can transfer the EAE disease. Circumstantial evidence includes the HLA-DR2 association with MS susceptibility and the finding of a higher T-cell response to myelin components in cerebral spinal fluid of MS patients than in control subjects.

TYPE I DIABETES MELLITUS. This form of diabetes involves *chronic inflammatory destruction of the insulin-producing β-islet cells* of the pancreas. The circumstantial evidence that type I diabetes is an autoimmune disease include the strong association with HLA. Susceptibility is associated with HLA-DR3 or DR4 and even a greater risk is associated with heterozygous individuals with HLA-DR3 and DR4, while resistance is associated with HLA-DR2. An experimental animal model, nonobese diabetic (NOD) mouse, shares many key features with the human disease, including the destruction of islet cells by lymphocytes, the association with susceptible MHC genes and the transmission by T cells. There are, however, notable differences including the predominance of T cells in NOD mice when compared with type I diabetes in humans and a greater bias towards females when compared with humans.

HASHIMOTO'S THYROIDITIS. Hashimoto's thyroiditis, which is a disease of the thyroid, most commonly found in middle-aged women, leads to the *formation of a goiter or to hypothyroidism,* which results from destruction of thyroid function. Once again, there is no known etiology. It appears that the disease is mediated by antibody and also by T cells.

Several target antigens appear to be involved in this disease process, including thyroglobulin, the major hormone made by the thyroid. Microsomal antigens from thyroid epithelial cells have also been implicated, and antibodies to both these types of antigen have been found in patients with Hashimoto's disease.

The evidence for mediation by T cells is, at best, indirect. The evidence rests, in part, on the histologic picture that accompanies this disease. There is an infiltration of predominantly mononuclear cells into the thyroid follicles, which is characteristic of other T cell-mediated delayed hypersensitivity reactions. However, the mononuclear infiltrates contain large numbers of B cells in addition to T cells and macrophages, indicating the possibility of the local synthesis of antibodies. Progressive destruction of thyroid follicles accompanies the presence of these infiltrates, and the gland attempts to regenerate and becomes enlarged. When destruction of follicles reaches a certain level, the output of thyroid hormone declines and the symptoms of hypothyroidism appear: dry skin, puffy face, brittle hair, and nails, and a feeling of being cold all the time.

Further evidence implicating T-cell-mediated responses comes from study of experimental autoimmune thyroiditis, which may be induced in animals either by immunization with thyroglobulin in complete Freund's adjuvant or by passively transferring by clones of T cells specific for thyroglobulin. An important distinction between the experimental and the naturally occurring autoimmune disease is that the former is acute and nonrecurring while the latter has a chronic, recurrent course. Thus, the precipitating event in the naturally occurring autoimmune disease is probably some ongoing process, rather than a single immunizing event.

Antibody- and T-Cell-Mediated Autoimmune Disease

RHEUMATOID ARTHRITIS. Rheumatoid arthritis is characterized by chronically *inflamed synovium, densely crowded with lymphocytes,* which may result in the destruction of cartilage and bone. The synovial membrane, usually one cell thick, becomes intensely cellular and mimics lymphoid tissue containing vessels, dendritic cells, macrophages, T, B, and NK cells, clumps of plasma cells and sometimes even secondary follicles. This condition causes the destructive joint erosion. The pathology in its most intense form is probably the consequence of a mixture of immunopathological mechanisms, specifically, antigen–antibody complexes, complement, polymorphonuclear neutrophils, inflammatory T cells, activated macrophages, and NK cells. This angry mix releases a variety of cytokines, enzymes, and mediators that results in the destruction of the cartilage integrity, exposure of chondrocytes, the cells of the cartilage, to the immune system and perpetuation of damage.

It has been suggested that inflammatory processes are initiated by abnormally produced antibody, generally IgM, called *rheumatoid factor (RF)*, which is specific for a determinant on the Fc portion of the patient's own IgG molecules. The complexes between rheumatoid factor and IgG are apparently deposited in the synovia of joint spaces, where they activate the complement cascade to release the chemotactic factors that attract granulocytes. The ongoing inflammatory response, accompanied by increased vascular permeability, induces joint swelling and pain as the exudate accumulates. Hydrolytic enzymes released by the neutrophils progressively break down the collagen and cartilage in the joints, with the eventual destruction of the sliding surfaces needed for proper function. After repeated bouts of inflammatory insult, with deposition of fibrin and replacement of the cartilage by fibrous tissue, the joint fuses (ankylosis), becomes immobile, and the inflammatory process subsides. However, the destructive consequences have also been observed in patients where no circulating RF have been detected. Thus, cell-mediated immune response may be initiated by other environmental insults (physical or infectious). It is clear that the cellularity of the synovium, however initiated, is responsible for the disease pathology in rheumatoid arthritis.

Autoimmune Diseases Arising From Deficiency in Components of Complement

Many patients with deficiencies in the early components of complement develop autoimmune diseases such as SLE. In addition, specific allotypes of some complement components predispose to the development of autoimmunity.

In the normal process of immune complex formation, such as occurs in infectious disease leading to antibody production, the complexes are very efficiently disposed of by the reticuloendothelial system. Complement-activating antigen–antibody complexes that form in the blood produce C3b, which noncovalently binds to these complexes. C3b bound to the complexes serves as a ligand for the C3b receptor on many cell types, including phagocytic cells as well as erythrocytes. The complexes bound to erythrocytes are rapidly transported to the liver and spleen where they are transferred to macrophages releasing the red cells to recirculate.

The *inappropriate deposition of immune complexes leading to disease can occur under several different circumstances:*

1. *Excessive immune complex formation* overwhelming the clearance mechanism as in serum sickness (see Chapter 15).

2. *Deficient antibody response* such that complement is poorly activated.

3. *Inherited deficiency* of a component of the classical complement pathway. A defect in any one of the C1, C4, or C2 complement components prevents the activation of the classical pathway, and deficiency of C4b and C3B would result in failure to clear immune complexes by macrophages.

4. *Abnormalities in complement or Fc receptors* on cells also leading to inefficient clearance of immune complexes.

It is of interest that SLE occurs in over 80% of individuals with complete deficiency of C1, C4, or C2. The sera of such patients are markedly deficient in their ability to deposit C3b on immune complexes and "processing" of even normal amounts of these complexes would be altered, thus permitting infectious agents to persist for extended periods.

SUMMARY

1. Autoimmunity is a condition in which the body makes an immune response to one or more of its own constituent.

2. Establishing a disease as autoimmune rests on several types of evidence: (a) direct proof made by transferring autoantibodies or self-reactive lymphocytes and reproducing the disease in an otherwise healthy individual; (b) indirect proof, which requires finding an experimental animal model to mimic the disease; (c) circumstantial evidence based on familial tendency and involvement of immune cells and antibodies; and (d) clinical improvement with immunosuppressive drugs.

3. Initiation of autoimmune diseases usually requires a combination of genetic and environmental events. It is believed that many autoreactive clones of T and B cells exist normally but are held in check by homeostatic mechanisms. It is the breakdown, by various mechanisms, of these controls that leads to the activation of autoreactive clones and autoimmune disease.

4. A multiplicity of organs and tissues is involved in autoimmune disease, and the type of immune response may involve antibody, complement, T cells, and macrophages.

REFERENCES

Bowman MA, Leiter EH, Atkinson MA (1994): Prevention of diabetes in the NOD mouse: implications for therapeutic intervention in human disease. Immunol Today 15:115.

Frank MM, Austen KF, Claman HN, Unanue ER (eds) (1995): Samter's Immunologic Diseases, 5th ed. Boston: Little, Brown.

Gill RG, Haskins K (1993): Molecular mechanisms underlying diabetes and other autoimmune diseases. Immunol Today 14:49.

Liblau RS, Singer SM, McDevitt HO (1995): Th1 and Th2 CD4$^+$ T cells in the pathogenesis of organ specific autoimmune diseases. Immunol Today 16:34.

Miller SD, Karpus WJ (1994): The immunopathogenesis and regulation of T cell mediated demyelinating diseases. Immunol Today 15:356.

Roitt I (1994): Essential Immunology, 4th ed. Oxford: Blackwell Scientific Publications.

Rose NR, Bona C (1993): Defining criteria for autoimmune diseases (Witebsky's postulates revisited). Immunol Today 14:426.

Theofilopoulos AN (1995): The basis of autoimmunity. Immunol Today 16:90 (Part I), 150 (Part II).

Zouali M, Kalsi J, Isenberg D (1993): Autoimmune diseases–at the molecular level. Immunol Today 14:473.

REVIEW QUESTIONS

Choose the ONE BEST answer or completion.

1. Most autoimmune diseases are caused by
   A) a single genetic defect
   B) a known infectious organism
   C) a constellation of genetic and environmental events
   D) a hormonal dysregulation
   E) a B-cell defect

2. The following is/are possible mechanism(s) for the recognition of self-components by the immune system in autoimmune diseases:
   A) alteration of a self antigen so it is recognized as foreign
   B) leakage of sequestered self antigen
   C) loss of suppressor T cells
   D) infection with a microorganism that carries a cross-reactive antigen
   E) any of the above

3. Rheumatoid factor, found in synovial fluid of patients with rheumatoid arthritis, is most frequently found to be
   A) IgM reacting with L-chains of IgG
   B) IgM reacting with H-chain determinants of IgG
   C) IgE reacting with bacterial antigens
   D) antibody to collagen
   E) antibody to DNA

4. The pathology in autoimmune diseases due to antibody may occur
   A) as a consequence of formation of antigen–antibody complexes
   B) as a result of antibody blocking a cell receptor
   C) as a result of antibody-induced phagocytosis
   D) as a result of antibody-induced complement mediated lysis
   E) as a result of any of the above

5. Hemolytic anemia may result from
   A) passive transfer of maternal anti-Rh antibody to the fetus

B) production of cold agglutinins after certain viral infections
C) transfusion of autologous stored red cells
D) A, B, and C
E) A and B

6. Lupus erythematosus
   A) is due to a mutation in double-stranded DNA
   B) has multiple symptoms and affects many organs
   C) is a classic example of a T-cell-mediated autoimmune disease
   D) results from antibodies specific to thyroid
   E) affects only skin epithelial cells

7. A patient is found to have a form of diabetes in which his immune system is destroying his pancreatic islet cells. He has been found to have an increased ratio of CD4$^+$/CD8$^+$ cells. Which is the most likely explanation for this disease state:
   A) the patient has an acquired immunodeficiency syndrome
   B) the patient's CD4$^+$ cells have been activated and are contributing to the pathology
   C) there is an increase in suppressor T cells
   D) CD8$^+$ T cells are being destroyed by pancreatic enzymes
   E) CD4$^+$ T cells are being destroyed by pancreatic enzymes

Case study: A 17-year-old boy suffered an injury to his left eye when, during a car crash, a sharp sliver of glass penetrated his eye, damaging his lens and uveal tract. The glass was removed and the injury repaired with complete recovery. However, 3 weeks later he noticed some redness in the left eye and photophobia, followed by pain and severe visual impairment. The left eye was removed, and histologic examination showed an extensively infiltrated uveal tract with abundant lymphocytes and mononuclear cells. Two weeks later the other eye began to show the same symptoms. What is going on, and what could be done?

ANSWERS TO REVIEW QUESTIONS

1. *C* The etiologies of most autoimmune diseases appear to be multifactorial and require a combination of genetic and environmental events to manifest themselves.

2. *E* Self-reactive T and B cells may be activated by any of the mechanisms listed.

3. *B* Rheumatoid factor is generally an IgM antibody that reacts with the determinants on the H chain.

4. *E* All are possible causes of antibody-induced autoimmune disease.

5. *E* Hemolytic anemia can be due to *A* and

B; *C* is not known to cause formation of autoantibody.

6. *B* Lupus erythematosus affects skin, kidneys, heart, and joints. Symptoms are due to immune complexes that lodge in those areas and induce damage via activation of complement and infiltration of leukocytes. DNA may be involved as an antigen, but mutation plays no role, and the disease is initiated primarily by antibodies and is not considered a classic T-cell disease.

7. *B* One of the currently favored mechanisms for type 1 diabetes is an autoimmune response in which CD4$^+$ T cells specific for islet-cell antigens are by a DTH reaction, leading to the destruction of islet cells.

Case study: The most likely diagnosis is of a rare case of sympathetic ophthalmia, an autoimmune disease in which trauma to uveal, retinal, and lens tissues releases antigens that induce T-cell-mediated responses. Once generated, these T cells attack the damaged eye and induce a granulomatous uveitis. They also have the potential for attacking the healthy eye, producing the same damaging effects. The diagnosis could be confirmed by the appearance of positive delayed-type reactions following skin testing with an extract of bovine uveal tissue, which cross-reacts immunologically with human uveal tissue. A safe procedure would be to look for an in vitro proliferative response of the patient's peripheral blood lymphocytes when exposed to the same antigen.

Immunosuppressive therapy with topical or systemic corticosteroids is useful in mild cases. Removing the damaged eye is the only way to prevent the onset of the autoimmune reaction. In these cases, clinicians must weigh the chances of maintaining useful vision in the injured eye against the risk of an autoimmune reaction with possible loss of both eyes.

IMMUNODEFICIENCY AND OTHER DISORDERS OF THE IMMUNE RESPONSE

INTRODUCTION

The acquired immune response is mediated by B lymphocytes (and antibody), T lymphocytes, phagocytic cells, and complement. The interaction of these components is tightly regulated in a variety of ways to ensure optimal function. Disorders in the development and differentiation of the cells, in the synthesis of their products, or in the regulation of these processes may lead to immunologic disorders that range in severity from mild to fatal. In this chapter, several of the most important disorders of the immune system are described. The chapter begins with disorders that result from immune deficiencies and concludes with a short description of some of the neoplastic disorders that result in the uncontrolled proliferation of immunocytes and the appearance, in serum, of high concentrations of their products.

In view of the present-day importance and general interest in acquired immune deficiency syndrome (AIDS), a special section is devoted to this disease.

IMMUNE DEFICIENCY DISORDERS

Immune deficiency disorders can roughly be divided into those disorders with a deficiency or malfunction of one or more of the major aspects of the immune response: (1) *B-cell-* or antibody-mediated immunity, (2) *T-cell-*mediated immunity, (3) both B- and T-cell-mediated immunity, (4) immunity mediated by the action of non-antigen-specific cells such as phagocytic cells and natural killer (NK) cells, and (5) immunity associated with the activation of serum *complement*. This classification provides a manageable way of dealing with the broad spectrum of immune disorders. It should be borne in mind that the expressed immune response is often the result of the interaction between several cell types and that a certain deficiency, for example, of a B-cell function, may be caused by a defect in the function of a T cell. Nevertheless, the classification of immune deficiency disorders given in the present chapter is based on the apparent expressed defect and not necessarily on its basic underlying cause (which is also discussed). Indeed, the basic underlying cause may be one of the many factors that control cellular differentiation, activation and interaction.

People with immunodeficiencies generally suffer from recurrent infections. Thus, an immune deficiency disorder should always be considered a possibility in a patient with recurrent infections. As we will see, the various disorders have their own particular characteristics and can be diagnosed by specific laboratory tests. The types of infection that occur as a result of an immune deficiency often facilitate the diagnosis of the deficiency. For example, recurrent bacterial otitis media and pneumonia are common in individuals with B-cell (antibody) deficiency; increased susceptibility to fungal, protozoan, and viral infections is common in individuals with deficiencies in T cells and cell-mediated immunity; systemic infections with bacteria, which are normally of low virulence, superficial skin infections, or infections with pyogenic (pus producing) organisms suggest deficiencies in phagocytic cells or their products; and recurrent infections with pyogenic microorganisms are associated with deficiencies in the complement system (Table 18.1).

Immune deficiency disorders are frequently divided into two major categories: (1) *primary immune deficiency disorders*, which may be hereditary or acquired, in which the immune deficiency is the cause of a disease; and (2) *secondary immune deficiency disorders*, in which the immune deficiency is a result of other disease(s).

TABLE 18.1 The Major Levels of Immune Disorders

Disorder	Associated disease
Deficiency	
B-lymphocyte deficiency—deficiency in antibody-mediated immunity	Recurrent bacterial infections, e.g., otitis media, recurrent pneumonia
T-lymphocyte deficiency—deficiency in cell-mediated immunity	Increased susceptibility to viral, fungal, and protozoal infections
T- and B-lymphocyte deficiency—combined deficiency of antibody- and cell-mediated immunity	Acute and chronic infections with viral, bacterial, fungal, and protozoal organisms
Phagocytic cell deficiency	Systemic infections with bacteria of usually low virulence; infections with pyogenic bacteria; impaired pus formation and wound healing
NK cell deficiency	Viral infections, associated with several T-cell disorders and X-linked lymphoproliferative symptoms
Complement component deficiency	Bacterial infections; autoimmunity
Unregulated excess	
B lymphocytes	Monoclonal gammopathies; other B-cell malignancies
T lymphocytes	T-cell malignancies
Complement components	Angioneurotic edema due to absence of C1 esterase inhibitor

Primary Immunodeficiency Disorders

The frequency of primary immune deficiency disorders is very low when compared to other diseases. It is estimated to be in the order of about 1 in 10,000, with antibody deficiency constituting about 50% of the cases. Approximately 20% of the cases are attributed to combined deficiency in both antibodies and cell-mediated immunity, 18% to phagocytic disorders, 10% to disorders of cell-mediated immunity, and 2% to complement deficiency. Although all of these disorders are relatively rare, trying to understand the defects in these diseases has contributed immensely to the elucidation of the role of T cells, B cells, phagocytes, and complement in the immune response and in protection against infectious diseases.

IMMUNODEFICIENCY DISEASES ASSOCIATED WITH B CELLS OR ANTIBODY. Immune deficiency diseases that are associated with deficiencies in B cells or antibody may range from defects in the development of B cells and the complete absence of all classes of immunoglobulins to deficiencies in a single class or subclass of immunoglobulin.

Laboratory tests for disorders of B cells or antibody immunodeficiency include analysis of the number and function of B cells and immunoelectrophoretic and quantitative evaluations to determine the presence and levels of the various classes and subclasses of immunoglobulin. These tests are usually prescribed for patients who are suspected of having immunodeficiency disorders because they suffer from recurrent or chronic infections.

X-Linked Infantile Agammaglobulinemia. First described in 1952 by Bruton, *X-linked infantile agammaglobulinemia* is also called *Bruton's agammaglobulinemia*. The disorder is X-linked, occurring only in *male infants*, and is relatively rare (1/100,000). It is expressed at approximately 5–6 months of age when the infant has lost most of the maternally derived IgG that had passed through the placenta. At that age, the infant with X-linked agammaglobulinemia begins to suffer from repeated *bacterial infections*. Analysis of the infant's serum immunoglobulins reveals a severe depression or virtual *absence of all classes of Ig*. In spite of the involvement of all classes of Ig, the disorder is still referred to as agammaglobulinemia, an old term used to encompass all immunoglobulins.

The major defect in X-linked agammaglobulinemia is the inability of pre-B cells, which are present at normal levels in these infants, to develop into mature B cells. It is associated with the failure of IgV gene rearrangement, specifically the rearrangement of the V_H region genes to the DJ_H junction (see Chapter 6). It appears that the underlying defect is the absence of enzymes specific for translocation of the V_H genes or a defect in regulatory genes necessary for the differentiation of the pre-B cell to a stage that can utilize these enzymes.

The limited number of B cells actually generated appear normal in their ability to become plasma cells. Analysis of the blood, bone marrow, spleen, or lymph nodes reveals a *near absence of mature B cells*, which, together with the relative *absence of plasma cells*, explains the depressed levels of Ig. Infants with X-linked agammaglobulinemia suffer from recurrent *bacterial* otitis media, bronchitis, septicemia, pneumonia, arthritis, meningitis, and dermatitis. The most common etiologic agents are *Haemophilus influenzae* and *Streptococcus pneumoniae*. Frequently, patients with this disorder suffer from malabsorption due to infestation of the gastrointestinal tract with *Giardia lamblia*. Infections that occur in infants with X-linked agammaglobulinemia do not respond well to antibiotics. The treatment of choice consists of periodic *injections of large amounts of IgG*, which is effective in varying degrees. Although such passive immunization has maintained several patients for 20–30 years, the prognosis for patients with X-linked agammaglobulinemia is guarded, as chronic lung disease due to repeated infections often supervenes.

Transient Hypogammaglobulinemia. At approximately 5–6 months of age, the maternal IgG that has been passively transferred through the placenta finally disappears, and the level of IgG synthesized by the infant then begins to rise. Infants born very prematurely who are not yet synthesizing immunoglobulins and after their mother's transferred immunoglobulins have disappeared, suffer from a transient IgG deficiency (other Ig classes are not placentally transferred). Occasionally, an infant born in term may fail to synthesize appropriate amounts of IgG, even when levels of IgM or IgA appear normal. The absence of IgG appears to be due to a deficiency in number and function of T helper cells, which are essential for synthesis of IgG. This results in the disorder known as *transient hypogammaglobulinemia*. The disorder may persist from a few months to as long as 2 years.

Transient hypogammaglobulinemia is not sex-linked and can be distinguished from the X-linked disease by the normal numbers of B cells in the blood. Patients with transient hypogammaglobulinemia usually recover by the first or second year of life. If a patient does not have severe recurrent infections, passive administration of immune serum globulin is not necessary or advisable. However, such treatment may be warranted in the rare cases where the patient suffers from severe recurrent infections. Routine immunizations given to infants should not be given during the period of transient hypogamomaglobulinemia. In fact, immunization with live viruses is very risky since the individual is unable to mount an immune response against the viruses, and immunization with killed or attenuated viruses is ineffective.

Common Variable Hypogammaglobulinemia. The cause of *common variable hypogammaglobulinemia*, which affects both males and females, is not entirely clear. The onset may occur at any age, with a somewhat higher frequency between the ages of 15 and 35 years. Affected patients suffer from an increased susceptibility to infection with *pyogenic bacteria* and, paradoxically exhibit a high incidence of *autoimmune diseases*, such as hemolytic anemia, thrombocytopenia, and systemic lupus erythematosus, which are associated with autoantibodies. A high percentage of patients also have disorders of cell-mediated immunity.

As with patients with transient hypogammaglobulinemia, patients with common variable hypogammaglobulinemia have ***B cells that fail to mature into antibody-secreting cells***. The nature of the defect in B cells is not uniform in all patients, and ranges from absence of proliferation of B cells in response to antigen to normal proliferation of B cells but secretion of only IgM, or to failure of glycosylation of γ-chains of IgG. In most cases, however, the disorder appears to be the result of diminished synthesis and secretion of immunoglobulins.

The treatment of common variable hypogammaglobulinemia depends on the severity of the disease. For severe disease, accompanied by many recurrent or chronic infections, treatment with immune serum globulin is indicated. Treated patients with this disorder can survive to age 70 or 80 years. Women with this disease have normal pregnancies, although, of course, no maternal IgG is transferred to the fetus (unless the mother receives globulins).

Selective Immunoglobulin Deficiencies. Several immunodeficiency syndromes are associated with the selective deficiency of a certain class or subclass of immunoglobulins. Some such deficiencies may be accompanied by compensatory elevated levels of other isotypes, as exemplified by the increased IgM levels in cases of IgG or IgA deficiency.

Selective ***IgA deficiency*** is the most common immunodeficiency disorder in this category, with an incidence of approximately 1 in 800. The cause of IgA deficiency is not known, but it appears to be associated with a decreased release of IgA synthesized by B lymphocytes. Patients with this disorder may suffer from recurrent sinopulmonary viral or bacterial infections. Increased incidence of celiac disease (defective absorption in the bowel) has been noted in patients with selective IgA deficiency. Paradoxically, most people with IgA deficiency remain generally healthy.

Treatment of symptomatic patients with IgA deficiency consists of administration of wide-spectrum antibiotics. Therapy with immune serum globulin is not useful because commercial preparations contain only low levels of IgA, and because injected IgA does not get to the local secretory areas where IgA is normally the protective antibody. Furthermore, the patients may mount an immune response of IgG or IgE antibodies to the IgA in the transferred immune serum, causing hypersensitivity reactions. In general, however, the prognosis is good, with many patients surviving to old age. There are other disorders that result from selective deficiencies in immunoglobulin isotypes. An example is IgM deficiency, a rare disorder, in which patients suffer from recurrent and severe infections with polysaccharide-encapsulated organisms, such as pneumonococci and

Haemophilus influenzae. Selective deficiencies in subclasses of IgG have been described but are very rare.

IMMUNODEFICIENCY DISORDERS ASSOCIATED WITH T CELLS AND CELL-MEDIATED IMMUNITY. Patients with T-cell-associated deficiency diseases (Table 18.1) are extremely susceptible to *viral, fungal, and protozoal* infections. Moreover, because T cells participate in the antibody response to T-dependent antigens, patients with T-cell defects exhibit various defects in the production of antibody after immunization or exposure to many microorganisms. Consequently, patients with T-cell deficiency suffer from diseases against which the body is normally protected by both T and B cells.

Congenital Thymic Aplasia (DiGeorge Syndrome). DiGeorge syndrome is the most notable of the T-cell deficiency diseases. The disease results from a defect in the embryonic development of the *third and fourth pharyngeal pouches*, which takes place during approximately the 12th week of gestation. Both the thymus and the parathyroids fail to develop, with consequent *thymic aplasia* and *hypoparathyroidism*. The newborns suffer from hypocalcemia during the first 24 hours of life, as well as from a variety of other congenital disorders, for example, of the heart and kidneys. DiGeorge syndrome is not hereditary. Babies with DiGeorge syndrome suffer from recurrent or chronic infections with *viruses, bacteria, fungi, and protozoa*. They have either no T cells or very few T cells in the blood, lymph nodes, or spleen. The few T lymphocytes that are present exhibit abnormalities involving cell-surface molecules. These abnormalities are also expressed by the inability of the T cells to respond to mitogens such as concanavalin A and phytohemagglutinin.

Although the B cells, plasma cells, and levels of serum immunoglobulins of patients with DiGeorge syndrome may be normal, many patients fail to mount an antibody response after immunization. Most notably absent is the IgG response, which requires helper T cells. Because of the absence of T cell responses and abnormal antibody responses, individuals with DiGeorge syndrome should never be immunized with live attenuated viral vaccines!

Treatment for DiGeorge syndrome consists of transplantation of fetal thymus. In many cases, the treatment brings about the appearance of T cells within a week after transplantation and may lead to permanent reconstitution of T-cell-mediated immunity. The fetal thymus used for transplantation should not be older than 14 weeks of gestation, to avoid *graft-versus-host (GVH)* reactions, which would occur if mature thymocytes were transferred from the donor into an immunoincompetent recipient, causing tissue damage in the recipient (discussed in Chapter 20). Donor fetal thymus of less than 14 weeks of gestation provides a sufficient number of thymic epithelial cells to permit successful development of T cells from bone marrow precursors in the recipient.

The prognosis for untreated patients is poor, but transplantation of fetal thymus has resulted in prolonged survival of patients with DiGeorge syndrome. Other disorders associated with the syndrome (such as congenital heart disorders), however, must also be dealt with, and these can complicate both the treatment and prognosis.

Chronic Mucocutaneous Candidiasis. Chronic mucocutaneous candidiasis, an infection of skin and mucous membranes by a *fungus* that is normally present but nonpathogenic (*Candida albicans*), is a poorly defined collection of syndromes associated with a *selective defect in the functioning of T cells*.

Patients with this disorder usually have a normal T-cell-mediated immunity to microorganisms other than *Candida* and normal B-cell-mediated immunity to all microorganisms including *Candida* (against which the patients mount a normal antibody response). This disorder affects both males and females, and there is some evidence that it may be inherited. Children are particularly affected. There is additional morbidity associated with this disorder because patients with chronic mucocutaneous candidiasis also suffer from various endocrine dysfunctions such as adrenal or parathyroid deficiencies, especially Addison's disease, which is the major cause of death.

Treatment of candidiasis is very difficult. It consists of the administration of antifungal agents. However, the general prognosis for the disease is guarded.

X-Linked Lymphoproliferative Syndrome (Duncan's Syndrome). Cases of this X-linked lymphoproliferative syndrome are very rare. They are associated with an abnormal response to Epstein–Barr Virus (EBV) infection which results in B-cell proliferation, T-cell depletion, and/or malignant lymphoma. This syndrome has been observed in six maternally related males of the Duncan family. Thus the syndrome has been named Duncan's syndrome.

SEVERE COMBINED IMMUNODEFICIENCY DISEASE. Combined immunodeficiency diseases (SCID) are a heterogeneous group of immune disorder diseases due to a failure of stem cells to differentiate into T and/or B cells and due to defects in cell function. These disorders exhibit a severe reduction in the number of circulating lymphocytes with either T- or B-cell markers; in some patients the lymphocytes that are present fail to express MHC class I or class II molecules (*"bare lymphocyte syndrome"*).

Individuals with SCID are susceptible to virtually any type of microbial (*viral, bacterial, fungal, and protozoal*) infection, most notably cytomegalovirus, *Pneumocystis carinii*, and *Candida*. Symptoms begin in early infancy, and untreated patients seldom survive beyond their first year. However, infants with this disorder can be cured by transplantation of bone marrow (see below).

The disease is inherited as either an *X-linked* or an autosomal recessive trait (the latter formerly known as *Swiss-type agammaglobulinemia*). Patients with this deficiency exhibit an absence of T and B cells, expressed by a marked *lymphopenia*. It must be emphasized that patients with SCID should not be vaccinated with attenuated live microorganisms. Vaccination could have disastrous results, since the patient is unable to mount an immune response against the inoculated microorganism.

A variant of SCID that is present in about 50% of patients with the autosomal recessive form of the disease is associated with a deficiency in the enzyme *adenosine deaminase (ADA).* The enzyme is absent from all the patient's cells. However, its absence from lymphoid cells is particularly harmful to these cells since toxic amounts of adenosine triphosphate (ATP) and deoxyATP accumulate within them without being destroyed by the enzyme. Early diagnosis is important if treatment is to be initiated before the appearance of irreversible complications. Treatment consists of transplantation with histocompatible or partially HLA-matched bone marrow from which mature T cells have been eliminated (see Chapter 20). The gene coding for ADA has been cloned, and gene insertion therapy for ADA deficiency has been successful. In fact, it represents the first gene therapy in humans.

In addition to the immunodeficiency diseases already described, there are several that are associated with other abnormalities. One such disease is *ataxia telangiectasia*, in which neurologic symptoms (staggering gait) and abnormal, spider-like vascular dilation (telangiectasia) accompany the lymphopenia and depressed levels of IgA, IgE, and sometimes IgG.

Another immunodeficiency disease, *Wiskott–Aldrich syndrome*, affects patients early in life and is associated with thrombocytopenia (low platelet level in blood), eczema, and recurrent infections. The patients suffer from bleeding, due to the thrombocytopenia, as well as from recurrent bacterial infections that cause otitis media, meningitis, and pneumonia.

The underlying defect in patients with Wiskott–Aldrich syndrome has not yet been conclusively defined. The immunologic defects are broad and involve the cellular as well as the humoral arm of the immune response. The patients have a normal number of circulating lymphocytes, but their response to antigen is low. They also have a defect in the generation of cytotoxic lymphocytes. Some of the immunologic disorders appear to be associated with the peculiar inability to respond to polysaccharide antigens.

Treatment consists of antibiotics and antiviral agents given promptly with each infection. Reconstitution of T and B cells has been reported following bone marrow transplantation. Without treatment, the average life of patients with Wiskott–Aldrich syndrome is approximately 3 years.

PHAGOCYTIC DYSFUNCTIONS. The immunodeficiency disorders discussed so far involve defects in the function or products of T cells, B cells, or both. Since polymorphonuclear leukocytes and monocytes also play an important role in both innate and acquired immunity, acting either alone or in concert with lymphocytes, defects in their activity may lead to disease.

Phagocytic dysfunction may be caused by *extrinsic factors*, such as deficiency of antibodies, complement components, or the lymphokines, which activate the phagocytic cells. It may also be caused by *defects in the metabolic pathways* of the phagocytic cells themselves, pathways that are essential for the killing of the pathogen. Such deficiencies include reduced or absent levels of glucose-6-phosphate dehydrogenase, myeloperoxidase, and alkaline phosphatase; abnormal functions of microtubules; and low levels of lysosomal enzymes (*Chediak-Higashi syndrome*).

Chronic granulomatous disease (CGD) is an important disease associated with a defective intracellular respiratory burst of phagocytes. It is inherited as an X-linked or autosomal recessive disorder and consists of a group of a heterogeneous *disorders of oxidative metabolism* affecting the pathways required for hydrogen peroxide production by phagocytic cells. The cells ingest bacteria but do not kill them; the intracellular survival of the organisms results in the formation of a granuloma, which is an organized structure consisting of mononuclear cells. Normally, activated neutrophils and mononuclear phagocytes have a respiratory burst—increased oxygen consumption leading to the generation of intracellular hydrogen peroxide and superoxide radicals. In patients with CGD, the generation of hydrogen peroxide and superoxide radicals required for the killing of ingested intracellular organisms does not take place. Most patients with CGD are males who lack cytochrome b_{245}, which is required for oxidase activity; female patients do have cytochrome b_{245}, but have a defect in another factor required for respiratory burst oxidase activation.

Symptoms begin to appear during the first 2 years of life. Patients suffer from a greatly enhanced susceptibility to infection with organisms that are normally of low virulence, such as *Staphylococcus aureus, Serratia marcescens*, and *Aspergillus*. Frequent abnormalities include lymphadenopathy, hepatosplenomegaly, and chronic draining lymph nodes due to the chronic and acute infections occurring in lymph nodes, skin, intestinal tract, liver, and bone.

Treatment consists of aggressive therapy with wide-spectrum antibiotics and with antifungal agents. Lately attempts have been made to treat CGD with interferon γ. Prognosis is poor, although in the past decade the prognosis has been significantly improved with the use of prophylactic antibiotics and improved education.

NK-CELL DEFICIENCY. Very little is known about NK (natural killer)-cell deficiency in humans, and only a few such cases have been reported. From animal studies it appears that NK-cell deficiency impairs allograft rejection and is linked to higher susceptibility to viral diseases and increase in spread of metastatic tumors. NK-cell deficiency has been detected in severe combined immunodeficiency disorders, in some T cell disorders, and in X-linked lymphoproliferative syndrome (Duncan's syndrome) mentioned earlier.

LEUKOCYTE ADHESION DEFICIENCY. *Leukocyte adhesion deficiency (LAD)* is an autosomal recessive trait resulting in deficiency of a component of several related glycoproteins on the surface of leukocytes that participate in adherence, such as LFA-1 (CD11a, CD18) (see Chapter 11). Those functions of granulocytes, monocytes, and lymphocytes that depend upon cell adhesion are impaired. LAD individuals suffer from recurrent bacterial infections, impaired pus formation, and impaired wound healing. Bone marrow transplantation constitutes the treatment of choice for LAD.

DISEASES DUE TO ABNORMALITIES IN THE COMPLEMENT SYSTEM. As we have seen (Chapter 13), complement components are important in the killing of bacteria, in opsonization, and in chemotaxis. They may also play a role in the prevention of immune aggregate diseases by participating in the elimination of antigen–antibody complexes. Thus, deficiencies in complement components may result in a variety of effects, ranging from *recurrent bacterial infections* to increased susceptibility to *autoimmune diseases*. Excess of a given component of complement or the absence of an appropriate inhibitor of the component may also result in disorders of varying severity. Certain genetic defects have been shown to be associated with most of the individual components of complement. The defects are inherited as autosomal recessive traits, with heterozygous individuals having half the normal level of a given component of the complement system.

Deficiencies in C1 as well as C4 and C2 have been associated with ***autoimmune diseases***, predominantly in patients with syndromes that resemble ***systemic lupus erythematosus (SLE)***. These patients also have increased susceptibility to ***bacterial*** infections. It is felt that these problems stem from a decreased ability to clear antigen–antibody complexes through the reticuloendothelial system, allowing them to accumulate inappropriately and induce pathology (see Chapter 17).

An important disorder associated with C1 is ***hereditary angioedema,*** alluded to in Chapter 13. Patients with this disease lack a functional ***inhibitor of C1 esterase***, the activated form of C1. The absence of this inhibitor leaves the action of C1 on C4 or C2 uncontrolled, generating large amounts of vasoactive peptides. C1 also controls the activity of the kallikrein system through which bradykinin, another vasoactive peptide, is formed. The vasoactive peptides cause increased blood vessel permeability. Patients with this deficiency suffer from local ***edema*** in various organs, which may become particularly life-threatening when it occurs in the larynx and obstructs the passage of air.

Treatment includes avoidance of the precipitating factors, usually trauma, and infusion of C1 esterase inhibitor. ϵ-Aminocaproic acid (EACA), an inhibitor of plasminogen activation, can be used effectively prophylactically before unavoidable trauma such as from surgery or dental work. Patients with deficiency in C3 experience recurrent bacterial infections. In some patients, the deficiency is also associated with chronic glomerulonephritis.

Patients with deficiencies in the latter complement components C5–C8 have a tendency to increased infections, most notably to recurrent infections with *Neisseria*.

Another disorder associated with complement regulation is ***paroxysmal nocturnal hemoglobulinuria (PNH),*** a disease in which red blood cell lysis may occur at night. These patients have a deficiency in DAF (decay accelerating factor of certain complement components; see Chapter 13), which leads to increased sensitivity to complement-mediated lysis of erythrocytes.

Secondary Immunodeficiency Diseases

In contrast to primary immunodeficiency diseases, in which there are hereditary or acquired defects in B or T lymphocytes, phagocytic cells, or complement, secondary immunodeficiency diseases are those in which the immune dysfunction is secondary to other disease states and generates further complications. Secondary immune deficiency diseases may result from the loss of T or B lymphocytes or their functions due to illnesses such as leukemia, in which malignant cells replace normal populations.

By far the most common cause of immunodeficiency disorders in developed countries is secondary to the use of ***chemotherapeutic agents*** in cancer therapy. Many of these agents are toxic to bone marrow cells and to T and B lymphocytes. Also, the deliberate ***immunosuppression*** induced during organ transplantation, in order to avoid immunologic rejection, may bring on the consequences of an immunodeficiency disease. Secondary immunodeficiencies are also associated with overwhelming infections by bacteria, leading to a swamping of the immune response. These are often refractory to antibiotic therapy and are generally fatal.

ACQUIRED IMMUNODEFICIENCY SYNDROME

An immune deficiency disease that has become the focus of much global concern and that is reaching epidemic proportions in some parts of the world is ***acquired immunodeficiency syndrome (AIDS)***. It is interesting to note that from the discovery of AIDS in 1981 until today, the scientific progress made in understanding the cause and the epidemiology of the disease was so rapid that it has no parallel with other infectious diseases. Nevertheless, what has been said in the previous edition of this book (1991) still holds true today, namely, that with much of the present-day understanding of the disease, vaccination and a cure for AIDS are not yet "around the corner."

The Disease and Its Epidemiology

Infection with a retrovirus, the human immunodeficiency virus, HIV, is the cause of AIDS. Two to 4 weeks after infection, some infected individuals experience fever, sore throat, general malaise and several other symptoms, all of which usually disappear within 1–2 weeks. This is usually followed by an asymptomatic period that may last for years. Finally, the infected individual develops overt disease (AIDS). The AIDS patient exhibits various manifestations of the syndrome, typically, immune dysfunction accompanied by the presence of ***opportunistic*** infections that become overwhelming in the absence of an effective immune response. A common opportunistic infection that often leads to death is *Pneumocystis carinii*. Infections by bacteria, viruses, fungi, and protozoa, particularly infections by cytomegalovirus, cryptococcus, mycobacteria, and toxoplasma, are commonly seen in AIDS patients. Often patients exhibit a pronounced susceptibility to ***Kaposi's sarcoma***, a rare skin cancer previously seen only in elderly individuals and individuals receiving immunosuppressive therapy. Patients may also exhibit an increased incidence of chronic lymphadenopathy and a rare lymphoma (diffuse, undifferentiated non-Hodgkin's lymphoma). About 35% of living AIDS patients show clinical symptoms of disease of the central and peripheral nervous system.

This collection of clinical conditions became recognized in 1982 as acquired immunodeficiency syndrome, or AIDS. As of 1986, over 90% of the AIDS cases in the United States were diagnosed in sexually active male homosexuals in large cities, but it is clear that the infection and the disease have no sexual preference: AIDS has spread into the heterosexual population through exposure to the blood or semen of infected individuals. It is estimated that, in the United States, as of 1994, over 50% of the AIDS cases were among homosexual or bisexual men, 26% were among intravenous drug users, 4% among heterosexual men and women, and the rest of the cases were mainly among hemophiliacs and other recipients of blood or blood products. A growing population of AIDS patients are children who were infected from their mothers before, during, or soon after birth.

Currently there are approximately 500,000 cases of AIDS in the United States. At the end of 1993 approximately 200,000 individuals had died from AIDS in the United States. This is alarming since generally no known recovery from AIDS has been reported and since over 90% of the diagnosed cases will result in death. Equally alarming are reports of the World Health Organization (WHO) about the worldwide spread of HIV infections, over half of which are in central Africa where the spread is primarily from heterosexual contact. Current WHO reports estimate that, worldwide, there are 14 million people infected with HIV. The projection for the year 2000 is 30 million infected people, worldwide. Other estimates for the year 2000 range from 40 million to 120 million infected individuals. Thus, although various estimates may differ, it is clear that HIV infection constitutes a serious threat to a significant portion of the world human population.

It is hoped that a better understanding of the disease, better application of effective social, behavioral, and public health measures to reduce HIV transmission, a better diagnosis of the disease, and, hopefully, some therapeutic modalities and vaccination against infection will make the general outlook less depressing.

Human Immunodeficiency Virus

It is now firmly established that AIDS is caused by human immunodeficiency virus (HIV). New and sensitive tests reveal the virus in every individual with AIDS. Moreover, over 90% of the patients with AIDS have antibodies to HIV.

HIV is a retrovirus; it is depicted diagrammatically in Figure 18.1. Like other viruses, it requires the synthetic apparatus of the host's cell for its replication. However, unlike other viruses, the retroviruses utilize a unique system by which the ordinary flow of genetic information from DNA to RNA is reversed. The entire

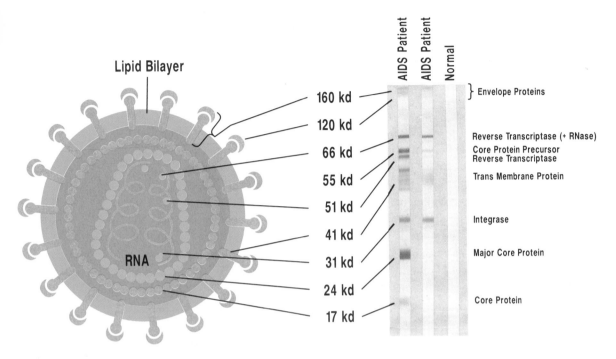

Figure 18.1

A diagrammatic representation of the human immunodeficiency virus (HIV) indicating the various viral proteins. (Adapted from B. Matija Peterlin and Paul A. Luciw, 1988: AIDS 1:S29–S40.) Also shown are Western blots performed on viral proteins, using sera from two AIDS patients and serum obtained from a normal, noninfected individual. (Courtesy of Dr. J.R. Carlson, AIDS Diagnostic Laboratory, University of California, Davis.)

process begins with the attachment of HIV to its target cell, mainly through a glycoprotein (gp120) [where gp stands for glycoprotein and the number refers to molecular weight in multiple of thousand] of the viral envelope protein to CD4 on the T lymphocyte. After attachment, the viral envelope fuses with the cell membrane and the viral core, which includes two identical strands of RNA as well as some structural proteins and enzymes, enters the host's cell. The viral information contained in the RNA is transcribed to DNA by the viral enzyme reversed transcriptase (also called **RNA-dependent DNA polymerase**). The enzyme first makes a single-stranded DNA copy of this viral DNA. After destruction of the viral RNA by the viral RNAse H activity, the polymerase uses the DNA as a template and makes a complementary copy of DNA forming a double-stranded DNA, which migrates into the nucleus of the host's cell and is inserted by the aid of yet another viral enzyme (integrase) into the host's cell genome. However, significant levels of integrated HIV

DNA persist in the cytoplasm of infected cells. Completion of the reverse transcription of viral genomic RNA is dependent on activation of the host cell. Moreover, activation of the host cell is required for the transcription of integrated viral DNA into viral RNA and mRNA, leading to the biosynthesis of new viral particles which can infect new cells. From the long and variable period called the *latent* or *asymptomatic phase* which exists between viral infection and the development of symptomatic AIDS, it is clear that the virus can remain with a rather minimal replication state for several years, until some events trigger cell activation, rapid replication, cell death, and further infection of other cells. (Just what triggers this rapid replication is still a mystery, but, as we shall see, several mechanisms may be offered.) Thus, HIV infection can be divided into three major phases: (1) the early or acute phase caused by the primary HIV infection, lasting from a few days to a few weeks, during which time the patient may have symptoms resembling acute mononucleosis with fever, sweats, sore throat, and fatigue; (2) the latent or asymptomatic phase, lasting years; and (3) the final or crisis phase with overt AIDS, lasting months or even years—during this phase, the patient is immunocompromised and is susceptible to various infections usually leading to death.

The precise origin of HIV is still not clear. Two strains of HIV have been described, HIV-I and HIV-II, the latter mainly confined to Africa. The virus is related to several other retroviruses that infect humans and other primates. However, while some of the retroviruses are highly pathogenic in several host species, they appear to be benign in other species and are able to coexist with their host. A good example is the simian immunodeficiency virus (SIV), a close relative of HIV. (HIV I and HIV II have about 50% nucleotide homology, while HIV I and SIV share about 80% homology.) SIV causes an immunodeficiency syndrome similar to AIDS in Asian macaques in various primate research centers. However, 30–70% of individuals in various African green monkey populations are infected with SIV, yet the infection does not lead to disease. It is, therefore, possible that the African green monkeys may serve as a reservoir for SIV.

The relationship between the geneology of the various strains of HIV and SIV is still not clear. It goes without saying that understanding the relationship between the host and the virus, whether SIV or HIV, is of critical importance in devising modalities to control AIDS.

Immunopathogenic Mechanisms of HIV Infection

It is now firmly established that a major mechanism in infectivity by HIV is through the attachment of the viral envelope glycoprotein of molecular weight

120,000 daltons (gp120) to CD4 molecules that serve as high-affinity receptors for the viral envelope protein. CD4 molecules are abundant primarily on helper T cells. However, cells such as the monocyte/macrophage lineage may be infected with HIV through ingestion of virus-antibody complexes, or through CD4 that they can express at low density on their cell surface.

In general, there is strong evidence that the CD4 molecule plays a crucial role in the pathogenesis of HIV and in the cytopathic effect of HIV. Whereas a wide range of cytopathicity is observed among various CD4$^+$ cells, it is apparent that cytopathicity is highest in those cells with the highest surface CD4 density: CD4$^+$ lymphocytes. Cell death can result from HIV infection, because of extensive lysis of the infected cell and the lysis of the cell by complement activated by antibody to gp120 and gp44 on the infected cell [gp44 is derived from the HIV envelope protein gp160 (see Fig. 18.1)]. Infected cells are also killed by ADCC, or by cytolytic T lymphocytes directed to viral proteins on the surface of the infected cell. Asymptomatic infected individuals exhibit a depletion of CD4$^+$ cells in spite of the finding that only 1 in 10^4 or 1 in 10^5 CD4$^+$ cells carries the virus, viral RNA or unintegrated viral DNA. This points to several possible pathogenetic mechanisms in AIDS. For example, HIV may infect and kill or impair CD4$^+$ cells that are required for the growth of the CD4$^+$ lymphoid pool. Also, CD4$^+$ cell depletion may result from HIV induction of certain CD4$^+$ cells to secrete substances toxic to CD4$^+$ T cells. It has been shown that the envelope protein gp120 present on the surface of HIV-infected cells may react with CD4 on noninfected cells, leading to fusion of the cell membranes and resulting in the formation of multinucleated giant cells *(syncytia),* which, within a short time, undergo cytolysis and death. It has also been suggested that the binding of free gp120, which is present in the circulation of infected individuals, with CD4 molecules on uninfected cells leads to autoimmunity, which eliminates by ADCC or by antibody-activated complement these gp120-complexed CD4$^+$ (but uninfected) cells. Several other possibilities have been suggested, all attempting to explain the phenomenon of the depletion of uninfected CD4$^+$ T cells.

These possibilities notwithstanding, it should be pointed out that with the decline in the number of peripheral CD4$^+$ cells, the proportion of CD4$^+$ cells infected with HIV increases dramatically with the progression of the disease to one infected cell in 100 CD4$^+$ cells. These findings strongly suggest that the killing of CD4$^+$ cells during HIV infection is mostly a direct result of virus expression rather than by the indirect mechanisms mentioned above to explain the depletion of non-infected cells.

The immune deficiency of AIDS patients is caused not only by the reduction of CD4$^+$ helper lymphocytes but also by the impairment of their function in the absence of any cytopathic effect. Early in the course of AIDS when infected individuals are seropositive for HIV, but are still totally asymptomatic, they may display a lack of responsiveness to tetanus toxoid and to some other test antigens. There is good evidence indicating that this lack of responsiveness is due to an impairment of antigen-specific CD4$^+$ function. This functional impairment, in the absence of significant CD4$^+$ cell infection, may be caused by HIV or its gp120 envelope protein blocking antigen-specific CD4$^+$ cell responses. This is caused by binding of HIV or its gp120 to CD4 molecules and, thus, preventing the interaction of these molecules with MHC class II molecules on the surface of antigen-presenting cells. Such an interaction is essential for the activation of CD4$^+$ cells by antigen. Indeed, a noncytopathic infection of CD4$^+$ cells by HIV has been shown to interfere with CD4 expression on the cells that would now lack the ability to interact with class II molecules of the antigen-presenting cells.

The impairment in CD4$^+$ T cell function is also expressed by the dramatic reduction in IL-2 that they produce. As discussed in earlier chapters, IL-2 is essential for the activation of many T-cell subpopulations, including T cytotoxic lymphocytes, which participate in the killing of virally infected cells.

The picture is further complicated by the fact that HIV is capable of infecting cells of the monocyte/macrophage line through several mechanisms such as engulfment of virus, free or complexed to antibodies, or attachment to the CD4 molecules that may be sparsely present on the surface of these cells. The cytopathic effect of HIV on monocytes is much smaller than on CD4$^+$ T cells. This raises the possibility that monocytes may act as a reservoir for HIV, transporting the virus to various parts of the body.

As mentioned earlier, one of the puzzling phenomena in HIV infection is how after years of latent or asymptomatic phase the virus begins to replicate rapidly, leading to infection of new cells and ultimately to fulminating disease. The answer to this mystery is beginning to appear. It has been shown that during the latent period the stimulation of T lymphocytes by mitogens and antigens results in cell activation accompanied by cytokine production and in extensive viral replication. Peripheral blood mononuclear cells, which include CD4$^+$ cells that had been activated by antigen before HIV infection, exhibit 10–100 times higher viral replication than similarly infected cells that had not been activated by antigen. This raises the possibility that the viral RNA or integrated DNA present in CD4$^+$ cells specific to certain antigens, such as those of various microorganisms, may become activated to replicate rapidly by a new exposure of these CD4$^+$ cells to these microorganisms and their antigens. Since activation of CD4$^+$ cells by antigen is highly dependent on various cytokines, it is possible that these cytokines can control the activation of the latent HIV. For example, it has been shown that progression of AIDS is characterized by less IL-2 and interferon γ production concomitant with an increase in IL-4 and IL-10, and that the cytokine controlled ratio between some Th-cell subpopulations (Th$_1$ and Th$_2$) is important in the etiology of HIV infection (see Chapter 11). Some experiments led to the speculation that coinfection with several DNA viruses, such as hepatitis B virus, Epstein–Barr virus, and cytomegalovirus, may contribute cofactors that dramatically increase transcription of HIV, leading to a high degree of destruction of CD4$^+$ cells and fulminating AIDS.

The induction of rapid HIV replication in the CD4$^+$ cells by antigenic stimulation or by cofactors contributed by other viruses may account for the previously mentioned epidemiologic observation that patients with active AIDS have a high incidence of cytomegalovirus, hepatitis B virus, and other viral infections.

Whatever the pathogenetic mechanisms, from the observations discussed above it is clear that infection with HIV results in a variety of immunopathogenic effects that ultimately translate into a continuous decline in the immunologic competence of the infected individual, a decline attributed to the destruction and functional impairment of CD4$^+$ lymphocytes. The vital role played by CD4$^+$ lymphocytes, not only in cell-mediated immunity but also in T cell-dependent antibody production and in immune regulation, explains the generalized immunodeficiency of AIDS patients, who are left defenseless to various opportunistic infections and certain malignancies.

Diagnosis of HIV Infection

As with other immunodeficiency syndromes, individuals, primarily high-risk individuals, who suffer from opportunistic infections or certain tumors, like Kaposi's sarcoma, should be suspected of being infected with HIV.

The diagnosis of HIV infection is performed primarily by *serologic means*. The ELISA test for the presence of anti-HIV antibodies is highly sensitive. It was first developed to screen for the presence of antibodies in donated blood. Today it is routinely used in the diagnostic workup for HIV infection. Confirmation of positive results is performed by *Western blot analysis* for the presence of antibodies to several HIV proteins (Fig. 18.1), specifically to p24 or p31, gp41, and gp120/gp160. The presence of antibodies to these four viral proteins is considered proof of HIV infection. However, a decrease in antibodies to p24 concomitant with an increase in free p24 in the blood indicates progression from the latent period to virus production and lytic infection, two indications of progression to overt AIDS.

In certain cases it is imperative to assess whether serum-positive babies born to serum-positive mothers are infected with virus or whether the antivirus antibodies are maternal antibodies transferred to the fetus. Also, there are reports of virally infected individuals who are serum-negative. Thus, it is important to test for the presence of the virus rather than of antibodies. Sensitive methods are now available to test for the viral gene, notably the method that utilizes gene amplification by *polymerase chain reaction (PCR)*.

Late manifestations of the disease include low $CD4^+:CD8^+$ ratios and poor delayed skin reactions to common recall antigens (antigens to which the individual was exposed in the past) such as tetanus toxoid. These manifestations are sometimes used to monitor progress of therapy.

Therapy and Vaccination

In spite of the enormous amount of information gathered in the past 15 years, the many gaps in our understanding of HIV infection and AIDS are reflected by the present-day lack of effective chemotherapy or immunotherapy and by the lack of an effective vaccine against HIV infection. There are, however, beginnings, albeit modest, in treatment and in immunoprophylaxis.

The first promising drug against AIDS is *AZT (azidothymidine),* also called Zidovudin. It was originally developed as an anticancer drug. AZT has been shown to improve several impaired immunologic mechanisms in patients with advanced AIDS and to lengthen median survival time. However, although to date it has an effect on several variants of HIV, resistance to AZT may develop in patients receiving the drug for long periods of time. Also, AZT, an inhibitor of reverse transcriptase, is highly toxic, especially to bone marrow cells. To reduce its toxicity it is being tried in combination with other drugs. A less toxic drug, *dideoxyinosine (DDI)*, is currently undergoing clinical trials. As more knowledge about the life cycle of HIV becomes available, more effective drugs and therapies can be expected. Another experimental modality of preventing infection of new cells is by the use of free CD4 molecules, the receptors for the virus. It is hypothesized that administered CD4 will react with the virus in the blood and prevent its attachment to cells. Since CD4 persists in the circulation for only a short period, various interesting methods, such as splicing it to the Fc fragment of IgG or glycosylating the molecule, are being employed to increase the in vivo half-life of CD4. To date, results of trials with these preparations are disappointing.

Various anti-HIV vaccines are being developed. These range from synthetic envelope peptides and recombinant viral subunit vaccines to anti-idiotypic vaccines, all attempting to induce antibodies and, lately, CMI. To date, no vaccine has yet been found effective in immunotherapy of AIDS, and none has yet been tried and found effective for immunoprophylaxis of human HIV infection. This failure may be due in part to the high mutation rate of the virus resulting in immune selection of viral genotypes that escape the immune response. Simian AIDS, caused by the simian immunodeficiency virus (SIV), a close relative of HIV, offers a powerful model for the development of prophylactic and therapeutic modalities for HIV infection. Indeed, several reports describe vaccines for SIV that are effective in immunoprophylaxis (prior to infection) but not immunotherapy (after infection). However, until prophylaxis and therapy become a reality for HIV infection, public health measures such as practicing safe sex, avoiding intravenous drug abuse, and testing donated blood or blood products for viral proteins or antibodies remain the main line of defense against AIDS.

IMMUNE DISEASES DUE TO ABNORMAL PRODUCTION OF IMMUNE COMPONENTS

Gammopathies

Several neoplastic diseases involve abnormal proliferation of B cells and plasma cells, the two types of cells that produce antibodies. These diseases are associated with an excessive production of whole immunoglobulins or immunoglobulin chains. Because the synthesis of these immunoglobulins takes place in clones that arise from a single cell, the synthesized immunoglobulins are referred to as *monoclonal immunoglobulins*, and the disorders are referred to as *monoclonal gammopathies*. There are three principal monoclonal gammopathies: multiple myeloma, macroglobulinemia, and heavy chain disease. A brief description of these diseases follows.

MULTIPLE MYELOMA. Multiple myeloma is the most common of the gammopathies and results from a malignant proliferation of plasma cells. The disease is associated with the synthesis of large amounts of *monoclonal immunoglobulins* (*M proteins*) of any given isotype, with either κ or λ light chains. Multiple myeloma may also be associated with the occurrence of large amounts of free κ- or λ-chains in the serum or the urine (these proteins are called *Bence-Jones proteins*).

Multiple myeloma may involve multiple organ systems (e.g., the skeletal system, the nervous system, the bone marrow, and the kidneys), predominantly as a result of the infiltration of malignant plasma cells into the organ. X rays of the skeletal system may show many well-demarcated, osteolytic lesions around such infiltrates.

Patients with multiple myeloma suffer from a suppression of the synthesis of normal antibodies and are, consequently, susceptible to recurrent bacterial and viral infections.

MACROGLOBULINEMIA. Macroglobulinemia, also referred to as *Waldenström's macroglobulinemia*, is associated with the synthesis and release of large amounts of *IgM*. The concentration of this macroglobulin in the serum can result in an increased viscosity of the serum that may, in turn, lead to slower blood flow, thromboses, disorders of the central nervous system, and bleeding. In addition to the overproduction of IgM, the disease is often characterized by decreased synthesis of other immunoglobulins, leading to *hypogammaglobulinemia* with all its harmful consequences.

HEAVY-CHAIN DISEASE. Heavy-chain disease is characterized by the appearance in the serum and urine of large amounts of a monoclonal protein with a molecular weight of approximately 55,000 daltons, similar in composition to the Fc fragment of IgG, IgA, or IgM.

Patients with this rare disease have recurrent bacterial infections, enlargement of the lymphoid organs, and anemias. The most frequent causes of death are recurrent infections, which proceed unchecked because of impairment of antibody synthesis.

Treatment of monoclonal gammopathies involves the reduction and elimination of the malignant cells that produce the proteins. Depending on the disease, this therapy usually includes local irradiation and/or cytotoxic chemotherapy with a variety of cytotoxic drugs.

B- and T-Cell Malignancies

Analogous to gammopathies, which are caused by malignancy of antibody-producing cells (B cells or plasma cells), are those diseases associated with malignancy of early B and of T cells. However, while a discussion of these malignancies is beyond the scope of this book, one aspect of their causation is directly attributable to some of the processes involved in the differentiation to normal B and T cells. It is therefore worth a brief discussion.

Oncogenes are genes felt to be directly involved in the development of malignancy. The exciting discovery (for which a Nobel Prize was awarded to Bishop and Varmus) that oncogenes code for the formation of normally occurring proteins was coupled with the finding that the control of the synthesis and function of these products has been lost through some genetic event. Thus in some cases the oncogene causes formation of a receptor or of a growth factor that is perpetually turned on, providing a constant growth stimulus to the cell.

Several cases have now been described in which B- and T-cell malignancies occur as the result of the translocation of a piece of chromosome to another chromosome, resulting in an abnormal pair in which one is shorter or longer than the homologous members. One of the best understood is the Burkitt lymphoma, a B-cell tumor occurring in some populations following Epstein–Barr virus (EBV) infection. Molecular DNA analysis has revealed that a piece of chromosome 8, containing an oncogene (c-*myc*), is translocated to chromosome 14. The c-*myc* oncogene codes for a nuclear binding protein that is involved in cell activation. What is most intriguing is that the translocation of this gene is to a D-J joining region or an S switch region in the immunoglobulin H-chain locus on chromosome 14 (see Chapter 8). Apparently this occurs while a pre-B cell is undergoing rearrangement prior to becoming a B cell with Ig receptors. Once the oncogene is translocated to the heavy chain locus, it comes under control of the more active regulatory elements for synthesis of immunoglobulin. Thus c-*myc* apparently gets turned on and made in abnormal amounts, driving the cell to repeated replication.

An analogous situation has been found for a class of T-cell tumors. These also involve translocation of the *myc* oncogene from chromosome 8 to chromosome 14. In contrast to Burkitt's lymphoma, however, the piece of chromosome 8 containing the oncogene joins to chromosome 14 higher up, in the D-J joining region of the α-chain of the T-cell receptor. Thus this translocation occurs in an early thymocyte making V gene rearrangements on the way to maturity. Again the *myc* gene comes under the control of elements in the α-chain locus, which drive its production and in turn lead to rapid proliferation of the affected cell.

The intersection of lines of investigation concerning the nature of oncogenes and the nature of immunoglobulin and TcR synthesis has yielded a detailed understanding of the causation of whole families of malignancies and give hope for devising strategies for their diagnosis and therapy.

SUMMARY

1. Immune deficiency disorders are called *primary* when the deficiency is the cause of a disease and *secondary* when the deficiency is a result of other diseases or the effects of treatment regimens.

2. Immune deficiency diseases may be due to disorders in the development or function of B cells, T cells, phagocytic cells, or components of complement, as shown in Table 18.1.

3. Immune deficiency disorders frequently predispose patients to recurrent infections. The association of various infections with deficiencies in B cells, T cells, phagocytes, or components of complement is also shown in Table 18.1.

4. Immune deficiencies constitute one type of defect or disorder of the immune system. Another aspect of such disorders is the unregulated proliferation of B lymphocytes, T lymphocytes, phagocytes, and their products, or the unregulated activation of components of the complement system.

5. Various infectious agents can significantly compromise the activity of the immune system by directly infecting cells of the immune system. Most notable is HIV, which, by infecting and killing CD4$^+$ lymphocytes, causes a massive immunosuppressive illness known as the acquired immune deficiency syndrome (AIDS).

REFERENCES

Ammann AJ (1994): Mechanisms of Immunodeficiency. In Stites DP, Terr AI, Parslow TG (eds): Basic and Clinical Immunology, 8th ed. Norwalk, CT: Appleton & Lange.

Anderson DC, Springer TA (1987): Leukocyte adhesion deficiency: an inherited defect in Mac-1, LFA-1, and p150, 95 glycoproteins. Annu Rev Med 38:175.

Baltimore D, Feinberg MB (1989): HIV revealed: towards a natural history of the infection. New Engl J Med 132:1673.

Clerici M, Shearer GM (1994): The Th1–Th2 hypothesis of HIV infection: new insights. Immunol Today 14:107.

Fahey JL (1993): Update on AIDS. The Immunologist 1:131.

Fauci AS (1993): Multifactorial nature of human immunodeficiency virus disease: implications for therapy. Science 262:1011.

Green WC (1993): AIDS and the immune system. Sci Am (Sept):99.

Helbert MR, Lage-Stehr J, Mitchison NA (1993): Antigen presentation, loss of immunologic memory and AIDS. Immunol Today 14:340.

Köhler H, Müller S, Nara P (1994): Deceptive imprinting in the immune response against HIV-1. Immunol Today 15:475.

Lusso P, Gallo RC (1995): Human herpes virus 6 in AIDS. Immunol Today 16:67.

Orkin SH (1989): Molecular genetics of chronic granulomatous disease. Annu Rev Immunol 7:277.

Rosenberg ZF, Fauci AS (1990): Immunopathogenic mechanisms of HIV infection: Cytokine induction of HIV expression. Immunol Today 11:176.

Schwartz DH (1994): Potential pitfalls on the road to an effective HIV vaccine. Immunol Today 15:54.

Scientific American (Oct 1988): What Science Knows About AIDS.

Steim RE (1989): Immunologic Disorders in Infants and Children, 3rd ed. Philadelphia: Saunders.

Waldman TA (1988): Immunodeficiency diseases: primary and acquired. In Samter M, Talmage DW, Frank MM, Austen KF, Claman HN (eds): Immunological Diseases, 4th ed. Boston: Little, Brown.

Wigzell H (1993): Will we have an HIV vaccine? The Immunologist 1:20.

REVIEW QUESTIONS

For each question, choose the ONE BEST answer or completion.

1. An 8-month-old baby has a history of repeated gram-positive bacterial infections. The most probable cause for this condition is that
   A) the mother did not confer sufficient immunity on the baby in utero
   B) the baby suffers from erythroblastosis fetalis (hemolytic disease of the newborn)
   C) the baby has a defect in the alternative complement pathway
   D) the baby is allergic to the mother's milk
   E) none of the above

2. A 50-year-old worker at an atomic plant who previously had a sample of his own bone marrow cryopreserved was accidentally exposed to a minimal lethal dose of radiation. He was subsequently transplanted with his own bone marrow. This individual can expect
   A) to have recurrent bacterial infections
   B) to have serious fungal infections due to deficiency in cell-mediated immunity

   C) to respond with antibodies to thymus-independent antigens only
   D) all of the above
   E) none of the above

3. Which of the following immune deficiency disorders is associated exclusively with an abnormality of the humoral immune response?
   A) X-linked agammaglobulinemia (Bruton's agammaglobulinemia)
   B) DiGeorge syndrome
   C) Wiskott–Aldrich syndrome
   D) chronic mucocutaneous candidiasis
   E) hereditary angioneurotic edema

4. A sharp increase in levels of IgG, with a spike in the IgG region seen in the electrophoretic pattern of serum proteins, is an indication of
   A) IgA or IgM deficiency
   B) multiple myeloma
   C) macroglobulinemia
   D) hypogammaglobulinemia
   E) severe fungal infections

5. Patients with DiGeorge syndrome may fail to produce IgG in response to immunization with T-dependent antigens because
   A) they have a decreased number of B cells, which produce IgG
   B) they have increased numbers of suppressor T cells
   C) they have a decreased number of helper T cells
   D) they have abnormal antigen-presenting cells
   E) they cannot produce IgM during primary responses

6. A 2-year-old child has had three episodes of pneumonia and two episodes of otitis media. All the infections were demonstrated to be pneumococcal. Which of the following disorders is most likely to be the cause:
   A) an isolated transient T-cell deficiency
   B) a combined T- and B-cell deficiency
   C) a B-cell deficiency
   D) transient anemia
   E) the child has AIDS

7. A healthy woman gave birth to a baby. The newborn infant was found to be seropositive, with serum IgG to the HIV-1 virus. This finding is most likely the result of
   A) the virus being transferred across the placenta to the baby
   B) the baby making antivirus antibodies
   C) the baby's erythrocyte antigens cross-reacting with the virus

   D) the mother's erythrocyte antigens cross-reacting with the virus
   E) none of the above

8. Immunodeficiency disease can result from
   A) a developmental defect of T lymphocytes
   B) a developmental defect of bone marrow stem cells
   C) a defect in phagocyte function
   D) a defect in complement function
   E) all of the above

9. A 9-month-old baby was vaccinated against smallpox with attenuated smallpox virus. He developed a progressive necrotic lesion of the skin, muscles, and subcutaneous tissue at the site of inoculation. The vaccination reaction probably resulted from
   A) B-lymphocyte deficiency
   B) reaction to the adjuvant
   C) complement deficiency
   D) T-cell deficiency
   E) B and T lymphocyte deficiency

10. The most common clinical consequence(s) of C3 deficiency is (are)
   A) increased incidence of tumors
   B) increased susceptibility to viral infections
   C) increased susceptibility to fungal infections
   D) increased susceptibility to bacterial infections
   E) all of the above

Case study: A 4-year-old child is brought to your office with a complaint of "failure to thrive," including loss of appetite, weight loss, and persistent cough. On physical examination the child appears pale and sickly, has a low-grade fever, but no other physical signs. His past history is unremarkable except for a fractured leg at 1 year of age that required a blood transfusion during surgery, but it healed without complication.

A battery of tests is performed to arrive at a diagnosis. X-ray examination showed some bilateral pulmonary infiltrates. Blood count is normal, with slightly reduced white cell numbers. Serum immunoglobulin assay showed elevated IgG, IgM, and IgA. Skin tests performed with mumps, tetanus, and candida antigens were negative. Antibiotic therapy is started, but on the next visit the child is sicker and now has enlarged lymph nodes, spleen, and liver.

What diagnosis would you be thinking of at this point and how would you confirm it?

ANSWERS TO REVIEW QUESTIONS

1. *E* None of the above is likely to be the underlying cause for the history. The baby is probably hypogammaglobulinemic. Hypogammaglobulinemia leads to recurrent bacterial infections. Viral and fungal infections are controlled by cell-mediated immunity, which is normal in hypogammaglobulinemic individuals. Answer *A* is incorrect because the mother's IgG, which passed through the placenta, would have a half-life of 23 days, and would therefore not be expected to remain in the baby's circulation for 8 months. At this age any Ig present in the baby's circulation is synthesized by the baby. Answer *B* is irrelevant since erythroblastosis fetalis is caused by the destruction of the newborn's Rh⁺ erythrocytes by the Rh⁻ mother's antibodies to Rh antigen. Answer *C* is unlikely since the classical complement pathway would still be protective; moreover, a defect in the alternative pathway would not result in the selective inability to protect from only gram-positive bacterial infections. Answer *D* is incorrect since, even if allergic to the mother's milk, the baby should not suffer from increased frequency of bacterial infections.

2. *E* The autologous bone marrow cells, which contain stem cells, will replicate, differentiate, and repopulate the hematopoietic-reticuloendothelial system, rendering the individual immunologically normal. As such, the individual is not expected to have bacterial, viral, or fungal infections or to respond to antigens differently from a normal individual.

3. *A* The only immune deficiency disorder that is associated with an abnormality exclusively of the humoral response is Bruton's agammaglobulinemia or X-linked agammaglobulinemia. DiGeorge syndrome results from thymic aplasia, where there is a

deficiency in T cells that may influence the IgG responses, which require helper T cells. Wiskott–Aldrich syndrome is associated with several abnormalities. Chronic mucocutaneous candidiasis is a poorly defined collection of syndromes associated with a selective defect in the functioning of T cells. Hereditary angioneurotic edema is associated with a deficiency of the inhibition of C1 esterase.

4. **B** This pattern is characteristic of multiple myeloma (IgG myeloma). Multiple myeloma may be recognized by the synthesis of large amounts of homogeneous antibody of any one isotype. Although patients with multiple myeloma may suffer from a decreased synthesis of other Ig isotypes, the electrophoretic pattern is not necessarily an indication of IgA or IgM deficiency.

5. **C** Patients with DiGeorge syndrome have a decreased number of T cells—in particular, helper T cells, which are essential for the IgG response to T-dependent antigens. These patients have normally functioning B cells and are capable of responding to T-independent antigens, or with only IgM responses (primary responses) to T-dependent antigens.

6. **C** The cause for the described case history is very likely due to B-cell deficiency which is characterized by recurrent bacterial infections leading to otitis media and pneumonia. T-cell deficiency would usually result in viral, fungal, and protozoal infections. The same is true for com-bined T- and B-cell deficiency. Answer **D** (transient anemia) is irrelevant in this case—anemia is not generally associated with increased infections. It is unlikely that with a history of only pneumococcal infections the child would have AIDS. The latter syndrome is associated more with characteristic infections such as with *Pneumocystis carinii* and various viral infections.

7. **E** None of the above is correct. The newborn does not synthesize IgG. The most likely explanation is that the "healthy" mother has been infected with HIV-1 and is making anti-HIV-1 IgG which is transferred to the fetus and newborn transplacentally. Answers **C** and **D** are false because this unlikely situation would result in the recognition of the viral antigen as "self" and the individual would not make anti-self antibodies.

8. **E** All are correct. Immunodeficiency disorders may result from defects in the development of bone marrow stem cells into lymphocytes and other cells that participate in the immune response. They can also result from defects in phagocyte functions, which are important in phagocytosis and presentation of antigen. Immunodeficiency disorders may also result from defects in complement function—an absence or malfunction of one or more of the complement components, their activators, or regulators.

9. **D** T-cell deficiency would result in the absence of the crucial immunological de-

fenses against viral infection, i.e., cell-mediated immunity. Cell-mediated immunity plays the major role in immunity to viral infections, much greater than the roles of antibody or complement. In fact, individuals with impaired T-cell-mediated immunity should not be vaccinated with live virus, which, even if attenuated, may cause a serious infection.

10. ***D*** Deficiency in C3 is associated with increased susceptibility to bacterial infec-

tions, since C3 plays an important role in the destruction of bacteria and their increased opsonization, by participating in the classical and the alternative pathways of complement activation. Cell-mediated immunity (CMI) is generally more important in the resistance of the host to viral and fungal infections. Also, in general, CMI is considered to be more important than complement in the resistance of the host to tumors.

Case study: This is a possible case of childhood AIDS, presumably attributable to the earlier transfusion with blood obtained from a blood bank. Until a few years ago, the test for anti-HIV antibodies (or for HIV components) present in blood was not sufficiently reliable to exclude viral transmission. Although present-day tests are highly reliable, there are still isolated cases of HIV transmission by blood transfusion. Following a long incubation period the child presented with a slightly lowered white cell count, somewhat elevated immunoglobulin levels, but a seriously compromised T-cell function. The latter was determined by the absence of skin reactions to mumps, tetanus toxoid, and candida antigens, all of which elicit T-cell-mediated delayed-type hypersensitivity reactions in normal individuals. A follow-up test of the levels of circulating CD4$^+$ and CD8$^+$ cells revealed a ratio of 0.4, indicating that helper CD4$^+$ cells, the target of the HIV virus, have declined markedly. Further study of the lung infiltrate, which failed to respond to antibiotic therapy, would be done by bronchoscopy and lavage. Microscopic examination of the washings would probably show an opportunistic organism such as *Pneumocystis carinii*, the most usual cause of death from AIDS. A final confirmatory evidence would come from an examination of the child's serum for the presence of antibody to HIV antigens, a clear indication of an infection with HIV virus, and from a test for the viral gene by PCR.

TRANSFUSION IMMUNOLOGY

INTRODUCTION

After the discovery of the circulatory system by Harvey in the seventeenth century, many attempts were made to transfuse blood, first from animals into humans and later from humans into other humans. These transfusions almost always had disastrous consequences.

The discovery in 1900 of the ABO blood group antigens by Landsteiner (a Nobel laureate) established the immunologic basis for transfusion reactions. This discovery, and the subsequent discovery by Landsteiner of the Rh antigens and the tests that were developed to determine the blood group antigens, made the transfusion of blood from one human to another a practical and useful clinical procedure.

In this chapter we discuss the major human erythrocyte ***alloantigens*** (antigens that differ between individuals of the same species), the problems they can cause, how they are detected, and how today, as a result of blood group typing, most blood transfusions proceed without any significant immunologic risk.

THE ABO SYSTEM

Investigations with various human sera and red blood cells (RBCs) led Landsteiner to conclude that, on the basis of the substances or antigens present on their surface, human RBC can be divided into four major groups: (1) erythrocytes with *group A* substance, (2) erythrocytes with *group B* substance, (3) erythrocytes with both *group A and B* substances, and (4) erythrocytes with *neither group A nor group B* substances. These blood group types were named A, B, AB, and O, respectively. Landsteiner further established that individuals with type A blood have serum antibodies that agglutinate group B erythrocytes; people with type B blood have antibodies that agglutinate type A erythrocytes; individuals with type AB blood have no antibodies to these alloantigens; and individuals with type O blood have antibodies that agglutinate type A, B, and AB erythrocytes. The antibodies that agglutinate the alloantigen-bearing cells are referred to as *isohemagglutinins*. The blood groups, their genotypes, their phenotypes, and the antibodies present in the sera of people with the RBC of a given blood group are shown in Table 19.1. It is clear that individuals with blood group O are universal donors (i.e., can give blood to any type recipient), while those with group AB can receive erythrocytes from any type donor.

The blood group antigens are controlled by three alleles (A, B, and O); A and B are dominant over O and codominant with respect to each other. These alleles produce transferase enzymes that add terminal sugar residues to a parent structure. While the A and B genes determine the presence of A and B substances, respectively, the O gene is inactive and does not code for any of the erythrocyte alloantigens. Nevertheless, blood group O erythrocytes do have a glycoprotein on

TABLE 19.1   The Genotype and Phenotype of the ABO Blood Groups and the Antibodies Present in the Sera of Individuals With the ABO Blood Groups

| Erythrocyte antigens | | Distribution (%) | | | | Antibodies present in sera |
| | | | | American | | |
Genotype	Phenotype	White[a]	Black	Indians	Asians	
AA AO	A	4	27	16	28	Anti-B (agglutinate with group B and AB RBC)
BB BO	B	11	20	4	27	Anti-A (agglutinate with group A and AB RBC)
AB	AB	4	4	1	5	No anti-A or anti-B (will not agglutinate A, B, or AB RBC)
OO	O	45	49	79	40	Anti-A and anti-B (agglutinate with A, B, or AB RBC)

[a]White, North American population.

the surface—the *H substance*—which can be recognized by antisera from different animals. This glycoprotein is not the product of the O gene since it is present on RBCs of people who are homozygous for the A or B genes.

The A, B, and H substances are related to each other, representing different determinants on the same molecule: during the synthesis of the blood group molecules, the parent molecule H substance is synthesized first. The H substance is a glycoprotein with L-fucose as the terminal epitope that is recognized by antibodies. The transferase enzyme coded by the A gene converts the H substance into the A substance by adding a terminal α-N-acetylgalactosamine group (which becomes the antigenic determinant group of blood group A). Similarly, the enzyme coded by the B gene converts the H substance into the B substance by adding a terminal α-D-galactosyl residue (which becomes the antigenic determinant of blood group B). Group O individuals do not make either enzyme and, thus, their erythrocytes have the unmodified H substance on their surface.

Since the H substance is common to groups A, B, AB, and O, none of the individuals in any of the blood groups have antibodies to the H substance. However, there are rare cases in which humans do form antibodies to the H substance of O type RBC. Because this rare antibody was first found in Bombay, the individuals who form anti-H antibodies are called *Bombay-type* individuals. They lack the gene that converts a glycolipid precursor to the H substance. Accordingly, they do not have the H (nor the A or B) substance, and they produce serum isoantibodies to the H substance (as well as to the A and B substances).

Distribution of A, B, and H Antigens

The blood group substances A, B, and H are present as *glycolipids* on the surface of *erythrocytes*, as well as on the surface of many *epithelial* cells and most *endothelial* cells. In approximately 80% of all humans, A, B, and H substances are also present as *mucopolysaccharides* in secretions (such as saliva, sweat, gastric juices) and become bound to red cells. These people are termed "*secretors*," and their secreted substances are immunologically but not chemically identical to those present on their erythrocytes. The secretion of these substances is controlled by alleles Se and se, with Se being dominant. Only homozygous recessive individuals (se/se) are nonsecretors. Thus, the individual oligosaccharide determinant, which accounts for the designation A, B, or O, may appear on different backbones, but it is recognized by the same antisera.

Approximately four-fifths of individuals have a high density of A antigen on their cells. Thus, the A group can be subdivided into A_1 (high density) and A_2 (low-density) groups. Probably because of the high density of the A antigen, some new epitopes are formed from adjacent molecules. Although of relatively rare occurrence, A_2 and especially A_2B individuals may have antibodies to A_1.

Isohemagglutinins

Because of their ability to agglutinate human RBC, and because they are of human origin, antibodies to the A and B antigens are called *isohemagglutinins*. They occur naturally, that is, without deliberate sensitization or immunization against them, and they are often referred to as *"natural antibodies."* Individuals with type O erythrocytes normally produce IgM isohemagglutinins, directed against A and B blood groups; individuals with type A blood have anti-B IgM isohemagglutinins, and those with type B blood have anti-A IgM.

It is still not certain what triggers the synthesis of these antibodies in the absence of prior exposure to the antigens. It is generally believed, however, that the antibodies have been induced by A, B determinant-bearing polysaccharides of intestinal bacteria or of other microorganisms that cause occult infections and induce antibodies that cross-react with the A and B blood group substances. Evidence in support of this hypothesis derives from the fact that isoantibodies are not present at birth but develop during the first year of life, as the gut is colonized by various bacteria. It should be pointed out that upon repeated transfusions of incompatible blood, IgG antibodies to A and B antigens may form in the recipient.

THE LEWIS GROUP

The Lewis group consists of two alleles, Le^a and Le^b, which code for substances structurally related to the ABO system but differing in two important aspects: (1) the genes regulating these blood group substances are not linked to the ABO locus and (2) the Le^a and Le^b substances are complex glycoproteins found free in saliva and serum and do not constitute part of the erythrocyte surface structure. Their presence on the surface of erythrocytes is due to their ability to adsorb to the cells. Antibodies to the Lewis blood group substances can occur naturally without prior exposure to heterologous erythrocytes. High anti-Le^a titers may cause transfusion reactions, while anti-Le^b antibodies are usually harmless.

Rh ANTIGENS

In the 1930s, after the discovery of ABO blood group antigens, Landsteiner and Weiner discovered that rabbit antisera raised against rhesus monkey RBC agglutinated the erythrocytes from approximately 85% of humans tested. These human erythrocytes had, on their surface, an antigen called **Rh antigen** (for rhesus), and the cells of these individuals were designated Rh^+ cells. The remaining 15% of humans had no such antigen on the surface of their erythrocytes and their cells were, therefore, designated Rh^- cells.

At approximately the same time as these investigations were undertaken, Levine and Stetson, who were obstetricians, not immunologists, described the case of a woman who had given birth to a baby with **hemolytic disease of the newborn (erythroblastosis fetalis)**, and who had suffered a severe transfusion reaction on receiving blood from her husband, who had the same ABO type. A collaboration between the obstetricians and Landsteiner and Weiner established that the father's RBC and the baby's RBC were Rh^+ but that the mother's RBC were Rh^-. It was subsequently established that in all cases of babies with hemolytic disease the mother was Rh^- and the baby was Rh^+ (fathered by an Rh^+ father).

It was also shown that the serum of the mothers of babies with hemolytic disease contained antibodies to the Rh antigens and that these antibodies were predominantly of the IgG isotype. This isotype passes through the placenta, so that maternal IgG, directed against fetal Rh antigens on fetal RBC, reacts with the fetal erythrocytes and causes hemolysis. In cases of ABO incompatibility, erythroblastosis fetalis is not a problem because the isohemogglutinins belong primarily to the IgM class and do not cross the placenta. However, even in cases where IgG antibodies are made, they tend to be absorbed by placental tissues, which themselves contain AB blood group substances, whereas Rh is present only on RBC.

Rh^- mothers become sensitized to Rh antigens when small numbers of fetal red blood cells enter the maternal circulation during pregnancy. This number is usually too low to induce significant titers of anti-Rh antibodies during the first pregnancy. However, during parturition (separation of the placenta) release of cord blood into the mother exposes her to massive numbers of Rh^+ cells from the fetus and she becomes immunized, producing high levels of anti-Rh IgG, which can affect the second pregnancy. Indeed, the more pregnancies an Rh^- woman goes through (with Rh^+ babies), the greater the likelihood of her receiving "booster" exposures to Rh antigens and the higher her anti-Rh titer.

Rh Genetics

From results of experiments with various anti-Rh sera, it now appears that there are more than 30 distinct antigenic specificities of Rh antigens. It appears that the Rh specificities are encoded by a single Rh locus with closely linked genes and with many alleles (Table 19.2).

It is now clear that the **D antigen** is by far the strongest immunogen and the most important of all the Rh antigens. Over 90% of all cases of hemolytic disease of the newborn are attributed to the D antigen. Thus, a mother who is phenotypically dXX is D⁻ and is therefore considered Rh⁻, and potentially capable of making anti-D antibodies. This is illustrated in Table 19.2 where the C, D, and E Rh antigens are compared.

TABLE 19.2   Rh Phenotypes and Their Frequencies in the United States

Phenotype (Fisher-Race nomenclature)	Frequency (%)	Reaction with anti-D	Rh group designation
DCe	54	+	Rh⁺
DCE	15	+	Rh⁺
DcE	4	+	Rh⁺
Dce	2	+	Rh⁺
dce	13	−	Rh⁻
dCe	1.5	−	Rh⁻
dcE	0.5	−	Rh⁻
dCE	Very rare	−	Rh⁻

Prevention of Rh Disease

The major event that sensitizes the Rh⁻ mother to D antigen and other Rh⁺ antigens appears to occur during parturition, when the mother is exposed to the baby's Rh⁺ erythrocytes. Thus, the administration of anti-Rh antibodies (human anti-Rh) within 72 hours of parturition is an effective way to "tie up" and cause the rapid clearance of Rh⁺ cells from the mother's circulation. One widely used preparation of anti-Rh antibodies is called **Rhogam** and consists of human IgG against the D antigen.

THE MN BLOOD GROUP

The MN blood group is a **minor blood group** that was discovered by use of rabbit antisera raised against human erythrocytes. This blood group is totally independent of the ABO system.

Regardless of the ABO blood type, the erythrocytes of each human individual have M or N, or both, antigens on their surface. These antigens are encoded by the codominant M and N alleles. The antigenic activity is related to the glycoprotein *glycophorin* (of molecular weight approximately 16,000 daltons), which is present on the membrane of all erythrocytes. There are at least two types of glycophorin molecules, which differ somewhat in their amino acid sequences and in the extent of glycosylation. Only their glycosylation products are related to the M or the N antigenicity.

Ss ANTIGENS

The S and s antigens are associated with the M and N antigens: the S antigen is associated predominantly with M; and the s, with N. The S and s antigens are encoded by two codominant alleles. Like the MN groups, the Ss group is a *minor blood group* that rarely plays a role in blood transfusion.

THE KELL AND DUFFY BLOOD GROUPS

The Kell and Duffy blood groups are *minor blood groups* that, nevertheless, on occasion can be responsible for transfusion reactions. The Kell system consists of two allelic forms, K and k. Approximately 10% of the population carries the K antigen, which is highly immunogenic, on their erythrocytes. Exposure to K antigen during pregnancy or transfusion induces the formation of anti-K IgG, which may cause lysis in the presence of complement.

The Duffy system has two allelic forms, Fy^a and Fy^b. Repeated transfusions (or repeated pregnancies) may induce anti-Fy^a IgG, which is a common cause of problems during transfusion. It is of some interest that the Fy antigen is apparently a receptor by which *Plasmodium vivax*, the parasite causing malaria, enters the red cell. Most blacks are $Fy(a^- b^-)$ and, lacking the receptor, are resistant to malaria caused by *Plasmodium vivax*.

TRANSFUSION REACTIONS

Transfusion reactions may cause the destruction of the transferred cells by hemolysis, opsonization, or enhanced phagocytosis. Most commonly they occur because of the reaction between the recipient's antibodies and the transfused cells from the donor. The amount of antibody against the recipient's cells, present in the donor's serum, is generally not important in transfusion, because the high dilution of these antibodies in the recipient's blood results in their low concentration, insufficient to affect the large number of red cells of the recipient. However, transfusion reactions have been known to occur when the donor's antibodies against the recipient's antigens were present at very high titers.

There are three types of immunologically mediated transfusion reactions: *hemolytic reactions, febrile reactions*, and *allergic reactions*.

Hemolytic Reactions

Hemolytic reactions are the most serious consequence of blood transfusions. They result mainly from (1) ABO incompatibility (usually due to clerical or laboratory error), (2) Rh incompatibility (the D antigen is the most immunogenic of all blood group antigens), and (3) incompatibility in minor blood group antigens, such as Kell or Duffy.

Severe hemolytic reactions occur within minutes of transfusion. The reaction is accompanied by diffuse muscle pain, headache, nausea, and sometimes vomiting. A rise in temperature is common. The reaction can result in a state of shock, and renal failure may develop. Also, because of the activation of the blood clotting factors by damaged erythrocytes, those factors become depleted and a generalized hemorrhagic tendency develops. Such a transfusion reaction, occurring immediately on transfusion, dictates the immediate discontinuation of the transfusion.

Febrile Reactions

Febrile reactions are often due to reaction of antibodies with minor blood group antigens. Therefore, repeated transfusions of the same blood type, mismatched for minor blood groups, which may lead to higher titer of antibodies directed against the minor blood groups, should be avoided.

Allergic Reactions

Allergic reactions ranging from mild urticaria to systemic anaphylactic shock may be seen. The patient may break out in hives and develop bronchoconstriction with dyspnea and wheezing, which may proceed to a cardiovascular collapse with a drop in blood pressure (symptoms typical of systemic anaphylaxis; see Chapter 14). It is not clear whether this is due to transfer of antigen to which the recipient is sensitive or whether the transfused blood contains IgE antibody.

TRANSFUSION TRANSMITTED INFECTIONS

Transfusion carries the risk of transmitting microorganisms from donor to recipient. This is especially true for microorganisms that are not detected by the standard donor screening procedures. In the developed countries the important and most frequent reported posttransfusion infections are hepatitis (approximately 1–2%) and cytomegalovirus, CMV (approximately 1–5%). With highly improved screening methods post transfusion HIV infections are now very rare with a risk factor of approximately one per 500,000 transfused units. Other infections while rare in the developed countries are more common in the developing countries. We can hope that with the rapid advances in biotechnology and efficient detection methods, post transfusion infections will become extremely rare.

SELECTION OF DONORS BY CROSS-MATCHING

In routine *blood typing*, tests for only the ABO and Rh (D) blood groups of donor and recipient are performed. Mismatch or incompatibility with respect to these antigens precludes transfusion between the pair.

Cross-matching between donor and recipient, which provides a more reliable measure of compatibility, consists of an agglutination test, which involves the mixing of donor's cells with recipient's serum in both the absence and presence of anti-immunoglobulins (the Coombs test). The rest of the cross-match (seldom performed in the United States or Canada) consists of mixing the donor's serum with a sample of the recipient's cells.

In cases of extreme emergency, when cross-matching is not possible, unmatched blood from the universal donor (type O, Rh$^-$) may be used.

SUMMARY

1. **The major erythrocyte alloantigens of humans, which are responsible for transfusion reactions, are as follows:**

   a) **The ABO blood group antigens are present on the surface of erythrocytes (and on the surface of many epithelial and endothelial cells). Isohemagglutinins are "naturally" occurring IgM antibodies against the ABO alloantigens. Individuals with type O blood have anti-A and anti-B IgM; individuals with type A blood have anti-B agglutinins; and individuals with type B blood have anti-A agglutinins.**

b) **MN, Ss, Lewis, Kell, and Duffy antigens constitute minor human blood groups.**

c) **Rh antigens are present on erythrocytes of 85% of the human population, referred to as Rh$^+$. The remaining 15% have no Rh antigens on their erythrocytes and are referred to as Rh$^-$. Rh$^-$ mothers, who are exposed to Rh antigens, make anti-Rh IgG antibodies which pass through the placenta and cause hemolytic disease of the newborn, erythroblastosis fetalis.**

2. **Transfusion reactions may result in the destruction of the transferred cells by hemolysis or by opsonization and increased phagocytosis. They can also result in fever and/or allergic reactions.**

3. **To avoid transfusion reactions, the donor and recipient blood groups are cross-matched, primarily for ABO and Rh compatibility.**

REFERENCES

Bowman JM (1988): The prevention of Rh immunization. Transfusion Med. Rev. 2:129.

Dodd RY (1992): The risk of transfusion-transmitted infection. New Engl J Med 327:419.

Donegan E, Bossom EL (1994): Blood banking and immunohematology. In Stites DP, Terr AI, Parslow TG (eds): Basic and Clinical Immunology, 8th ed. Norwalk, CT: Appleton & Lange.

Mollison PL (1983): Blood Transfusion in Clinical Medicine, 7th ed. Oxford: Blackwell Scientific Publications.

REVIEW QUESTIONS

For each question, choose the ONE BEST answer or completion.

1. Blood from group AB donors can be transfused to a recipient without causing a transfusion reaction if
   A) the recipient is AB
   B) the recipient is A
   C) the recipient is B
   D) the recipient is O
   E) the recipient and donor are siblings

2. Transfusion between donors and recipients with different ABO blood group antigens
   A) should not be attempted
   B) should be performed only after treatment with immunosuppressive drugs
   C) should be followed by giving the recipient epinephrine or antihistamines

D) will induce a mixed lymphocyte reaction
E) recipient and donor have different MHC antigens

3. The following statements regarding hemolytic disease of the newborn are correct *except*:
   A) Administration of anti-Rh globulins to an Rh$^-$ mother soon after delivery of an Rh$^+$ baby can suppress the induction of anti-Rh globulins by the mother.
   B) It is an example of type II hypersensitivity reaction.
   C) If the newborn is Rh$^-$ and the mother is Rh$^+$, the fetus becomes tolerant to Rh antigens.
   D) The mother forms antibodies against Rh antigens that she lacks.
   E) D antigen is the most important Rh antigen in hemolytic disease of the newborn.

4. A type A, Rh$^+$ woman gave birth to a type O, Rh$^-$ baby. Therefore, all of the following statements are true *except*:
   A) The mother must be heterozygous for Rh antigen.
   B) The mother does not have the AA genotype.
   C) The father could have the BO, Rh$^+$ genotype.
   D) A type AB, Rh$^+$ man could not be the father.
   E) The baby may have the AO genotype.

5. If IgG antibodies to the A and B erythrocyte antigens are formed, hemolytic disease of the newborn would occur in the children of
   A) AB mothers and O fathers
   B) O mothers and AB fathers
   C) A mothers and A fathers
   D) O mothers and O fathers
   E) AB mothers and AB fathers

6. Intentional protection of a future newborn against Rh disease involves

A) passive immunization of the newborn to remove the Rh antigen
B) passive immunization of the mother to remove Rh antigen
C) active immunization of the mother to produce transplacental IgG
D) active immunization of the mother with Rh antigen to induce antibody
E) use of steroids to reduce maternal immune reactivity

7. If a patient with red blood cell phenotype B Rh$^-$ MSs Fy^b K requires a transfusion, the most likely donor would be someone with phenotype
   A) AB Rh$^+$ MNSs, because type AB is a universal recipient
   B) O Rh$^+$ Fy^b, because type O is the universal donor
   C) A Rh$^+$ Fy^a, because the donor phenotype should be complementary to the recipient
   D) B Rh$^-$ K, because ABO and Rh antigens are the most important
   E) AB Rh$^-$ MSs, because MN, S and Rh antigens are the most important

8. Blood group incompatibility usually poses a transfusion risk because
   A) the donor's immunoglobulins react with the recipient's erythrocytes
   B) a mixed lymphocyte reaction takes place
   C) the recipient's T lymphocytes will become activated by the donor's antigens
   D) the recipient's immunoglobulins react with donor's erythrocytes
   E) only A and C are correct
   F) only B and D are correct

9. The structural units that confer immunologic specificity to ABO blood group substances
   A) contain no galactose

B) are oligosaccharides

C) are small peptides attached to a polysaccharide backbone

D) contain fucose and N-acetylhexosamine

E) only A and C are correct

F) only B and D are correct

10. John (blood type AB, Rh⁻) is married to Julie (type AB, Rh⁺). After some years Julie gives birth to Jane, who is brought to the hospital for a transfusion 3 years later. The blood-typing lab results on hemagglutination assays are as follows (+ = hemagglutination; = no hemagglutination):

Saline + Jane's RBC	−
Anti-A + Jane's RBC	−
Anti-B + Jane's RBC	+
Jane's serum + A-RBC	+
Jane's serum + B-RBC	−
Jane's serum + O-RBC	−

What conclusions are valid?

A) A mistake was made in the lab.

B) John could not be the natural parent.

C) Julie could not be the natural parent.

D) Jane can be the natural offspring of these parents.

E) only A and C are correct

F) only B and D are correct

Case study: A patient entered the hospital in late August for a bleeding ulcer that required multiple blood transfusions over several days. While recovering about a week later he walked out into the garden for the first time. Within 15 minutes his nose began to run, his eyes itched, and he began to sneeze in paroxysms. No fever, joint pain, urinary protein loss, or other symptoms were noted, and he told his physician he had never experienced anything like this before. What would be a possible explanation for his symptoms?

ANSWERS TO REVIEW QUESTIONS

1. *A* If the donor's blood group is AB, the donor's blood can be transfused into a type AB recipient because the recipient does not make antibodies against his or her own blood group. Type AB cells cannot be transfused to a type A individual because the recipient has anti-B antibodies. Similarly, type AB cells cannot be transferred into a type B individual because he or she has antibodies against type A. Finally, AB cells cannot be transfused into a type O individual because that individual has both anti-A and anti-B antibodies. Unless they are homozygous twins, even brothers and sisters can have different blood groups.

2. *A* Transfusion should not be performed if donor and recipient differ in their ABO blood group antigens. A mixed lymphocyte reaction between donor's and recipient's lymphocytes may occur, but this reaction is not the one responsible for the transfusion reaction, in which recipient's antibodies destroy the donor's erythrocytes. MHC differences do not play a role in the transfusion reactions.

3. *C* All the statements are correct except *C*: hemolytic disease of the newborn (erythroblastosis fetalis) occurs when the mother is Rh⁻ and the fetus is Rh⁺; thus, statement *C* is untrue.

4. *E* All the statements are true except statement *E*. A type O individual must be homozygous for O, since both A and B are dominant over O.

5. *B* The only situation where hemolytic absence could be induced would be when an O mother made IgG antibodies to fetal erythrocytes with surface A or B antigens.

6. *B* The protection against Rh disease of the newborn is done by administration of human anti-Rh antibodies (e.g., Rhogam) to the Rh⁻ mother within 72 hours of parturition. The administered antibodies "tie up" and cause the rapid clearance of baby's Rh⁺ cells from the mother's circulation, thus preventing further exposure and immunization of the Rh⁻ mother to Rh antigens. Statement *A* is wrong—such a procedure will only harm the newborn. The same is true for statements *C* and *D*—these procedures will induce in the mother anti-Rh antibodies which are harmful to the newborn. Administration of steroids to the mother would be harmful—it will reduce her general immunity.

7. *D* A match of the ABO and Rh blood groups is most important for transfusions. Any of the minor groups may be mismatched without harm.

8. *D* The transfusion risk arises mainly because the recipient's immunoglobulins (the isohemagglutinins, which are IgM, or the IgG antibodies if the recipient has been previously transfused with cells that contain the donor's antigens) react with the donor's erythrocytes. The reaction of the donor's immunoglobulins with the recipient's erythrocytes is *usually* not of clinical significance because of the dilution of the donor's antibodies in the recipient's blood. However, if the donor's blood contains high titers of antibodies against the recipient's erythrocytes, a transfusion reaction may occur in which the donor's antibodies destroy the recipient's erythrocytes. Although donor blood contains lymphocytes, which may participate in a mixed lymphocyte reaction with a recipient's lymphocytes, this reaction poses no transfusion risk. Also, the possibility that the recipient's lymphocytes will become activated by donor antigens does not pose a potential transfusion risk when donor and recipient are incompatible.

9. *F* The structural units of ABO blood group antigens are oligosaccharides (*B*) which contain fucose and *N*-acetylhexosamine (*D*). Also, the A and B substances contain galactose; thus *A* is incorrect. There are no peptides involved in the immunological specificity of the ABO blood groups; thus *C* is incorrect.

10. *D* The child Jane types as B by agglutination of her red cells with anti-Bserum as well as the presence of anti-A antibody in her own serum. This is compatible with her being a homozygous B having received a B allele from each parent. Rh antigens are not relevant here because no typing for them was done.

Case study: This could be a rare incident in transfusion therapy in which an individual having severe clinical allergy was used as a donor. The passive transfer of the donor IgE antibody to the patient sensitized his mast cells to the ragweed pollen present at that time of year, producing typical anaphylactic symptoms of hay fever. Since this was passive immunization, sensitivity persisted only as long as the transferred IgE and was gone by the next year's ragweed pollen season.

TRANSPLANTATION IMMUNOLOGY

INTRODUCTION

The immune response has evolved as a way of discriminating between **"*self*"** and **"*nonself.*"** Once "foreignness" has been established, the immune response proceeds toward its ultimate goal of destroying the foreign material, be it a microorganism or its product, a substance present in the environment, or a tumor cell. The triggering of the immune system in response to such foreign substances is, of course, of great survival value.

The same discriminating power of the immune response between "self" and "nonself" is undesirable in instances that are highly artificial, such as the transplantation of cells or organs from one individual to another for therapeutic purposes. Indeed, results of such transplantations have been disastrous, culminating in the rejection of the transplanted tissue.

With the current understanding of the mechanisms involved in transplant rejection, transplantation for therapeutic purposes has become commonplace. For example, transfusions of blood are routine, and over 10,000 kidneys are transplanted annually worldwide with a high degree of success. Transplantations of heart, lungs, cornea, liver, and bone marrow that were considered spectacular and were widely publicized as recently as 20 years ago, have become commonplace—

they are now seldom mentioned in the media (although rejection episodes have been reduced but not eliminated).

Transfusion refers to the transfer of blood from one individual to another. The transfer of any other tissue or organ is referred to as *transplantation. Antibodies are responsible for transfusion reactions; the rejection of transplanted tissue is mediated predominantly by T cells.*

Transfusion immunology was dealt with in Chapter 19; transplantation immunology is the subject of the present chapter.

RELATIONSHIP BETWEEN DONOR AND RECIPIENT

Various gradations in relationships of transplantation from donor to recipient are shown in Figure 20.1 and are described below.

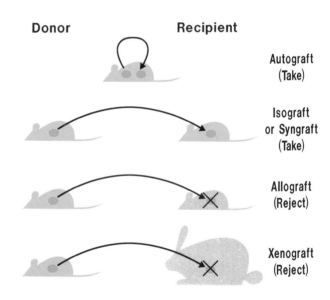

Figure 20.1.
Situations of tissue transplantation.

1. An *autograft* is a graft or transplant from one area to another on the same individual such as would occur in the transplantation of normal skin from one area of an individual to a burned area of the same individual. The graft is recognized as *autochthonous* or *autologous* ("self"), and no immune response is induced against it. Barring technical difficulties in the transplantation process, the graft will survive or "*take*" in its new location.

2. An *isograft* or *syngraft* is a graft or transplantation of cells, tissue, or organ from one individual to another individual who is *syngeneic* (genetically identical) to the donor. An example of an isograft is the transplantation of a kidney from one identical (homozygotic) twin to the other. As in the case of an autograft, the recipient who is genetically identical to the donor recognizes the donor's tissue as "self" and does not mount an immune response against it. The two individuals (i.e., donor and recipient), are described as *histocompatible*.

3. An *allograft* is a graft, or transplant, from one individual to a genetically dissimilar individual of the same species. Since all individuals of a given outbred species, except monozygotic twins, are *allogeneic* (genetically dissimilar), regardless of how closely they may be related, the graft is recognized by the recipient as "foreign" and is immunologically rejected. The donor and recipient, in this case, are *nonhistocompatible* or *histoincompatible*.

4. A *xenograft* is a graft between a donor and a recipient from different species. The transplant is recognized as foreign, and the immune response mounted against it will destroy or reject the graft. Donor and recipient are again described as *histoincompatible*.

THE ROLE OF THE IMMUNE RESPONSE IN ALLOGRAFT REJECTION

The role of the immune response in graft rejection is a proven fact: the most direct evidence is provided by experiments in which skin is transplanted from one individual to a genetically different individual of the same species, namely, between allogeneic donor and recipient. Mouse skin with black hair transplanted onto the back of a white-haired mouse appears normal for 1 or 2 weeks. However, after approximately 2 weeks, the transplant begins to be rejected, and is completely sloughed off within a few days. This process is called *first-set rejection*. If, after this rejection, the recipient is transplanted with another piece of skin from the *same* initial donor, the process of *rejection is accelerated*, and the graft is sloughed quicker, within about a week of the second transplant. This accelerated rejection is termed a *second-set rejection*. In contrast, a piece of skin from a genetically different strain grafted onto this same mouse is rejected with first-set kinetics. Thus, second-set rejection is an expression of specific *immunologic memory* for antigens expressed by the graft. The participation of T cells in the rejection response can be shown by transferring T cells from an individual sensitized to an allograft into a normal syngeneic recipient. If the second recipient is transplanted with the same allograft that was used on the original T-cell donor, a second-set rejection ensues. This establishes that T cells primed in the initial grafting mediate the accelerated rejection in the second host.

Many other lines of evidence establish the immunologic nature of graft rejection. For example, (1) histologic examination of the site of the rejection reveals *lymphocytic and monocytic cellular infiltration* reminiscent of the delayed-type hypersensitivity reaction (see Chapter 16); both CD4$^+$ and CD8$^+$ cells are present at the site (and, as we shall see later, both play a crucial role in graft rejection); (2) individuals that lack T lymphocytes (such as athymic, or "nude," mice or humans with DiGeorge syndrome; see Chapter 18) do not reject allografts or xenografts; and (3) the process of rejection slows down considerably or does not occur at all in immunosuppressed individuals. It has been conclusively demonstrated that specific *T cells* and *circulating antibodies* are induced to an allograft or a xenograft. However, although antibodies are responsible for the rejection of red blood cells during the transfusion reaction (see Chapter 19), T cells constitute the major immunologic component responsible for the rejection of allograft tissues (it has been demonstrated in several in vitro instances that certain antibodies that are not effective in the process of graft rejection compete with T cells for the transplantation antigens, thereby *blocking* the process of rejection mediated by T cells and enhancing the survival of the graft. Because of this phenomenon, these antibodies are described functionally as *enhancing antibodies*. The relevance of this phenomenon in vivo is still not clear).

CLINICAL CHARACTERISTICS OF ALLOGRAFT REJECTION

Clinically, allograft rejections fall into three major categories: (1) *hyperacute rejection*, (2) *acute rejection*, and (3) *chronic rejection*. The following are descriptions of the rejection reactions as might be observed, for example, after transplantation of a kidney; they also apply for rejection of other tissues.

Hyperacute Rejection

Hyperacute rejection occurs within a few minutes to a few hours of transplantation. It is a result of destruction of the transplant by *preformed antibodies* such as in ABO blood group incompatibility, in which case no transplantation will be performed, or preformed antibodies to the graft, synthesized as a result of previous transplantations, blood transfusions, or pregnancies. These antibodies activate the *complement* system, followed by platelet activation and deposition causing *swelling* and *interstitial hemorrhage* in the transplanted tissue, which decrease the flow of blood through the tissue. ***Thrombosis*** with ***endothelial injury*** and ***fibrinoid necrosis*** are often seen in cases of hyperacute rejection. The recipient may have ***fever, leukocytosis***, and produce ***little or no urine***. The urine may contain various cellular elements, such as erythrocytes. Cell mediated immunity is not involved at all in hyperacute rejection.

At present there is no therapy for successful prevention or termination of hyperacute rejection.

Acute Rejection

Acute rejection is seen in a recipient who has not previously been sensitized to the transplant. Cell-mediated immunity mediated by T cells is the primary cause of acute rejection. It is the common type of rejection experienced by individuals for whom the transplanted tissue is a mismatch, or who receive an allograft and insufficient immunosuppressive treatment to prevent rejection. For example, an acute rejection reaction may begin a few days after transplantation of a kidney, with a complete loss of kidney function within 10–14 days. Acute rejection of a kidney is accompanied by a rapid ***decrease in renal function. Enlargement and tenderness*** of the grafted kidney, a ***rise in serum creatinine levels***, a ***fall in urine output, decreased renal blood flow***, and presence of blood ***cells*** and ***proteins in the urine*** are characteristic. Histologically, cell-mediated immunity, manifested by intense infiltration of lymphocytes and macrophages, is taking place at the rejection site. The acute rejection reaction may be reduced by immunosuppressive therapy, for example, with antilymphocytic serum, corticosteroids, or other drugs, as we shall see later in this chapter.

Chronic Rejection

Chronic rejection caused by both antibody and cell-mediated immunity occurs in allograft transplantation months after the transplanted tissue has assumed its normal function. In cases of kidney transplantation, chronic rejection is characterized by ***slow, progressive renal failure***. Histologically, the chronic reaction is accompanied by ***proliferative inflammatory lesions*** of the small arteries, ***thickening of the glomerular basement membrane***, and ***interstitial fibrosis***. Because the damage caused by immune injury has already taken place, immunosuppressive therapy at this point is useless, and little can be done to save the graft.

While the preceding example is for kidney transplantation, it is important to point out that the rate, extent, and underlying mechanisms of rejection may vary, depending on the transplanted tissue and site of the transplanted graft. The recipient's circulation, lymphatic drainage, expression of strong antigens on the graft, and several other factors determine the rejection rate. For example, bone marrow and skin grafts are very sensitive to rejection compared to heart, kidney, and liver grafts.

HISTOCOMPATIBILITY ANTIGENS

Antigens that evoke an immune response associated with graft rejection are referred to as *transplantation antigens*, or *histocompatibility antigens*. These antigens are cell-surface molecules encoded by histocompatibility genes (H genes) situated at a histocompatibility locus (H locus). Since different alleles encoding allelic forms of the histocompatibility antigens exist at each H locus in different individuals, the antigens are also referred to as *alloantigens*.

If there were only one H locus with two alleles, for example, A and B, the possible genotypes and phenotypes of the alloantigens would be

Genotype	Phenotype
AA	A
AB	AB
BB	B

Transplantation between individuals with the above genotypes would be accepted or rejected as follows:

	Donor		Recipient	Accept/Reject	Reason
1)	AA	→	AA	Accept	A recognized as self
2)	BB	→	AA	Reject	B recognized as foreign
3)	AB	→	AA	Reject	B recognized as foreign
4)	AA	→	BB	Reject	A recognized as foreign
5)	BB	→	BB	Accept	B recognized as self
6)	AB	→	BB	Reject	A recognized as foreign
7)	AA	→	AB	Accept	A recognized as self
8)	BB	→	AB	Accept	B recognized as self
9)	AB	→	AB	Accept	A or B recognized as self

In reality, there are many H loci containing many alleles. For example, in mice there are about 40 H loci. However, while transplantation antigens may be encoded by various loci, each species contains one major region that is of prime immunologic importance for that species. This region is the ***major histocompatibility complex (MHC)***. It codes for major transplantation antigens; minor transplantation antigens are encoded by other loci. As described in Chapter 10, in the mouse, this region is called H-2. It consists of a segment of chromosome 17, and contains the genes encoding for class I molecules encoded by K, D, and L genes and class II molecules encoded by I region genes. In humans, the MHC is situated on chromosome 6. Since it contains genes encoding the strong histocompatibility antigens present on human leukocytes, the human MHC is known as HLA (for ***human leukocyte antigens***).

As we have already seen in Chapter 10, the human HLA gene complex (see Fig. 10.1A) consists of several closely linked genes (loci), known as A, B, C MHC class I), and DP, DQ, and DR genes (MHC class II). Each locus has many different alleles. The particular combination of alleles at the same locus or at closely linked loci on the same chromosome is termed the ***haplotype:*** two haplotypes, one from each parent, constitute the genotype of the individual. In a sense, the haplotype is the genotype of linked loci on each of the parental chromosomes.

Recalling the structure and genetics of MHC class I and class II molecules (Chapter 10), class I molecules consist of an α chain encoded by the MHC and β_2 microglobulin, encoded by a gene on a completely different chromosome. The *A, B* and *C* loci in humans (K, D, and L loci in mice) code for the α chain (heavy chain) of MHC class I molecules, which contain a variable region. This accounts for the polymorphism exhibited by MHC class I molecules. MHC class I molecules are present on all *nucleated* cells of the body.

The DP, DQ, and DR genes of the D locus in humans (the I region in mice) code for class II molecules which may be expressed on the surface of ***B lymphocytes, monocytes, Langerhans cells*** of the skin, and certain ***endothelial*** cells. Again, as described in Chapter 10, each class II molecule consists of an α chain and a β chain. Both chains exhibit extensive allelic variability.

The structure and major function of class I and class II molecules in the presentation of antigen to T cells have been discussed in Chapters 10 and 11. In the present chapter, we shall discuss their role in inducing transplantation reactions.

MHC Class I and Class II Molecules as Targets in Allograft Rejection

As we have seen, graft rejection is the consequence of a T-cell-dependent immune response: the recipient's T cells are activated by antigen, in particular by the non-self or foreign MHC molecules expressed on the graft. The key initiating event in graft rejection is the direct activation of the recipient's CD4$^+$ T cells by nonself MHC class II molecules expressed on specialized cells of the graft. (These non-self MHC molecules may have peptides derived from either the graft or the recipient's proteins bound in their peptide-binding groove.) The recipient's CD8$^+$ T cells may also be directly activated by nonself MHC class I molecules expressed on many cells in the graft.

Nonself MHC molecules are highly potent transplantation antigens, activating an enormous number of T-cell clones in the recipient. It is estimated that up to 5% of all clones in the body may respond to a nonself MHC molecule, orders of magnitude higher than the response to a conventional protein antigen. Presumably, the combination of nonself MHC molecule plus bound peptides cross-reacts with T-cell receptors on many different T cells. As we described in Chapters 9 and 10, the "everyday" specificity of the T cell within an individual is restricted by self-MHC, the allelic specificity seen in the thymus during T-cell differentiation. Thus, the exposure of an individual to nonself MHC molecules expressed on the graft represents an artificial but clinically relevant situation.

Another mechanism that contributes to host T-cell activation is that the antigen-presenting cells of the recipient that encounter the graft take up the alloantigens (major and minor), process the molecules, present the resulting peptides on self (recipient) MHC molecules to T cells, and activate them.

Sensitization of the recipient by donor-cell antigens activate the immune response by triggering both CD4$^+$ and CD8$^+$ cells. As a result, cytokines are synthesized and T cells cytotoxic for the graft are activated. The most important cytokines generated are IL-2, IFN-γ, and TNF-β as happens in delayed-type hypersensitivity (see Chapter 16). IL-2 is important for T-cell proliferation and differentiation into cytotoxic T lymphocytes (Tc) and T cells participating in DTH (T$_{DTH}$), IFN-γ is important for the accumulation and activation of macrophages in the graft area, and TNF-β is cytotoxic to the graft. Moreover, IFN-α, β, and γ as well as TNF-β and TNF-α increase the expression of class I molecules, while IFN-γ increases the expression of class II molecules on allograft cells, thus amplifying the reaction and enhancing graft rejection.

The MHC class II molecules or antigens coded by the DR locus play the most important role in tissue rejection, so much so that there is a good agreement among transplant immunologists that the better the match (parity) in HLA-DR between donor and recipient, the higher the probability of graft survival. In general, the graft does not survive if the donor and recipient do not share any DR haplotype.

It should be pointed out that although molecules coded for by the MHC are mainly responsible for graft rejection, weak antiallograft reactions may be generated by minor transplantation antigens, and the combined response to several minor antigens may result in eventual graft rejection. In fact, as we will discuss later in this chapter, minor transplantation antigens appear to be important in bone marrow transplantation and have been implicated in graft-versus-host (GVH) disease (discussed later in this chapter) in cases of HLA-matched bone marrow transplantations.

Xenogeneic Transplantation

To address the critical shortage of donated human organs for transplantation, studies are under way in the use of nonhuman organs. For ethical and practical reasons, species closely related to the human, such as the chimpanzee, have not been widely used. Attention has focused on the pig, some of whose organs are anatomically similar to the human. Interestingly, the human T-cell response to xenogeneic MHC antigens is not as strong as to allogeneic MHC molecules.

The major problem with using pig organs, and organs from other species, in human recipients, however, is the existence of natural or preformed antibody to carbohydrate moieties expressed on the graft's endothelial cells. As a consequence, the activation of the complement cascade occurs rapidly and hyperacute rejection ensues.

TESTS FOR HISTOCOMPATIBILITY ANTIGENS

Tissue typing consists of the analysis of histocompatibility antigens of donor and recipient and allows a determination of the degree of foreignness between the two individuals, thus serving to predict the outcome of a transplant procedure. With the advent of new and better immunosuppressive drugs and modalities, analysis of histocompatibility antigens and attempts to match donor and recipient by the similarity of their HLA antigens is becoming less and less essential. Nevertheless in many instances, such as bone marrow transplantation, HLA analyses are being performed and are therefore discussed below.

There are several ways to determine the degree of parity or disparity between transplantation antigens. One way is the serologic detection of cell-surface antigens; the other way is measuring the reaction between leukocytes from the donor and recipient [primarily detecting differences (or showing parity) of class II antigens].

Serologic Detection of Transplantation Antigens

A panel of antisera that react differently with different histocompatibility antigens is used to define transplantation antigens. The antisera are obtained from people who have had multiple transplantations or transfusions and from multiparous (multiple birth) women. Monoclonal antibodies are also used for defining HLA antigens. These antisera and monoclonal antibodies are used in a *lymphocytotoxicity test* in which the sera, in the presence of complement, are monitored for ability to damage the target cells, which are lymphocytes. Thus, lymphocytes of the donor and recipient, which carry MHC class I and class II antigens, are reacted with a panel of antibodies. The reaction with the various antibodies establishes the *serologic type* of each transplantation antigen on the cells. Similarity of donor and recipient transplantation antigens is indicated by similarity in the specific antisera with which the two sets of cells react (or do not react).

Serologic *tissue typing* provides a fairly reliable measure of parity (or disparity) between transplantation antigens of the donor and the recipient. However, because the number of antisera available for such a test is finite, there is always the possibility that, although the panel of sera shows a "match" (i.e., the identity of antigens on the donor's and recipient's leukocytes) differences would be found if the panel of antisera were enlarged.

Genotyping of Transplantation Epitopes

A relatively new approach to tissue typing is to type epitopes on HLA molecules rather than the entire molecule. Such comparison may be performed serologically, or better yet, on the genomic level. Thus, DNA segments are amplified by the polymerase chain reaction (PCR) to obtain DNA quantities that afford sequencing oligonucleotides and sequence comparison. This highly sensitive, rapid, and accurate method is far more accurate than serological typing because it can detect differences on the level of a single amino acid. Indeed, typing on the genomic level has shown differences in instances where complete "match" has been shown by serological means.

Detection of Transplantation Antigens by Mixed Leukocyte Reaction

In the *mixed leukocyte reaction (MLR)*, leukocytes from donor and recipient are cultured together for several days. The donor leukocytes contain T cells with specificity directed against the alloantigens on the recipient cells, and those *T cells* will therefore be triggered to ***proliferate*** in the presence of these antigens. The same is true for recipient leukocytes, which will proliferate in the presence of alloantigens on the donor cells. The proliferation is usually measured by introducing a radioactively labeled precursor to DNA, such as *^{3}H-thymidine*, into the culture. The greater the extent of proliferation, the more DNA is synthesized by the proliferating cells, and the more radioactivity is incorporated into the cells' DNA. The radioactivity incorporated in DNA is then calculated to provide a measure of the proliferative response.

In comparison to the serologic test, which defines the specific antigens of the MHC of the donor and recipient, the MLR measures the total parity (or disparity) between donor and recipient cells, a parameter that is important for transplantation: the stronger the MLR (the greater the extent of proliferation), the higher the disparity between donor and recipient. Conversely, a mixed lymphocyte culture (see Table 20.1), in which cellular proliferation is not induced, in-

TABLE 20.1   Cases of Mixed Lymphocyte Reaction Associated With Different Transplantation Situations

Transplantation situation	HLA relationship	Treatment of reacting leukocytes	MLR
Tissue between identical twins	HLA identical (syngeneic)	No treatment	(−) No reaction
Tissue between nonrelated donor and recipient	HLA different (allogeneic)	No treatment	(+) Reaction intensity depends on the degree of HLA difference between donor and recipient
Tissue between nonrelated donor and recipient	HLA different (allogeneic)	Donor's cells are treated with a mitotic inhibitor, thus testing reactivity of only recipient cells (performed to test for donor–recipient match)	(+) This is a one-way MLR; reaction intensity depends on the degree of HLA difference between donor and recipient
Bone marrow transplantation, or tissue grafting to an immunoincompetent recipient	HLA different (allogeneic)	Recipient's cells are treated with a mitotic inhibitor, thus testing reactivity of only donor's cells (performed to avoid graft-versus-host reaction)	(+) This is a one-way MLR; reaction intensity depends on the degree of HLA difference between donor and recipient

dicates complete parity or histocompatibility between donor and recipient, as when it is performed on cells from identical twins. It is important to emphasize that disparity in class II antigens is the most important factor in transplant rejection.

In most cases, it is essential to ascertain whether the recipient lymphocytes will react against the donor histocompatibility antigen (rather than whether the donor lymphocytes will react against the recipient alloantigens). For this purpose, a mixed lymphocyte culture is set up in which the donor cells have been treated with mitomycin C or X irradiation to prevent their proliferation. In this way, the only cells with the ability to proliferate are the recipient leukocytes. Such a reaction is called a ***one-way mixed leukocyte reaction.*** In this one way MLR $CD4^+$ cells proliferate to foreign MHC class II molecules and $CD8^+$ cells develop into T cytotoxic cells specific for the foreign class I molecules.

The MLR is also performed when transplants are to be made into an immunosuppressed individual. It is essential that such transplantation be performed between well-matched individuals in order to avoid a reaction by any inadvertently transplanted immunocompetent cells directed against the recipient's tissue, a few of which can produce an intense graft-versus-host (GVH) reaction, which we will discuss later. As we shall see toward the end of this chapter, when bone marrow, which may contain immunocompetent T cells, is transplanted into an immunologically incompetent host, it is essential to remove all competent mature T cells before transplantation to avoid this reaction.

Although MLR testing for histocompatibility is a highly effective indicator of the degree of parity between donor and recipient, it is a lengthy procedure and requires several days, whereas the serologic test takes only a few hours. Thus, the use of MLR and/or serologic testing is dictated by the speed with which an organ must be transplanted after its removal from the donor. While transplantation of organs from a living donor can await the results of the MLR test, sufficient time for this test may not be available in cases of organs obtained from recent cadavers. This is one reason why organ banks are set up to select the best-matched recipient when an organ becomes available.

As has been pointed out earlier, tissue or organ transplantation is relying more and more on immunosuppressive agents to prolong graft survival and less and less on tissue typing. In fact, recent results comparing graft survival with immunosuppressive agents show that, depending on the transplanted tissue, there is little difference in graft survival regardless of whether tissue typing or cross matching indicated a "match" between donor and recipient, as long as an immunosuppressive regiment was used.

PROLONGATION OF ALLOGRAFTS

Since transplantation between identical twins is a rare event, allotransplantation must usually be done with all its risks of allograft rejection. The higher the degree of disparity between donor and recipient, the faster will be the rejection of the graft.

Several measures are taken during transplantation that are aimed at prolonging graft survival; mostly they suppress the entire immune response in a non-antigen-specific way. This leaves the patient almost defenseless against infection by many microorganisms. Accordingly, chemoprophylaxis is given to patients undergoing nonspecific, generalized immune suppression.

Several of the major immunosuppressive agents used in transplantation cases are given below. Commonly they are used in various combinations with each other to ensure graft "take".

Anti-inflammatory Agents

Corticosteroids, such as prednisone, prednisolone, and methyl prednisolone, are anti-inflammatory agents. The immunosuppressive action of these steroids is due to several effects. These include their ability to stabilize lysosomal membranes, thus preventing the release of harmful lysosomal enzymes. They therefore inhibit the activity of inflammatory cells that are responsible for destruction of the graft. Corticosteroids can also inhibit T-cell cytokine production as well as directly inducing lysis of lymphocytes. In addition, they reduce phagocytosis and killing by neutrophils and macrophages and reduce expression of MHC class II molecules and IL-1 production by macrophages. In this way corticosteroids inhibit T-cell activation and T-cell function.

Antimetabolites

Antimetabolites that suppress the immune response include the purine antagonists ***azathioprine*** and ***mercaptopurine***, which interfere with the synthesis of RNA and DNA by inhibiting inosinic acid, the precursor for the purines adenylic and guandylic acids. ***Chlorambucil*** and ***cyclophosphamide***, compounds that alkylate DNA, also have antimetabolic activity and interfere with the metabolism of DNA.

Cytotoxic and Blocking Agents

Among the cytotoxic agents that suppress the immune response are many that are specifically cytotoxic to lymphocytes. Such agents include *antilymphocytic serum (ALS)* or *antilymphocytic globulins (ALGs). Steroids, alkylating agents, X rays*, and *antibiotics* such as actinomycin D are less specific, but they are particularly effective against proliferating cells, such as the lymphocytes that proliferate in response to alloantigens.

Antibodies, especially monoclonal antibodies, are gaining use as somewhat more target-specific (not transplantation-antigen-specific) than the immunosuppressants. OKT3, a monoclonal antibody to the CD3 part of the TcR, antibodies to IL-2 receptor, and antibodies to CD4 and several other molecules important for T-cell activation are being tested for efficacy in graft enhancement when given before, during, and immediately after transplantation.

Cyclosporine and FK 506

Cyclosporine is a compound that has become important and widely used for immunosuppression during allotransplantation. In fact, it is being increasingly used in allotransplantation. In many instances, enhancement in survival of an allograft between "unmatched" donor and recipient cyclosporine was almost as effective as when transplantation was performed between "matched" individuals.

Cyclosporine is a cyclic peptide derived from a soil fungus. It greatly enhances graft survival by interfering with cytokine gene transcription in T cells. It suppresses production of IL-2, IL-4, and IFN-γ as well as the synthesis of IL-2 receptors. Cyclosporine is effective when administered prior to transplantation but is ineffective in suppressing ongoing rejection. However, cyclosporine is nephrotoxic and has also been associated with increased incidence of B-cell lymphoma.

FK 506 is a relatively new immunosuppressive drug. Although its structure is considerably different from that of cyclosporine, its biological and immunosuppressive activity is similar. Like cyclosporine its affect is on T cells, preventing T-cell activation and the accompanying cytokine production.

Total Lymphoid Irradiation

Total lymphoid irradiation (TLI) constitutes another approach, still mainly experimental, to induce immunosuppression prior to transplantation. While shielding the bone marrow, the recipient's thymus, spleen, and lymph nodes are X-irradiated during several sessions until 3400 rads have been given. This irradiation destroys many cells, most importantly the highly radiation-sensitive T cells. Following irradiation and transplantation, which is performed immediately, bone marrow stem cells differentiate and repopulate the lymphoid tissue. The newly immunocompetent individual is now highly tolerant to the allograft.

It is important to note that, when immunosuppression is induced by the agents mentioned, it is not antigen-specific. In fact, it results in a generalized suppression of the entire immune response, including the response against infectious microorganisms. Thus, the immunosuppressed individual is highly susceptible to infections. Furthermore, because immunosuppression is associated with an increased incidence of lymphoproliferative disorders, management of the transplant patient must take into account the immunosuppressed state of the individual.

BONE MARROW TRANSPLANTATION

Transplantation of bone marrow constitutes a special transplantation situation because it is performed mostly between an immunocompetent donor and an immunoincompetent recipient. Examples are patients with severe combined immunodeficiency (SCID), patients with Wiskott–Aldrich syndrome (see Chapter 18), or patients with advanced leukemia who receive bone marrow from identical siblings. Today such transplantations are performed with a fair degree of success. In the past few years, transplantation of bone marrow from donors who are nonidentical but who are HLA-matched or partially matched is gaining success and acceptance. Specifically, haploidentical bone marrow (parental bone marrow that is only half MHC-identical) has been successfully used. Indeed, such bone marrow transplantation constitutes the treatment of choice of children with SCID.

Whereas bone marrow transplantation between identical twins can be performed with relatively low immunologic risk, transplantation of bone marrow from an immunocompetent donor to an HLA-matched or partially matched recipient is highly risky due to the presence of competent T cells in the donor's marrow, which may result in a graft-versus-host reaction (see below). To reduce this risk, it is imperative to remove the T cells from the transferred bone marrow. This removal, which can be achieved by a number of ways (e.g., treatment with monoclonal anti-T-cell antibodies and complement), widens the choice of bone marrow donors.

GRAFT-VERSUS-HOST REACTIONS

Transplantation of immunocompetent lymphocytes from a donor to a genetically different recipient can result in a reaction mounted by the grafted lymphocytes against the recipient's tissue. This *graft-versus-host (GVH)* reaction is particularly important in cases where immunocompetent lymphoid cells are transplanted into individuals who are *immunologically incompetent* and therefore cannot reject the transplanted cells. This situation is best exemplified in cases where immunocompetent cells are transferred into individuals with various immunodeficiency disorders or in cases of bone marrow transplantation into an immunosuppressed recipient. It is interesting that GVH disease may occur in bone marrow transplant recipients even if the donor and recipient are perfectly HLA-matched. This is probably due to minor, non-HLA-coded, transplantation antigens recognized by donor T cells.

In experimental animals, a GVH reaction may lead to a *wasting syndrome* in the recipient; in humans, GVH reactions may produce *splenomegaly* (enlarged spleen), *enlarged liver and lymph nodes, diarrhea, anemia, weight loss*, and other disorders in which the underlying causes are inflammation and destruction of tissue. The GVH reaction is initiated by the transferred T lymphocytes from the donor, which recognize the recipient's transplantation antigens as foreign. Donor T cells thus become activated as in an allograft response. In GVH disease, however, most of the inflammatory cells that participate in the reaction, and that are mainly responsible for destruction of tissue, are host cells recruited to the site of the reaction by lymphokines released by the donor's lymphocytes.

FETAL–MATERNAL RELATIONSHIP

One of the puzzling phenomena associated with allograft rejection is why the fetus, which expresses maternal and paternal histocompatibility antigens, is not rejected by the mother as an allograft. On one hand, it is clear that the mother can mount an antibody response against fetal antigen, as exemplified by anti-Rh antibodies produced by Rh$^-$ mothers. More importantly, women who experienced multiple births have antibodies to the father's MHC. It appears, however, that in most cases the antibodies are harmless to the fetus, and what is important is the mother's ability—or, better yet, inability—to respond with the production of cytotoxic T cells against the fetus. There is evidence that fetal trophoblast cells that constitute the outer layer of the placenta that come in contact with maternal tissue do not express MHC class I or class II molecules. Thus, the fetal trophoblast does not prime for a cellular immune response associated with allograft rejection.

Another factor that appears to operate in the survival of the fetus—the "allograft"—is *α-fetoprotein*, a protein synthesized in the yolk sac and fetal liver. α-Fetoprotein has been demonstrated to have immunosuppressive properties. Other factors that affect the immune response and may be involved in the fetal–maternal relationship include cytokines, complement inhibitory proteins, and other as yet unknown factors. All in all, the fetus and several other tissues in the body that do not initiate an immune response or are not affected by immune components are termed *immunologically privileged* sites. Overall, it appears that multiple factors are responsible for one of the most spectacular immunologically privileged sites: the fetus.

SUMMARY

1. **Transplantation rejection is immunologically mediated.**

2. **Both T cells and circulating antibodies are induced against allografts of xenografts. While antibodies are responsible for rejection of erythrocytes, T cells are mainly responsible for the rejection of most other tissue.**

3. **The most important transplantation antigens, which cause rapid rejection of the allograft, are found on cell membranes and are encoded by genes in the major histocompatibility complex (MHC), which is called H-2 in mice and HLA in humans. The structures encoded by these genes, MHC class I and class II molecules, are involved in determining the discrimination between "self" and "nonself" and in cellular interactions.**

4. **The degree of histocompatibility between donor and recipient can be determined serologically, by genotyping, or by mixed lymphocyte reaction.**

5. **Survival of nonmatched allografts is prolonged by anti-inflammatory agents, cytotoxic agents, antimetabolites, and other modalities aimed at immunosuppressing the recipient. These approaches to enhancing graft survival are gaining acceptance and wide use in human tissue and organ transplantation.**

REFERENCES

Armitage JO (1994): Bone marrow transplantation. New Engl J Med 330:827.

Auchincloss H Jr, Sachs D (1993): Transplantation and graft rejection. In Paul WE (ed): Fundamental Immunology, 3rd ed. New York: Raven Press.

Charlton B, Auchincloss H Jr, Fathman CG (1994): Mechanisms of transplantation tolerance. Annu Rev Immunol 12:707.

Ferrara JLM, Deeq HJ (1991): Graft versus host disease. New Engl J Med 324:667.

Garovoy MR, Stock P, Baumgardner G, Keith F. Linker C (1994): Transplantation. In Stites DP, Terr AI, Parslow TG (eds): Basic and Clinical Immunology, 8th ed. Norwalk, CT: Appleton & Lange.

Hunt JS (1992): Immunobiology of pregnancy. Curr Opinion Immunol 4:591.

Lechler RI, Lombardi G, Batchelor JR, Reinsmoen N, Bach FH (1990): The molecular basis for alloreactivity. Immunol Today 11:83.

Roopenian DC (1992): What are the minor histocompatibility loci? A new look at an old question. Immunol Today 13:7.

Schreiber SL, Crabtree GR (1992): The mechanism of action of cyclosporin A and FK 506. Immunol Today 13:136.

Sherman LA, Chattopadhyay S (1994): The molecular basis of allorecognition. Annu Rev Immunol 11:385.

Suthanthiran M, Strom TB (1994): Renal transplantation. New Engl J Med 331:365.

Winkelstein A (1994): Immunosuppressive therapy. In Stites DP, Terr AI, Parslow TG (eds.): Basic and Clinical Immunology 8th ed. Norwalk, CT: Appleton & Lange.

REVIEW QUESTIONS

For each question, choose the ONE BEST answer or completion.

1. Kidney transplantation was performed using a kidney from a donor who was matched to the recipient by serologic tissue typing. However, within a few months the kidney was rejected. Assuming no technical problems with the surgical procedure, one reason for the rejection may be that
   A) there was insufficient blood supply to the graft
   B) there could have been a mismatch, which would have been detected by a mixed lymphocyte reaction
   C) the recipient developed blocking antibodies
   D) the recipient also suffered from Wiskott–Aldrich syndrome
   E) the donor was agammaglobulinemic

2. Currently, the best indicator for predicting compatibility for transplantation of tissue from donor A to recipient B is obtained by
   A) one-way mixed lymphocyte reaction between B cells and mitomycin C-treated A cells

B) one-way mixed lymphocyte reaction between A cells and mitomycin C-treated B cells
C) serologic typing and cross-matching of A and B cells
D) two-way mixed lymphocyte reaction between A and B cells
E) matching for blood group antigens

3. The MHC complex contains the following *except*:
A) genes that encode transplantation antigens
B) genes that encode immunoglobulins
C) genes that regulate immune responsiveness
D) genes that encode some components of complement
E) genes that encode class I and class II antigens

4. The most common serologic test used for the detection of HLA antigens on lymphocytes is
A) the complement fixation test
B) double gel diffusion
C) complement-dependent cytotoxicity test
D) mixed lymphocyte reaction
E) radioimmunoassay

5. Which of the following regarding GVH disease is incorrect?
A) requires MHC differences between donor and recipient
B) requires immunocompetent donor cells
C) may result from infusion of blood products that contain viable lymphocytes into an immunologically incompetent recipient
D) requires suppressor T cells
E) may occur in an immunosuppressed individual

6. Transplant rejection may involve the following:
A) cell-mediated immunity
B) type III (immune aggregate) hypersensitivity
C) complement-dependent cytotoxicity
D) the release of IFN-γ
E) all are correct

7. Which of the following statements concerning the mixed lymphocyte reaction (MLR) are correct?
A) specific responding cells are B lymphocytes
B) MLR results in clonal expansion of specific, alloantigen-reactive cells
C) MLR between unrelated individuals who differ according to HLA serology is usually negative
D) stimulation of proliferation is controlled primarily by the HLA-D region alleles
E) only A and C are correct
F) only B and D are correct
G) all are correct

8. In clinical transplantation, cytotoxic antibodies
A) cause delayed rejection of the transplant
B) are responsible for hyperacute rejection
C) cause rejection when present in the donor
D) may be directed against HLA antigens
E) only A and C are correct
F) only B and D are correct

9. A candidate for a kidney graft is tested against a panel of potential donors by performing a one-way MLR. Which donor(s) represents the best chance of a take:

Donor	Recipient cells alone	Donor cells alone	Donor and recipient cells
A	120	2	22,376
B	119	5	17,982
C	99	3	76,427
D	102	1	477

³H-Thymidine incorporation (cpm)

Case study: A child is brought to the hospital suffering from an aplastic bone marrow after ingestion of benzene. All blood elements are at low levels and death is imminent. The child and a sibling were rapidly typed as both being A^+ Rh^+ HLA-A3,7: B4,8, and bone marrow was transfused. Within a few days the RBC count rose, indicating a successful take. However, 3 weeks later the child began to experience diarrhea and a skin rash on the palms and soles of the feet, spreading to the trunk. This was followed by jaundice and enlarged liver and spleen. Administration of an anti-T-cell serum plus cyclosporine produced some improvement. What went wrong, and why?

ANSWERS TO REVIEW QUESTIONS

1. **B** The most probable reason for the rejection is that, although serologically the donor and recipient were matched, this was an incomplete measure. The accuracy of serologic matching is predicated on the number of sera used in the test. There is always the possibility that a mismatch would have been detected if additional sera were used. In genotyping by PCR, the transplantation epitope is highly sensitive and accurate. Even the mixed lymphocyte reaction is more reliable, since it can detect mismatches that may not be detected serologically. Answer *A* is not correct, since it is stated that there were no problems due to the surgical procedure. Answer *C* is incorrect since blocking antibodies, if indeed developed by the recipient, would be expected to enhance the survival of the transplant. Answer *E* is incorrect because the immune status of the kidney donor is, in this case, irrelevant to the outcome of the transplantation.

2. **A** Compatibility can be reliably predicted by the one-way mixed lymphocyte reaction between the recipient's B cells and mitomycin C-treated cells from the donor. In this test, only the reactivity of the recipient cells against the donor antigens is measured. The reverse—i.e., reaction between A cells and mitomycin C-treated recipient B cells—is of no practical importance, because A is not the recipient. Serologic typing and cross-matching of A and B are of value, since those tests are more rapid than the MLR. However, there is always the possibility that the panel of antisera used is not complete and that if more antisera were used a mismatch would be found. The two-way MLR is important in assessing the total degree of parity (or disparity) in transplantation antigens, but it does not determine if the reaction is that of the donor to the recipient cells, or of the recipient to donor cells, or both. Matching for blood group anti-

gens is imperative but not sufficient. Nevertheless, if you answered **D**, it is also acceptable.

3. **B** The MHC complex contains all genes mentioned except genes that encode immunoglobulins. They are on different chromosomes.

4. **C** The most common serologic test used for detection of HLA antigens on lymphocytes is the complement-dependent cytotoxicity test. The mixed lymphocyte reaction, especially the one-way MLR, is an excellent test for HLA-D antigens, but it is a test based on cellular reactions and not on the reaction of serum antibodies.

5. **D** The GVH disease is caused by the destruction of cells or tissue of an immunoincompetent recipient by immunocompetent lymphoid cells transferred from a histoincompatible donor. The GVH reaction does not require suppressor T cells.

6. **E** All are correct. The important process in the rejection of an allotransplant is cell-mediated immunity. Here, T cells, which recognize the alloantigens, become activated; the T cells release cytokines, one of which is IFN-γ, which recruits and activates phagocytic cells that, together with cytotoxic T cells, destroy the graft. However, the reaction to the allotransplant may also involve antibodies (IgM and IgG), which can cause damage to tissue via activation of complement and the recruitment of polymorphonuclear cells to the site of the reaction. The polymorphonuclear cells would damage the graft by the release of their lysosomal enzymes.

7. **F** The MLR results in the clonal expansion of specific T cells, which recognize the alloantigens in the D region of the HLA. Although clones of B cells may also expand, the major cellular expansion is that of the T cells. The MLR between unrelated individuals who differ according to HLA serology is usually positive (rather than negative). Thus only **B** and **D** are right.

8. **F** Cytotoxic antibodies, such as IgM and IgG, cause hyperacute rejection by complement-mediated cell lysis or by opsonization and subsequent destruction of the transplant by phagocytic cells. The cytotoxic antibodies may be directed against blood group antigens or to HLA antigens on transferred cells (e.g., leukocytes). The presence of cytotoxic antibodies in the donor is usually of no clinical importance since, even if they are transferred to the recipient with the donor's blood, they become highly diluted in the recipient. Thus only **B** and **D** are correct.

9. **D** A one-way mixed lymphocyte response measures the reactivity of host T cells against donor MHC antigens. The lowest reactivity (as measured by thymidine incorporation) would represent the best possibility for a successful take in a graft of donor tissue. Donors **A**, **B**, and **C** all give high levels of ^{3}H-thymidine incorporation and are therefore most likely to provoke graft rejection reactions.

Case study: The symptoms are typical of GVH disease. The hasty matching presumably involved serologic typing only and matching for MHC class II molecules by PCR genotyping, or by MLR, was not done. In addition, care was not taken to deplete the donor bone marrow of mature T cells. Presumably, histoincompatibility between the donor and recipient triggered the donor's T cells to attack the recipient's cells, resulting in the symptom complex seen. Therapy aimed at destroying or inhibiting activated donor T cells is not as effective as eliminating them to begin with.

TUMOR IMMUNOLOGY

INTRODUCTION

The existence of an immune response against a tumor is based on changes in the surface components of the malignant cell that do not occur in its normal counterpart, and that give rise to structures that are antigenic. In 1943 Gross observed that when tumor cells were transplanted into the skin of syngeneic (genetically identical), histocompatible mice, the cells formed nodules that grew for a few days and then regressed. When identical tumor cells were reinjected into the mice, they did not produce nodules or grow. These findings were interpreted to mean that the mice that rejected the tumor did so because they had become immunologically resistant—or immune—to the tumor. Subsequently, ***tumor-specific transplantation antigens (TSTAs)***, which have the ability to induce antitumor immune responses, have been demonstrated for many tumors in a variety of animal species, including humans.

The goals of tumor immunology are (1) to elucidate the immunologic relationship between the host and the tumor and (2) to utilize the immune response to tumors for the purpose of ***diagnosis, prophylaxis,*** and ***therapy***. In the present chapter we discuss various approaches to meeting these goals.

TUMOR ANTIGENS

Some antigens on the surface of malignant cells may consist of structures that are unique to the cancerous cells and are not present on their normal counterparts. These are termed *tumor-specific transplantation antigens (TSTAs)* or simply *tumor-specific antigens (TSAs)*. Other tumor antigens may represent structures that are common to both malignant and normal cells but that are "masked" on the normal cells and become "unmasked" on malignant cells. Still other antigens on tumor cells represent structures that are qualitatively not different from those found on normal cells but that are "overexpressed"—present at significantly increased numbers on the cancer cell as products of cellular oncogenes. These antigens are referred to as *tumor-associated antigens (TAAs)*. An example is the high levels of a growth factor receptor due to increased expression of the *neu* oncogene products found in a number of human breast cancer cells, and the elevated *ras* oncogene products present on some human prostate cancer cells. Still other antigens on malignant cells represent structures that are present on fetal or embryonic cells but disappear from normal adult cells. These latter antigens are referred to as *oncofetal* or *oncodevelopmental antigens*.

CLASSIFICATION OF TUMOR ANTIGENS

Tumor antigens may be classified into four major categories. The categories differ in both the factors that induce the malignancy and the immunochemical properties of the tumor antigens.

Antigens of Tumors Induced by Chemical or Physical Carcinogens

Antigens of tumors induced by chemical carcinogens exhibit *little or no immunologic cross-reactivity*; each tumor exhibits a *unique antigenic specificity*. Thus, cells of a given tumor, arising from a single transformed cell, all share common antigens, but different tumors, even if induced by the same carcinogen, are antigenically distinct from one another. For example, if the chemical carcinogen methylcholanthrene is applied in an identical manner to the skin of two genetically identical animals, or on two similar sites on the same individual, the cells of the developing tumors (sarcomas) will exhibit antigens unique to each tumor, with no immunologic cross-reactivity between the tumors. As with chemically induced tumors, there is little or no cross-reactivity between physically induced tumors, such as those induced by ultraviolet light or by X irradiation. This absence of cross-reactivity is probably due to the ***random mutations*** induced by the chemical or physical carcinogens, leading to a large array of different antigens.

Since most human and animal tumors are attributed to chemical and physical environmental factors such as radiation, smoke, and tar, these tumors, which lack immunologic cross-reactivity, are unfortunately not expected to be amenable to diagnosis, prophylaxis, or therapy by immunologic means.

Antigens of Virally Induced Tumors

Animal studies have shown that tumors induced by DNA or RNA oncogenic virus exhibit ***extensive immunologic cross-reactivity***. This is because any particular oncogenic virus induces the expression of the same antigens in a tumor, regardless of the tissue of origin or the animal species.

For example, DNA viruses such as polyoma, SV40, and Shope papilloma virus induce tumors that exhibit extensive cross-reactivity within each virus group. Many leukemogenic viruses, such as Raucher leukemia virus, induce the formation of tumors that exhibit cross-reactivity not only within each virus group but also between some groups. In this connection, there is considerable circumstantial evidence to suggest that several human cancers, such as ***Burkitt's lymphoma, nasopharyngeal carcinoma***, ***T-cell leukemia,*** and ***hepatocellular carcinoma*** are caused by viruses. Thus, although the viral etiology of these human cancers remain to be conclusively established, the immunologic cross-reactivity in these, as well as in some other human malignancies, is similar to the cross-reactivity seen in animal tumors induced by viruses. For example, cross-reactivity is well established for cell surface antigens of Burkitt's lymphomas or of ***neuroblastomas*** from different patients. ***Colon carcinoma*** cells obtained from different patients also exhibit immunologic cross-reactivity, as do ***melanoma*** cells from different patients.

Some antigens of virally induced tumors are encoded by the virus, but they are distinct from virion antigens and are referred to as ***tumor-associated antigens (TAA)***. Occasionally, virally induced tumors may express oncofetal antigens, encoded by the host genome.

Oncodevelopmental Tumor Antigens

Many tumors express on their surface, or secrete into the blood, products that are normally present during embryonic and fetal development, but that are either absent or present at very low levels in normal adult tissue. These structures are not immunogenic in the ***autochthonous*** (native or original) host. Their presence can be detected by antisera prepared against them in allogeneic or xenogeneic animals. One such oncofetal antigen is the ***carcinoembryonic antigen (CEA)***, found primarily in serum of patients with ***cancers of the gastrointestinal tract***, especially cancer of the colon. Elevated levels of CEA have also been detected in the circulation of patients with some types of ***lung cancer, pancreatic cancer***, and some types of ***breast and stomach cancer***. However, it should be noted that elevated levels of CEA have also been detected in the circulation of patients with nonneoplastic diseases, such as emphysema, ulcerative colitis, and pancreatitis, as well as in the sera of alcoholics and heavy smokers.

Another oncodevelopmental antigen is α-fetoprotein (AFP), which is normally present at high concentrations in fetal and maternal serum (see Chapter 20) but absent from serum of normal individuals. AFP is rapidly secreted by cells of a variety of cancers and is found particularly in patients with ***hepatomas*** and ***testicular teratocarcinomas***.

The association of oncodevelopmental antigens with a wide variety of tumor types strongly suggests that the derepression of normal genes that are usually repressed in the normal adult individual is a concomitant of malignancy.

Antigens of "Spontaneous" Tumors

"Spontaneous" tumors are those tumors that are induced by unknown causes. Until recently, for most "spontaneous" tumors, it was difficult to discern an immunologic response in the autochthonous host, and antigens on the surface of cells from spontaneous tumors could be detected only with the aid of allogeneic or xenogeneic antiserum. However, with the recent advent of sensitive detection techniques, antibodies to autochthonous tumors have been found in patients with some tumors, most notably ***malignant melanoma***. In some cases, the antigens exhibit immunologic cross-reactivity; in other cases they do not. Thus, antigens of spontaneous tumors seem to resemble those of chemically or virally induced tumors with respect to immunologic specificity.

THE IMMUNE RESPONSE TO TUMORS

Until recently most of the information concerning humoral and cellular antitumor immune effector mechanisms and their capacity to destroy tumor cells has been derived from experiments with transplantable tumors in animals or from in vitro experiments. There is now ample presumptive evidence to suggest that the immune response plays an important role in the relationship between the host and the tumor in humans as well.

Humoral and *cellular* immune effector mechanisms capable of destroying tumors in vitro are summarized in Table 21.1. In general, destruction of tumor cells by these mechanisms is more efficient in the case of *dispersed tumors* (i.e., when the target tumor cells are in single-cell suspension) than in the case of solid tumors, probably because dispersed cells are more accessible to immune action.

TABLE 21.1   Humoral and Cellular Effector Immune Mechanisms in Tumor Cell Destruction

A. Humoral mechanisms

    1. Lysis by antibody and complement

    2. Antibody-mediated and complement-mediated opsonization

    3. Antibody-mediated loss of tumor cell adhesion

B. Cellular mechanisms

    1. Destruction by cytotoxic T cells

    2. Antibody-dependent, cell-mediated cytotoxicity (ADCC)

    3. Destruction by activated macrophages

    4. Destruction by natural killer (NK) cells

Humoral Responses

LYSIS OF TUMOR CELLS MEDIATED BY ANTIBODY AND COMPLEMENT. Both *IgM* and *IgG* antibodies have been shown to destroy tumor cells in vitro in the presence of complement. Several studies conducted with mice indicate that, in the presence of complement, antitumor antibodies are effective in vivo in destroying some leukemia and lymphoma cells and in reducing metastases in several other tumor systems. Other studies in vivo and in vitro, however, show that the same antibodies, in the presence of complement, are ineffective in destroying the cells of the same tumor in a solid form.

DESTRUCTION OF TUMOR CELLS BY OPSONIZATION AND PHAGOCYTOSIS. Destruction of tumor cells by phagocytic cells has been demonstrated in vitro, but only in the presence of antitumor immune serum and complement. The relevance of this finding in vivo is unknown.

ANTIBODY-MEDIATED LOSS OF ADHESIVE PROPERTIES OF TU-MOR CELLS. It appears that metastatic activity of certain kinds of tumors requires the adhesion of the tumor cells to each other and to the surrounding tissue. Antibodies directed against tumor cell surfaces may interfere with the adhesive properties of the tumor cells. The relevance of this mechanism in vivo is also unknown.

Cell-Mediated Responses

DIRECT DESTRUCTION OF TUMOR CELLS BY CYTOTOXIC T LYMPHOCYTES. Destruction of tumor cells in vitro by specific immune T lymphocytes has been demonstrated numerous times for a variety of tumors, both dispersed and solid. Moreover, from many studies with experimental animals (primarily but not exclusively mice), there is good evidence that tumor-specific, cytotoxic T cells are responsible for destruction of tumor in vivo. Although helper T cells participate in the induction and regulation of cytotoxic T cells, the destruction of the tumor cell is achieved by the CD8$^+$ *cytotoxic T lymphocytes (CTL)* with specificity for the antigens on the surface of the tumor cell.

It should be remembered that CD4$^+$ helper T cells are MHC class II antigen restricted, and CD8$^+$ cytotoxic T cells are MHC class I restricted. It is therefore important to note that cytokines such as tumor necrosis factor (TNF) and IFN-γ have an anti-tumor effect because, among other functions, they upregulate MHC class I and class II antigens on some tumor cells, which originally had a decreased expression of these antigens, thereby evading the action of CD8$^+$ killer cells.

ANTIBODY-DEPENDENT, CELL-MEDIATED CYTOTOXICITY. Antibody-dependent, cell-mediated cytotoxicity (ADCC) involves (1) the binding of tumor-specific antibodies to the surface of the tumor cells; (2) the interaction of various cells, such as granulocytes and macrophages, which possess surface receptors for the Fc portion of the antibody attached to the tumor cell; and (3) the destruction of the tumor cells by substances that are released from these cells that carry receptors for the Fc portion of the antibody. The importance of this mechanism in the destruction of tumor cells in vivo is still not clear.

DESTRUCTION OF TUMOR CELLS BY ACTIVATED MACRO-PHAGES. Macrophages may become highly cytotoxic (Figs. 21.1, 21.2) when they become "activated" by cytokines, most notably IFN-γ produced by an activated population of T lymphocytes, which, by themselves, are not cytotoxic.

These T lymphocytes (CD4$^+$) are tumor-specific: they release IFN-γ after activation by tumor antigen. Other cytokines released by these antigen-activated T lymphocytes attract macrophages to the area of the antigen. IFN-γ also prevents migration of macrophages away from the antigen. The mechanism of activation of macrophages by T cells specific for tumor antigen, leading to destruction of tumor cells, is similar to mechanisms involved in delayed-type hypersensitivity reactions in allograft rejection or in the killing of microorganisms: antigen-specific T cells become activated by antigen, and they release lymphokines, which attract and activate macrophages. These activated macrophages are cytotoxic to the microorganism, to tumor cells, and even to "self" cells in the vicinity of the activated macrophages. The damaging and killing activity of activated macrophages is due to several products that they release, notably ***lysosomal enzymes*** and ***tumor necrosis factor*** α ***(TNF-α)***. Mounting evidence to indicate that destruction of tumor cells by activated macrophages occurs in vivo includes the following observations: (1) resistance to a tumor can be abolished by specific depletion of macrophages, (2) increased resistance to tumor accompanies an increase in the

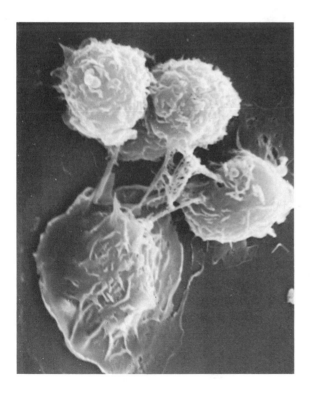

Figure 21.1.

A scanning electron micrograph showing an activated macrophage with filopodia extending to the surface of three melanoma cells. ×4,500. (Photo courtesy of Dr. K.L. Erickson, School of Medicine, University of California, Davis; reproduced with permission of Lippincott/Harper and Row.)

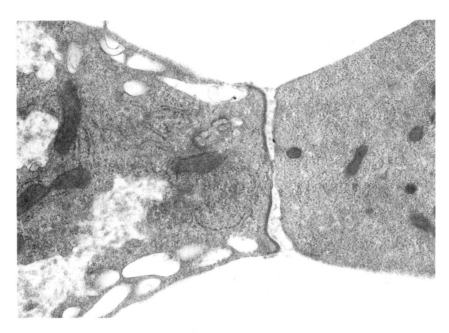

Figure 21.2.

"The kiss of death." An electron micrograph showing a contact point between an activated macrophage (left) and a melanoma cell after 18 hours of coculture leading to cytolysis of the melanoma target cell. Flocculent material is found between the cells; a dense plate is associated with the cell membranes of the macrophage process; microtubules also appear in these projections. ×26,000. (Photo courtesy of Dr. K.L. Erickson, School of Medicine, University of California, Davis; reproduced with permission of Lippincott/Harper and Row.)

number of activated macrophages, (3) administration of TNF-α into tumor bearing animals causes hemorrhage and tumor necrosis, and (4) activated macrophages are frequently found at the site of regression of a tumor. However, the relationship between the tumor and the tumor associated macrophages is quite complex. On one hand, macrophages can and, indeed, do kill tumor cells; on the other hand, macrophages and tumor cells have been shown to produce reciprocal growth factors leading to an almost symbiotic relationship. Thus, changes in the delicate balance between macrophages and tumor cells may drastically affect the fate of the tumor.

DESTRUCTION OF TUMOR BY NATURAL KILLER CELLS AND LYMPHOKINE-ACTIVATED KILLER CELLS. As we have seen in Chapter 2, *natural killer (NK) cells* are lymphoid cells found in spleen, lymph nodes, bone marrow, and peripheral blood of nonimmune animals and normal humans. These cells can lyse a variety of target cells, such as virally infected cells, antibody-coated cells, undifferentiated cells, and cells from a number of different tumors. The NK cells in humans are part of a population of large granular lymphocytes (LGL), so called because of their size and content of cytoplasmic granules. They lack most of the characteristic cell-surface markers of mature T lymphocytes, B lymphocytes, or macrophages, and their activity is not increased after immunization. NK cells do have receptors for the Fc region of IgG and, as we have seen in Chapter 5, can participate in ADCC (antibody-dependent cell-mediated cytotoxicity). They do not use this mechanism to kill tumors, however, since NK-mediated tumor killing can still occur even when their Fc receptors are blocked. ***Activation of NK cells does not involve immunologic memory.*** Like activated macrophages, NK cells secrete TNF-α that induces hemorrhage and tumor necrosis; however, the exact mechanism by which NK cells recognize and kill the tumor cells is still not clear.

There is circumstantial evidence to suggest that NK cells play an important role in the host–tumor relationship and may be particularly important in the host's defense against early stages of tumor growth, before the development of cytotoxic T cells and T-cell-mediated activated macrophages.

Lymphokine-activated killer (LAK) cells are tumor-specific killer cells obtained from the patient. The cells are grown in vitro in the presence of interleukin-2 (IL-2) and then given back to the same patient. LAK cells constitute a heterogenous population of lymphocytes that include NK cells. However their activity cannot be attributed solely to NK cells since they can kill, in vitro, tumor cells that are not killed by NK cells. Nor are LAK cells the classic cytolytic T lymphocytes since, unlike T lymphocytes, the killing by LAK cells is not MHC restricted. Although the natural biologic function of LAK cells is still obscure, they are now being tested for efficacy in tumor immunotherapy in humans (a topic discussed later in this chapter). A more recent innovation is the use of T cells isolated from the tumor and expanded and activated with IL-2. These ***tumor-infiltrating lymphocytes (TIL)*** show promise of greater specificity.

ROLE OF THE IMMUNE RESPONSE IN THE RELATIONSHIP BETWEEN HOST AND TUMOR

The foregoing discussion dealt with immune effector mechanisms, which have been shown to have the ability, in vitro and in some instances in vivo, to destroy tumor cells. However, a question may be raised about the degree to which the immune response plays a role in the host–tumor relationship. There are several phenomena that strongly suggest that the immune response has a profound effect on this relationship. These are described below.

Tumors in Immunosuppressed Individuals

There is evidence that tumors occur more frequently in immunosuppressed individuals than in their normal counterparts. Such tumors are predominantly but not exclusively *lymphoproliferative* malignancies. The 50- to 100-fold increase in the incidence of lymphoproliferative tumors in victims of radiation or in patients subjected to deliberate immunosuppression, and the elevated incidence of a wide range of tumors in older individuals whose immune response is reduced, strongly suggest that the immune response plays an important role in the relationship between a tumor and its host.

Tumors in the Immunocompetent Host

An involvement of the immune response in the host–tumor relationship is suggested by the correlation between the appearance of various immunologic effector mechanisms and the state of resistance to transplanted tumors in experimental animals. Furthermore, there is a correlation between the appearance of immune components at the site of the tumor and the regression of tumors in animals and humans. Moreover, there are examples in experimental animals to indicate that the primary tumor may induce a state of acquired "concomitant immunity" in the host. *Concomitant immunity* is expressed by the host's ability to reject newly arising or transplanted tumors of the same type, despite the progression of the primary tumor.

Immune Surveillance

The *theory of immune surveillance*, propounded by Thomas in the 1950s and expanded by Burnet (a Nobel Prize winner) later in the same decade, proposes that the immunological mechanisms that operate in the rejection of an allograft, in particular cell-mediated immunity, have evolved as a primary and specific defense against neoplastic cells, which arise continually in the normal organism as a result of somatic mutations. There are many examples, both experimental and clinical, that support the theory of immune surveillance, in particular those cases in which the incidence of cancer is high in the immunodeficient or immunosuppressed host. However, doubt is cast on the validity of the theory of immune surveillance by the finding that the incidence of tumors in athymic mice, which have no T-cell-mediated response, is no higher than in their normal counterparts. It should be noted, however, that such athymic mice have normal or, in some instances, increased numbers of NK cells. Furthermore, surface antigens on tumor cells of "spontaneous" tumors are generally of weak immunogenicity. Thus, to date, the theory remains controversial and unproven.

Limitations of the Effectiveness of the Immune Response Against Tumors

Whether or not the theory of immune surveillance is correct, there is no question that an immune response can be induced against tumors. Then, why, in spite of the immune response, does the tumor continues to grow in the host? Several possible mechanisms may be operational; either alone or in combination with each other (Table 21.2). Factors that may influence the escape of tumor cells from destruction by the immune system are described in the paragraphs that follow:

TABLE 21.2   Limitations of the Effectiveness of the Immune Response to Tumors

1. Tumor resides in immunologically privileged site
2. Antigenic modulation of tumor antigens
3. Presence of enhancing or "blocking" factors
4. Suppressor T lymphocytes
5. Immune suppression by tumor cell products
6. Excessive tumor mass

PRIVILEGED SITES. Certain areas of the body, such as parts of the eye and tissues of the central nervous system, are immunologically "privileged" sites: they are inaccessible to effector cells of the immune response or their products. Consequently, tumors arising in such immunologically privileged sites escape destruction by the immune response.

ANTIGENIC MODULATION. Tumor cells may change their antigenic characteristics or lose their antigens altogether, thus escaping destruction by the immune response. In fact, it is conceivable that the immune response destroys all the antigen-bearing tumor cells, thereby selecting for nonantigenic tumor cells.

ENHANCING AND BLOCKING FACTORS. On theoretical grounds, destruction of tumor cells by immune components may be "*blocked*" by circulating, *soluble antigens* derived from the tumor, which would bind with tumor-specific antibodies or cells and would prevent the binding of these antibodies and cells with the same antigens present also on the surface of the tumor cell. In addition, various immune components may interfere with each other. For example, protection of tumor cells and enhancement of tumor growth may be achieved in vivo by first reacting the tumor cells with *tumor-specific antibodies*. If these antibodies do not destroy the tumor, they can, in fact, inhibit its destruction by tumor-specific T lymphocytes directed against the same or adjacent epitopes on the surface of the tumor cell. Thus, antibodies, as well as circulating antigen and also *antigen–antibody complexes*, may constitute "*blocking*" factors, which prevent the destruction of the tumor and may even enhance its growth. Moreover, several studies have indicated that, through mechanisms not yet clear, some tumor-specific cell-mediated immune responses may even enhance the metastasis of a tumor. In addition, as mentioned earlier, the interrelationship between the tumor and tumor-associated macrophages may contribute to tumor enhancement rather than regression.

SUPPRESSOR T LYMPHOCYTES. Antigen-specific *suppressor T cells* may play a role in the regulation of the immune response to that antigen. Tumor-specific suppressor T cells have been demonstrated in many experimental systems. In humans, a generalized decrease of immune competence has been observed during advanced malignancy. Whether this decrease can be attributed to immunologically specific suppressor mechanisms or to a more generalized suppression mediated by tumor cells (see below) is unknown.

NONSPECIFIC SUPPRESSION MEDIATED BY TUMOR CELLS. Certain types of tumors synthesize various compounds, such as *prostaglandins*, which reduce many aspects of immune responsiveness. However, the role of this mechanism in the escape of tumors from destruction by the immune response is still unclear.

LARGE TUMOR MASS. The immune response and its various components have a finite capacity for the effective destruction of tumors (or, for that matter, of invading microorganisms). Thus, while immunization may result in effective protection against an otherwise lethal dose of tumor cells, it is ineffective if the dose of tumor cells is sufficiently large. The progression of the growth of a tumor in an immunocompetent host, in the face of an immune response, may be due to a rapid increase in the mass of the tumor, which outstrips the increase in immune responsiveness, until the large mass of the tumor overwhelms any effects of the immune response.

IMMUNODIAGNOSIS

Immunodiagnosis of tumors may be performed to achieve two separate goals: (1) the immunological detection of *antigens* specific to tumor cells and (2) the assessment of the host's *immune response* to the tumor (Table 21.3). Obviously, immunodiagnosis is predicated on immunologic cross-reactivity, and immunological methods may be used to detect tumor antigens and other "markers" in cases where tumor antigens exhibit similarities from individual to individual. In the presence of such immunologic cross-reactivity, antibody or lymphocytes from individuals with the same type of tumor would be expected to react with the cross-reactive tumor antigens, regardless of the individual from which they have been derived.

TABLE 21.3   Tumor Immunodiagnosis

A. Detection of tumor cells and their products by immunological means

   1. Myeloma and Bence-Jones proteins (e.g., plasma cell tumors)
   2. α-Fetoprotein (AFP) (e.g., liver cancer)
   3. Carcinoembryonic antigen (CEA) (e.g., gastrointestinal cancers)
   4. Prostate-specific antigen (PSA)
   5. Immunological detection of other tumor cell "markers" (e.g., enzymes and hormones)
   6. Detection of tumor-specific antigens (in the circulation or by immunoimaging)

B. Detection of anti-tumor immune response

   1. Anti-tumor antibodies
   2. Anti-tumor cell-mediated immunity

Immunologic Detection of Tumor Antigens

Tumor cells may express cytoplasmic, cell-surface, or secreted products that are different in nature and/or quantity from those produced by their normal counterparts. Because of the generally weak antigenicity of the tumor-specific markers, most such differences, either qualitative or quantitative, have been demonstrated by the use of antibodies produced in xenogeneic animals. In the past few years, the use of *monoclonal antibodies* has greatly enhanced the specificity of immunodiagnosis of tumor cells and their products. Some of the most widely used and reliable immunodiagnostic procedures for the detection of malignancies are described below.

DETECTION OF MYELOMA PROTEINS PRODUCED BY PLASMA CELL TUMORS. Abnormally high concentration in serum of monoclonal immunoglobulins of a certain isotype, or the presence of light chains of these immunoglobulins (*Bence–Jones proteins*) in the urine, is indicative of *plasma cell tumors*. The concentration of these *myeloma proteins* in the blood or urine is a reflection of the mass of the tumor. Consequently, the effectiveness and duration of therapy for this tumor may be monitored by measurement of the concentration of myeloma proteins in the serum and urine.

DETECTION OF α-FETOPROTEIN. α-Fetoprotein (AFP) is a major protein in fetal serum. After birth, the level of AFP falls to approximately 20 ng/ml. Levels of AFP are elevated in patients with *liver cancer*, but they are also elevated in noncancerous hepatic disorders such as cirrhosis and hepatitis. Nevertheless, concentrations of AFP of 500–1000 ng/ml are generally indicative of the presence of a tumor that is producing AFP, and monitoring AFP levels is indicative of regression or progression of the tumor.

CARCINOEMBRYONIC ANTIGEN. Carcinoembryonic antigen (CEA) is a term applied to a glycoprotein produced normally by cells that line the gastrointestinal tract, in particular the colon. If the cells become malignant, their polarity may change, so that CEA is released into the blood instead of the colon. Concentrations in the blood of CEA exceeding 2.5 ng/ml are generally indicative of malignancy, and monitoring CEA levels is helpful in monitoring tumor growth or regression. Here again, however, higher than normal levels of CEA in blood may be due to noncancerous diseases, such as cirrhosis of the liver or inflammatory diseases of the intestinal tract and lung.

DETECTION OF PROSTATE-SPECIFIC ANTIGEN. Prostate-specific antigen (PSA) is currently widely used for screening and early detection of prostate cancer. Levels above 8–10 ng/ml blood are suggestive of prostate cancer. Confirmatory tests are required since prostatitis and benign prostate hypertrophy also may result in the release into the bloodstream of the prostate-specific antigen derived from glandular prostate epithelium. The test is especially useful for monitoring significant increases or decrease of blood levels of PSA that correlate with increase or decrease of tumor size.

There are other "markers" associated with malignancies, such as enzymes and hormones, that can be detected by immunologic methods. Qualitative as well as quantitative determinations of all tumor markers are useful in monitoring the extent of malignancy and the effect of therapy on it.

The immunologic detection of tumors has recently been vastly improved by the availability of highly specific, antitumor monoclonal antibodies. Monoclonal antibodies are currently gaining use not only in the detection of antigens and products associated with the presence of tumor cells but also for their efficacy in the localization and *imaging* of tumors. Injection of *radiolabeled* tumor-specific antibodies (radioimmunoconjugates) into the tumor-bearing individual permits *visualization* by computer-assisted tomography (CAT) of the radiolabeled antibodies attached to the tumor. This method allows the detection of small metastases as well as the primary tumor mass.

Assessment of the Host's Immune Response to Tumor

It has been demonstrated in experimental animals and in humans that individuals with certain tumors have cell-mediated immunity and/or antibodies directed against tumor antigens. For example, antibodies to *Epstein–Barr virus (EBV)* have been demonstrated in patients with Burkitt's lymphoma, and antibodies reacting with melanoma-specific or sarcoma-specific antigens have been detected in patients with the respective malignancies. Thus, in cases of cross-reacting tumors, the assessment of an immune response against tumor antigens may be potentially useful.

To date, with a few exceptions, immunodiagnosis of cancer still does not constitute a reliably accurate method of choice for the early detection of malignancy. It is, however, proving useful clinically in monitoring the progression (or regression) and imaging of certain tumors.

TUMOR IMMUNOPROPHYLAXIS

Immunization against an oncogenic virus would be expected to provide prophylaxis *against the virus* and, hence, against the subsequent induction of tumor by the virus. Indeed, this approach has been successful in the protection of chickens against *Marek's disease*, and a significant degree of protection against *feline leukemia* and *feline sarcoma* has been achieved by immunizing cats with the respective oncogenic viruses. Immunization *against the tumor* itself requires that the tumor possess specific antigens and that these antigens cross-react immuno-logically with any prepared vaccine. There are literally thousands of reports of effective immunization against transplantable animal tumors, using as immunogens (1) sublethal doses of live tumor cells, (2) tumor cells in which replication has been blocked, (3) tumor cells with enzymatically or chemically modified surface membranes, and (4) extracts of antigens from the surface of tumor cells, either unmodified or chemically modified. In spite of these reported successes in the protection of experimental animals against transplantable tumors, the efficacy of immunoprophylaxis for protection of humans and animals against spontaneous tumors has not been sufficiently evaluated. This lack of complete study relates to the need for appropriate immunogens and the danger of inducing the production of immunological elements, such as the blocking factor or factors that enhance metastasis, that may be detrimental to the host.

IMMUNOTHERAPY OF TUMORS

Numerous attempts have been made in the past 30 years to treat cancers in animals and humans by immunologic means. Although some reports of successful immunotherapy in experimental animals, and of seemingly successful immunotherapy of human cancers, are sparsely scattered in the literature, to date cancer immunotherapy has not been proved to be an effective treatment of cancer, either when used as the sole treatment or as an adjunct to other forms of therapy such as chemotherapy, radiotherapy, or surgery.

Vaccination and Adjuvant Therapy

Attempts at immunotherapy of animal and human malignancy were aimed at the augmentation of specific anticancer immunity, utilizing various preparations of tumor antigens. Also, the nonspecific enhancement of the immune response, particularly of macrophages, using BCG (bacille Calmette-Guérin) or *Corynebacterium parvum* was attempted. Very recently interest is growing for the possibility of cancer vaccines directed against specific epitopes present on cancer antigens.

Cytokine Therapy

Trials are also in progress on the effects of various cytokines, such as ***interferon α, β, and γ, IL-1, IL-2, IL-4, IL-5, IL-12, tumor necrosis factor (TNF)***, and others either singly or in combination on tumor regression. To date, these trials are mostly inconclusive. A recent development is the use of *lymphokine-activated killer (LAK) cells*. As we have seen in Chapter 11, lymphokines are cytokines produced by lymphocytes. As mentioned earlier, LAK cells are produced in vitro by cultivation of the patient's own peripheral lymphocytes with interleukin-2 (IL-2). Upon reinfusion into the patient, dramatic improvement has been recorded in a number of cases.

A variation of this approach is the use of *tumor-infiltrating lymphocytes (TILs)*. These lymphocytes, removed from biopsied tumor, expanded in vitro, with IL-2 and given back to the tumor bearing individual have an anti-tumor activity many times higher than LAK, thus less is needed for therapy.

Anti-idiotype Antibody Therapy

An interesting approach for immunotherapy of B-cell lymphoma was to administer monoclonal anti-idiotypic antibodies directed against the idiotype of the surface immunoglobulin. Dramatic regressions have recently been reported in several lymphoma patients. More recently some patients were actively immunized with preparations containing their own individual idiotype. The patients developed idiotype-specific cellular and/or humoral immune responses with long lasting regressions in several patients.

Immunotoxin Therapy

With the advent of monoclonal antibodies, trials of cancer immunotherapy are under way in which toxins, such as ricin, or radioactive isotopes attached to tumor-specific antibodies are delivered specifically to the tumor cells for direct killing. The extent to which these "*immunotoxins*" will prove effective in the treatment of cancer remains to be established.

SUMMARY

1. Tumor immunology deals with (a) the immunological aspects of the host–tumor relationship and (b) the utilization of the immune response for diagnosis, prophylaxis, and treatment of cancer.

2. Tumor antigens of chemically or physically induced tumors do not

cross-react immunologically. On the other hand, extensive cross-reactivity is exhibited with virally induced tumor antigens; antigens of some spontaneous tumors show cross-reactivity while others do not. Several types of tumors produce oncofetal substances, which are normally present during embryonic development.

3. The immune response to tumors involves both humoral and cellular immune responses. Destruction of tumor cells may be achieved by (a) antibodies and complement; (b) phagocytes; (c) loss of the adhesive properties of tumor cells caused by antibodies; (d) cytotoxic T lymphocytes; (e) antibody-dependent, cell-mediated cytotoxicity (ADCC); and (f) activated macrophages, NK cells, and LAK cells.

4. The role of the immune response to tumors appears to be important in the host–tumor relationship, as indicated by increased incidence of tumors in immunosuppressed hosts and by the presence of immune components at sites of tumor regression. However, the immune response to a tumor may not be effective in eliminating the tumor because of a variety of possible mechanisms, which include enhancing and blocking factors, rapid growth of tumor, and large tumor mass.

5. Immunodiagnosis may be directed toward the detection of tumor antigens or the host's immune response to the tumor.

6. Immunoprophylaxis may be directed against oncogenic viruses or against the tumor itself.

7. Immunotherapy of malignancy employs various preparations for the augmentation of tumor-specific as well as nonspecific immune responses. "Immunotoxins" made with monoclonal antibodies are currently being tested. To date, in most cases, immunotherapy of cancer has proved to be marginal.

REFERENCES

Epenetos AA, Spooner RA, George AJT (1994): Application of monoclonal antibodies in clinical oncology. Immunol Today 15:559.

Goldenberg DM, Schlom J (1993): The coming of age of cancer radioimmunoconjugates. Immunol Today 14:5.

Herberman RB (ed) (1983): Basic and Clinical Tumor Immunology. Boston; Martinus Nijhoff.

Hellstrom KE, Hellstrom I (1989): Oncogene-associated tumor antigens as targets for immunotherapy. FASEB 3:1715.

Hsu FJ, Kwak L, Campbell M, Liles T, Czezwinski D, Hart S, Sysengelas A, Miller R, Levy R (1993): Clinical trials of idiotype specific vaccine in B-cell lymphomas. Ann NY Acad Sci 690:385.

Kuby J (1992): Immunology. New York: Freeman.

Langernecker BM, Maclean G (1993): Prospects for mucin epitopes on cancer vaccines. The Immunologist 1:89.

Lotze MT, Finn OJ (1990): Recent advances in cellular immunology: implications for immunity to cancer. Immunol Today 11:190.

Mantovani A, Bottazzi B, Colatta F, Sozzani S, Ruco L (1992): The origin and function of tumor associated macrophages. Immunol Today 13:265.

Schreiber H (1993): Tumor immunology. In Paul WE (ed): Fundamental Immunology, 3rd ed. New York: Raven Press.

Vitteta ES, Thorpe PE, Uhr JW (1993): Immunotoxins: magic bullets or misguided missiles? Immunol Today 14:252.

REVIEW QUESTIONS

For each question, choose the ONE BEST answer or completion.

1. The appearance of many primary lymphoreticular tumors in humans has been correlated with
   A) hypergammaglobulinemia
   B) acquired hemolytic anemia
   C) BCG treatment
   D) resistance to antibiotics
   E) impairment of cell-mediated immunity

2. Tumor antigens have been shown to cross-react immunologically in cases of
   A) tumors induced by chemical carcinogens
   B) tumors induced by RNA viruses
   C) all tumors
   D) tumors induced by irradiation with ultraviolet light

   E) tumors induced by the same chemical carcinogen on two separate sites on the same individual

3. Blocking factors formed during tumor growth
   A) bind to T lymphocytes and induce lysis of tumor cells
   B) block the stimulation of tumor-specific B cells
   C) block cell growth of tumor cells in vitro
   D) block the action of cytotoxic T lymphocytes on tumor cells in vitro
   E) only A and C are correct
   F) only B and D are correct

4. Rejection of a tumor may involve which of the following?
   A) T cell-mediated cytotoxicity
   B) ADCC

C) complement-dependent cytotoxicity
D) destruction of tumor cells by phagocytic cells
E) only A and C are correct
F) only B and D are correct
G) all are correct

5. Tumor progression is favored by
   A) cytotoxic T lymphocytes
   B) suppressor T lymphocytes
   C) presence of interferon
   D) presence of "blocking" factors
   E) only A and C are correct
   F) only B and D are correct
   G) all are correct

6. Immunotoxins are
   A) toxic substances released by macrophages
   B) lymphokines
   C) toxins completed with the corresponding antitoxins
   D) toxins coupled to antigen-specific immunoglobulins
   E) toxins released by cytotoxic T cells

7. It has been shown recently that a B-cell lymphoma could be eliminated with anti-idiotypic serum. The use of this approach to treat a plasma cell tumor would not be warranted because
   A) plasma cell tumors have no tumor-specific antigens
   B) plasma cell tumors are not expected to be susceptible to ADCC
   C) plasma cell tumors can be killed, in vivo, only by cytotoxic T lymphocytes which bear the same A, B, and C transplantation antigens
   D) the plasma cells do not have surface Ig
   E) the idiotype on the plasma-cell surface is different from that on the B-cell surface

8. B-cell lymphomas in mice, when experimentally treated with anti-idiotype sera, show regression. However, they frequently recur and now show no reactivity with the same anti-idiotype sera. Likely explanation(s) for this change could be
   A) a change in idiotype expressed by the B-lymphoma cells
   B) production of anticomplementary substances by the lymphoma cells
   C) a loss of surface Ig receptor on the B-lymphoma cells
   D) production of Ig splitting enzymes by the lymphoma cells
   E) only A and C are correct
   F) only B and D are correct

ANSWERS TO REVIEW QUESTIONS

1. *E* There is a nearly 100-fold increase in the incidence of lymphoproliferative tumors in individuals with impaired immunity, in particular with impaired cell-mediated immunity. Hypergammaglobulin-emia, acquired hemolytic anemia, or resistance to antibiotics are not correlated with increases in lymphoproliferative tumors; neither is BCG treatment, which in some instances has even been shown to

influence favorably the course of some leukemias.

2. **B** Immunologic cross-reactivity has been demonstrated only in cases of virally induced tumors (caused by either RNA or DNA viruses). Tumors induced by chemical or physical carcinogens do not exhibit cross-reactivity, even if induced by the same carcinogen on separate sites on the same individual.

3. **D** Blocking factors, formed during tumor growth, may consist of free circulating antigen, circulating anti-tumor antibodies, or antigen–antibody complexes. Blocking by tumor antigens is achieved through the binding of these antigens with tumor-specific T lymphocytes, thereby preventing the binding of the lymphocytes to antigens on the tumor cells. Tumor-specific antibodies may combine with tumor antigens on the tumor cells, thereby blocking the binding of cytotoxic T lymphocytes to these cells. Similar types of blocking can be achieved by circulating antigen–antibody complexes. The blocking factors do not perform any of the functions listed in options *A, B*, and *C*.

4. **G** All are correct. Destruction of tumor cells may be mediated by T-cell-mediated cytotoxicity, by antibody-dependent cell-mediated cytotoxicity (ADCC), by complement-mediated cytotoxicity, and by phagocytic cells, which are attracted to the tumor by T-cell lymphokines and/or complement components, and which become activated by the lymphokines or

perform enhanced phagocytosis as a result of the present of opsonins on the target cells.

5. **F** Tumor growth may be enhanced by suppressor T cells, which suppress the immune response to the tumor. Growth can also be enhanced by blocking factors, such as circulating tumor antigens, anti-tumor antibodies, or antigen–antibody complexes, all of which may compete with effector elements, such as cytotoxic T lymphocytes, for the tumor antigen on the tumor cell. The presence of interferon will not prevent the effector elements from destroying the tumor cell.

6. **D** Immunotoxins consist of toxic substances (or radioactive atoms) conjugated to immunoglobulin molecules specific for tumor cells or other target cells.

7. **D** The only relevant statement is that plasma cells do not have surface immunoglobulins and would therefore not be susceptible to treatment with anti-idiotypic antibodies. Plasma cell tumors do have tumor-specific antigens and would be susceptible to ADCC with antibodies to these antigens. Statement *C* is wrong and totally irrelevant.

8. **E** Treatment of tumors with antibody to surface antigens may induce antigenic modulation, causing them to lose these antigens (*C*). In addition, a variant with a changed surface phenotype may take over when the major cell type is killed off (*A*).

IMMUNOPROPHYLAXIS AND IMMUNOTHERAPY*

INTRODUCTION

Protection against infectious diseases by ***immunoprophylaxis*** (immunization) represents an immense, if not the greatest, accomplishment of biomedical science. One disease, smallpox, has been totally eliminated by the use of immunization, and the incidence of other diseases has been significantly reduced, at least in areas of the world where immunization can be practiced correctly.

If a large enough number of individuals can be immunized, "herd immunity" is achieved and the transmission of communicable diseases between persons is interrupted. Although deliberate immunization alone can sometimes reduce the incidence of a disease to a very low level, successful immunization programs require the intelligent practice of other measures, both hygienic and sanitary, which contribute to general improvements in public health.

Immunity results from either ***active*** or ***passive*** immunization. Active and passive immunizations are exemplified in Table 22.1.

In the present chapter we will discuss various aspects of conferring immunity to prevent infection (***immunoprophylaxis***) and to fight an on going infection

---

*Contributed by Demosthenes Pappagianis, University of California, Davis.

TABLE 22.1   Examples of Active and Passive Immunization

Type of immunity	How acquired
Active	
Natural (unintended)	Infection
Artificial (deliberate)	Vaccination
Passive[a]	
Natural	Transplacental or colostral transfer of antibody, mother to infant
Artificial	Administration of immune human globulin

[a]Passive immunity is generally of shorter duration than active immunity.

(***immunotherapy***). Included in this chapter are specific immunization procedures practiced in present-day medicine.

OBJECTIVES OF IMMUNIZATION

Protection generated prior to possible exposure to an infectious agent is the objective in the usual active immunizations in childhood. Protection through passive immunization is the objective achieved by injections of immune globulin to protect a traveler against hepatitis A virus (HAV) in countries where that disease is common. Protection against development of disease can also be afforded by post-exposure immunization, for example, by administration of rabies vaccine and immune globulin against rabies virus, toxoid and antitoxin against diphtheria and tetanus toxins, and immune serum globulins against HAV and hepatitis B virus (HBV). Great effort is being put into therapeutic vaccines that would hopefully forestall the relentless progression of AIDS.

The potential for use of vaccines to prevent certain cancers in humans is discussed in Chapter 21. For example, the association between primary carcinoma of the liver and infection by hepatitis B virus (HBV) is strong enough to suggest that use of the inactivated or recombinant HBV vaccine in high-risk groups may provide protection against development of hepatoma, as well as hepatitis due to this virus.

HISTORICAL ASPECTS OF IMMUNIZATION

Protective active immunity (immunoprophylaxis) may result from natural, unintended, or deliberate exposure to infectious agents or their components. This was evident to the ancients of Asia, who intentionally exposed people to the scabs and fluid from the lesions of smallpox, a disease known in the Western world as "variola major." The practice, termed *variolation*, was introduced into England and its American colonies in 1721.

Successful protection against smallpox was dependent on the presence of viral antigens in the lesions. The crudeness of the preparation assured the presence not only of inactive virus, but also of active (and virulent) virus in sufficient concentration to produce smallpox, so that some unfortunate individuals died of the disease. As a result, the practice was soon discontinued in the West.

Later in the eighteenth century it was noted that milkmaids who were exposed to cowpox (vaccinia), a disease of cattle, appeared to escape infection with smallpox. It was then that Jenner, an English physician, showed that deliberate administration to humans of lymph from a cow with vaccinia led to protection against smallpox. It is evident from this cross-protection by vaccinia that the viruses of smallpox and cowpox share an antigen(s). (The vaccinia virus used in modern times is known to differ genetically from the cowpox virus.)

Approximately a century later (1879) Roux, working in Pasteur's laboratory, demonstrated that bacteria that caused chicken cholera or anthrax could be weakened *(attenuated)* by certain cultivation practices in the laboratory, so that they could no longer cause disease but still retained enough antigenicity to induce immunity. Pasteur and his collaborators also showed that storage in the laboratory of tissue infected with rabies virus yielded an agent that was markedly less virulent than the parent rabies virus, but still antigenic. Pasteur termed these protective antigens "*vaccines*" in commemoration of Jenner's work on the use of vaccinia to protect against smallpox.

Toward the end of the nineteenth century, it was discovered that certain bacteria cause disease (diphtheria, tetanus) through their release of potent exotoxins. Fortuitously, it was demonstrated that treatment of these (protein) *exotoxins* with formaldehyde and other chemicals eliminated their toxicity but left their antigenic properties unaffected. Formaldehyde appears to effect this change by providing methylol derivatives at the amino groups. These modified toxins, or "*toxoids*" (see Chapter 3), have been the mainstays of immunization for many decades.

Successful cultivation of viruses in the laboratory, separate from the intact mammal, was not achieved until the 1930s, when tissue-culture techniques permitted replication and attenuation of the yellow fever virus so that it could be used for a vaccine. The most significant advance, however, followed the discovery, in 1949 by Enders, Weller, and Robbins (all Nobel laureates), that poliomyelitis virus could be grown in vitro in human embryonic cells or monkey kidney cells. Recovery of sufficient quantities of virions permitted preparation of inactivated (noninfective) polio vaccine and, later, modified, attenuated viral vaccines. "Subunit" vaccines, which contain particular fractions of viruses (or bacteria), have been introduced more recently. Moreover, recent advances in vaccine technology discussed later in this chapter will, undoubtedly, result in effective vaccines against many infectious diseases afflicting mankind and domestic animals.

ACTIVE IMMUNIZATION

Recommended Immunizations

The present, customary, active immunizations are indicated below (additional specific examples will be cited later).

The usual recommended schedule in the United States for active immunization at various ages is shown in Table 22.2. The schedule in the United Kingdom is similar for children, except that the age at which vaccines are administered may be slightly different, and BCG (bacille Calmette-Guérin, attenuated *Mycobacterium bovis*) vaccine is recommended for the 10–14-year-old age group.

In other parts of the world, the immunization schedule may be different. The World Health Organization, for example, recommends administration of BCG and oral polio vaccines at the time of birth, and measles vaccine as soon as possible after the ninth month of age (see section on age and immunization below).

SELECTIVE APPLICATION. In addition to the usual schedule of immunizations shown in Table 22.2, some individuals receive additional vaccinations as follows (see also Table 22.4).

Viral. *Influenza virus* (inactivated) is given to persons over 60 years of age and to those with cardiorespiratory ailments. *Hepatitis B* (inactivated virus or viral proteins produced by recombinant DNA technology) is given to medical personnel who are exposed to human blood. *Hepatitis A* (inactivated virus) has been approved for use in children and adults. *Varicella* (attenuated) is given to patients with acute lymphocytic leukemia and has recently been approved for broader use in healthy individuals. (Vaccination against smallpox, no longer recommended for civilians, is still given to selected military personnel.)

Bacterial. A polyvalent vaccine consisting of several antigenic types of capsular polysaccharides from *Streptococcus pneumoniae* is given to individuals

TABLE 22.2 Recommended Usual Schedule for Active Immunization

Age	Vaccine
Birth	Hepatitis B (HBV) vaccine
1–2 months	HBV vaccine
2 months	Diphtheria, tetanus, pertussis (DTP-1),[a] trivalent oral polio (TOP-1),[b] HbCV[c]
4 months	DTP-2, TOP-2, HbCV
6 months	DTP-3, HbCV
	TOP-3 (optimal in certain areas of high risk)
15 months	Measles, mumps, rubella (MMR),[d] DTP-4, TOP-3
4–6 years	DTP-5, TOP-5
14–16 years (and each 10 years thereafter)	Td (tetanus, reduced adult dose of diphtheria toxoid)
18–24 years	Measles, mumps,[e] rubella
25–64 years	Measles,[e] rubella[f]
> 65 years	Influenza, pneumococcal disease

[a]DTP is administered with alum adjuvant (see Chapter 3). DTP includes acellular fractions of *Bordetella pertussis.*
[b]DTP and TOP can be initiated as early as 4 weeks after birth in areas of endemicity.
[c]*Haemophilus influenzae* type b polysaccharide conjugated to protein.
[d]MMR should be given upon entry to middle or junior high school.
[e]Especially for susceptible males.
[f]Mainly for females up to 45 years of age.
For specific details see Morbidity and Mortality Weekly Report, 1994 (Jan), 43:No. RR-1.

with cardiorespiratory ailments, to anatomically or functionally asplenic individuals, and to patients with sickle-cell anemia, renal failure, alcoholic cirrhosis, or diabetes mellitus. These individuals have limited capability to mount the antibody/complement/phagocytic activity required against the encapsulated *S. pneumoniae. Haemophilus influenzae* (type b capsular polysaccharide) is recommended for 18-month-old children and for anatomically or functionally asplenic individuals. An *H. influenzae* type b polysaccharide–diphtheria toxoid conjugate is now available for use in younger children (first dose at 2 months of age). *Neisseria meningitidis* vaccine (several serogroups of capsular polysaccharide) is given to military recruits and to children in high-risk regions. Both live, attenuated *Salmonella typhi,* and inactivated vaccines are available against typhoid fever. Because of some unique needs or limited efficacy, some vaccines are recommended only under limited circumstances. These vaccines and appropriate circumstances are described in Table 22.3.

TABLE 22.3   **Vaccines Recommended Under Limited Circumstances**

Occupational or other exposure	Vaccine
Health care personnel	Hepatitis B
Health-care personnel in close contact with tuberculosis patients	BCG
Veterinarians,[a] animal handlers,[a] and victims of certain animal bites	Rabies
Handlers of imported animal hides, furs, bonemeal, wool, and animal bristles	Anthrax
Military personnel	Meningococcus, yellow fever
Homosexual males, intravenous drug users	Hepatitis B
Travel to certain areas	Meningococcus, yellow fever, cholera,[b] typhoid fever,[b] plague, Japanese B encephalitis, polio

[a]In some parts of the world (e.g., USSR) attenuated *Brucella* vaccine has been administered to humans.
[b]The duration and efficacy of these is limited.
For a tabulation of available vaccines, see table 21.7.

BASIC MECHANISMS OF PROTECTION

Anatomic Location of Host Immune Response

There are differences in the intravascular-extravascular distribution of immunoglobulins (see Table 5.1). For example, local synthesis of secretory IgA in the lamina propria, beneath a mucous membrane, yields antibody at the epithelial surface (respiratory or intestinal), an area through which certain pathogens or their toxins may enter. IgA is the predominant Ig in secretions of the nasal, bronchial, intestinal, and genitourinary tracts, and in saliva, colostrum, and bile. *Oral administration* of attenuated (Sabin) polio vaccine leads to demonstrable antipolio IgA in nasal and duodenal secretions, whereas *parenteral injection* of inactivated (Salk) polio vaccine does not. The local antibodies generated by the Sabin vaccine provide the advantage of intercepting of the polio virus at the portal of entry. However, some IgG and IgM may be found in local secretions, so that serum Ig may also play a role at an epithelial surface (while IgM appears to have restricted access to extravascular areas, both IgG and IgM can be found in inflammatory exudates). In addition, the hematogenous (viremic or bacteremic) stage of several infections that are acquired through a mucous membrane can lead to an encounter between infectious agent and antibody in the circulating as well as the extravascular fluid. Thus, the Salk vaccine given parenterally induces immunity to polio virus during its viremic stage.

There are some unique, but still poorly understood, differences in the partitioning of immunoglobulins in serum and secretions. For example, while IgG$_4$ represents only 3.5% of the plasma IgG, it constitutes 15% of IgG in colostrum. In the cerebrospinal fluid, IgG and IgM may be found as a result of local production in the central nervous system due to the stimulus by infectious agents.

Significance of the Primary and Secondary Responses

The rapidity of the *anamnestic response* to a reencounter with antigen provides the host with potential protection upon repeated exposures to an infectious agent. This anamnestic response is relevant in at least two significant ways in the application of immunoprophylaxis. First, it may be of particular importance in those infections with a relatively long incubation period (>7 days), as is illustrated in Figure 22.1. Thus, an individual infected by agent B, which causes disease after a 3-day incubation period, would produce a *primary* immune response some time (e.g., 7–14 days) after onset of the infection. On a second encounter with agent B,

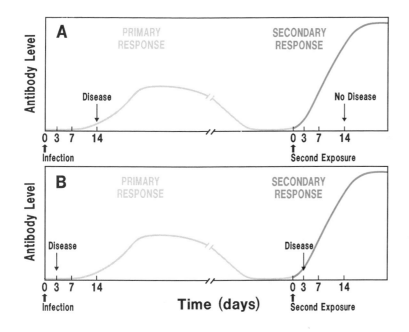

Figure 22.1.

The relationship between the primary and secondary immune responses and disease produced by infection with agent **A** or **B.** [After Macleod CM (1953): J Immunol 70:421.]

the individual may again develop disease, because an anamnestic response may not be sufficiently rapid to inhibit agent B (Fig. 22.1B). The individual infected with agent A, which causes disease after a 14-day incubation period, would produce a primary response (e.g., some 7–14 days after infection). On a second encounter with agent A, the anamnestic response occurring within 7 days would be sufficient to reduce the severity or prevent the disease with the 14-day incubation period (Fig. 22.1A).

The second influence of the anamnestic response concerns the *level* to which the immune response has been raised. In the example cited above, agent B, which causes disease in 3 days, may be prevented from causing disease after a reexposure if there is a persisting high enough level of antibody. Such a level can be achieved deliberately by a series of immunizations (especially applicable with nonviable antigens). Thus, it is customary to give several injections of tetanus toxoid (as DTP) over a period of 6 months in childhood immunizations. Such a "primary series" of injections generates anamnestic secondary responses that successively raise the concentration of antitoxin to protective levels, which are sustained in the serum for 10–20 years.

Protective Effect of the Immune Response

Acquired immune responses may exert their effects essentially independently of certain innate defense mechanisms, for example, neutralization of bacterial exotoxin by antitoxic antibody. Alternatively, these acquired responses may function in concert with other components of the host defense apparatus, for example, when antibody functions to opsonize infectious particles, or when antibody interacts with complement and an infectious agent leading to lysis of the agent.

ANTITOXIC IMMUNITY. Antitoxic immunity is predominantly associated with *IgG*, although IgA may also neutralize exotoxins such as cholera enterotoxin. Because the exotoxins bind firmly to their target tissue, they generally cannot be displaced by subsequent administration of antitoxin. Hence, in those diseases mediated by exotoxins (e.g., diphtheria) prompt administration of antitoxin is necessary to prevent attachment of (additional) exotoxin and the damage caused by the exotoxin. This can be illustrated by the effectiveness of antitoxin given at varying times as protection against the lethal effects of diphtheria toxin in humans (Table 22.4).

Exotoxic enzymes, such as the lecithinase of the bacterium *Clostridium perfringens* or of snake venom, may be neutralized by antibody. However, the enzy-

TABLE 22.4   Protection of Humans by Diphtheria Antitoxin Given on Indicated Day of Disease

Day	Number of cases	Fatality rate (%)
1	225	0
2	1,441	4.2
3	1,600	11.1
4	1,276	17.3
5 (or later)	1,645	18.7

From Pappenheimer AM Jr (1965): The diphtheria bacilli and the diphtheroid [sic]. In Dubos RJ, Hirsch JG (eds): Bacterial and Mycotic Infections of Man, 4th Ed. Philadelphia: Lippincott.

matically active sites of some enzymes may not be inhibited by enzyme-specific antibody.

The presence of antitoxic activity in IgG means that an adequately immunized mother can transmit antitoxin to her fetus and thus afford protection to the infant in its first days or weeks after birth. This protection is extremely important in areas of the world where an unclean obstetric environment can lead to ***tetanus neonatorum*** (of the newborn).

ANTIVIRAL IMMUNITY. The antiviral response can be complex, with several factors involved, such as the route of entry, site of attachment, and other aspects of pathogenesis by the infecting virus; induction of interferon; antibody response; and cell-mediated immunity. Thus, intracellular infection of the epithelium of the respiratory tract by influenza virus leads to production of virus in epithelial cells and spread of the virus to adjacent epithelial cells. An appropriate and sufficient immune response would involve action of antibody at the epithelial surface. This action might be effected through locally secreted *IgA*, or local extravasation of *IgG* or *IgM*. On the other hand, some viral diseases, such as measles or poliomyelitis, begin by infection at a mucosal epithelium (respiratory or intestinal, respectively) but exhibit their major pathogenic effects after being spread hematogenously to other target tissues. Antibody at the epithelial surface could protect against the virus, but circulating antibody could do likewise.

Interferons are antiviral proteins or glycoproteins produced by several different types of cell in the mammalian host in response to viral infection (or other inducers such as double-stranded RNA). Interferons appear before detectable activated macrophages or antibody and serve as an early protective device. The antibody response to viruses can be demonstrated, ***in vitro***, to involve Igs that (1) *neutralize* (impede) infectivity of viruses for susceptible host cells, (2) *fix complement*, and (3) *inhibit adherence to and agglutination of erythrocytes* by some viruses (hemagglutination inhibition). IgG appears to be the most significant of the antiviral antibodies, but once a virus has attached to a host cell, it is not displaced by antibody.

The effects of *antiviral Ig in vivo* include (1) *neutralization*; (2) *complement-mediated lysis of infected host cells*, which carry viral antigen on the cell membrane; (3) *inhibition of critical viral enzymes* (e.g., neuraminidase of influenza virus); and (4) *opsonization*. Opsonization represents a convergence of humoral and cellular immune mechanisms. IgG, which has combined, through its Fab portion, with viral antigens on the surface of infected host cells, links also to Fc receptors on macrophages, polymorphonuclear cells (PMNs), or killer (K) cells. These cells then can phagocytose and/or damage the virus-infected cell—a phenomenon termed *antibody-dependent cell-mediated cytotoxicity (ADCC)* (see Chapter 5).

Cell-mediated immune responses usually precede the antibody-mediated mechanisms. T cells interacting with virus may produce lymphokines (e.g., IFN-γ), causing accumulation of macrophages, which then inhibit the formation of intercellular bridges and, thus, the intercellular transfer of viruses. In addition, such macrophages can phagocytose antibody-coated viruses (the phagocytosis may not lead to destruction of the virus, but rather serve as means of disseminating the virus, as happens in the case of measles virus, and the T-cell lymphotrophic human immunodeficiency virus [HIV] associated with acquired immune deficiency syndrome [AIDS]). *Cytotoxic cells* may act directly against viral antigen associated with class I molecules of the MHC on the surface of host cells.

ANTIBACTERIAL IMMUNITY. Antibacterial immune responses include *lysis*, via antibody and complement, *opsonization*, and *phagocytosis*, with elimination of phagocytosed bacteria by the liver, spleen, and other components of the reticuloendothelial system.

Opsonization and phagocytosis, especially of gram-positive bacteria, involves the action of *IgG* and *IgM* alone or in concert with *C3b*, which promotes phagocytosis of bacteria by PMN. The *alternative complement pathway* may be triggered nonspecifically by the lipopolysaccharide endotoxin found in the walls of gram-negative bacteria, or by the polysaccharide capsule of gram-negative and gram-positive bacteria acting on C3. This alternative pathway leads to formation of the chemotactic molecules C3a and C5a and the opsonin C3b. In addition, the activation of the alternative pathway may result in *immune adherence* and bacteriolytic action of C5–C9. Because the opsonized and phagocytosed bacteria are cleared by the spleen, anatomically or functionally asplenic patients are particularly vulnerable to encapsulated bacteria, even though the alternative complement pathway may be activated by the bacteria. The classical lytic complement pathway operates in conjunction with IgM against gram-negative bacteria.

Cell-mediated immunity is also active against certain bacteria, characterized by their intracellular habitat, e.g., *Mycobacterium tuberculosis.*

ANTIFUNGAL, ANTIPROTOZOAL, AND ANTIHELMINTHIC IMMUNITY. Immune responses to fungi, protozoa, and helminths involve humoral and/or cellular immunity, as is the case for immunity to viruses and bacteria. There are also, however, unique aspects of the response to these organisms dependent on the various stages of their life cycles.

AGE AND TIMING OF IMMUNIZATIONS

The various mechanisms involved in protection, described in the preceding section, can be affected by several factors, including nutritional status, presence of underlying disease (which affects levels of globulin or cell-mediated immunity), and age.

In utero, the human fetus normally appears well insulated from antigens and most infectious agents, although certain pathogens (e.g., rubella virus) can infect the mother and seriously injure the fetus. The immunity of the mother protects the fetus by permitting interception and removal of infectious agents before they can enter the uterus, or it protects the newborn by virtue of transplacental or mammary gland antibody.

The fetus and neonate have poorly developed lymphoid organs, with the exception of the thymus, which at the time of birth is largest in size relative to the body size at any age. The fetus appears capable of synthesizing mainly IgM, which becomes apparent after 6 months of gestation. Levels of IgM gradually increase to about 10% of the adult level at the time of birth.

IgG becomes detectable in the fetus at about the second month of gestation, but it is IgG of maternal origin. The level of IgG increases significantly at about 4 months of gestation and markedly in the last trimester. At the time of birth the concentration of IgG slightly exceeds the maternal concentration of IgG. Thus, the fetus is provided with maternally synthesized IgG antibodies, which can provide antitoxic, antiviral, and some kinds of antibacterial protection. The levels of these maternal antibodies gradually decline as the infant begins to synthesize its own antibodies, so that total IgG at 2–3 months of age is less than 50% of the lev-

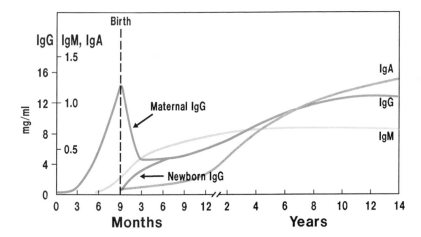

Figure 22.2.
Concentration of immunoglubulin in the serum during human development. [After Bennich H, Johanssen SGO (1971): Adv Immunol 13:1.]

el at birth. The serum concentrations of immunoglobulins during human development are shown in Figure 22.2.

Some aspects of the immune response of the newborn, for example, against some infectious agents (Toxoplasma, Listeria, herpes simplex virus) in which cell-mediated immunity is critical, are not well developed. But the newborn can produce antibody to various antigens, such as parenterally administered toxoid, inactivated poliomyelitis virus, orally administered attenuated poliomyelitis virus, and others. However, administration of pertussis vaccine (whole, killed bacteria) very soon after birth not only fails to induce a protective response but also creates an impaired response (tolerance?) to the vaccine when it is given again later in infancy. Therefore, in most industrialized countries initial administration of vaccines are deferred until the child is 2 months old. However, the WHO provides for earlier commencement of immunization (at 6 weeks) in developing countries.

Maternal antibody, while capable of providing protection to the neonate against a variety of infectious agents or their toxins, may also reduce the response to antigen. For example, a sufficient quantity of maternal measles antibody persists in the 1-year-old infant to interfere with the active response of the infant to the vaccine, so that vaccination in the United States against measles has for some time been carried out at 15 months of age rather than at 12 months.

Children less than 2 years of age have a general inability to produce adequate levels of antibody in response to injection of bacterial capsular polysaccharides, such as those of *Haemophilus influenzae* type b, various serogroups of *Neisseria meningitidis*, and *Streptococcus pneumoniae* serotypes. It has been suggested that this inability arises because infants do not respond to T-cell-independent antigens, despite their early (in utero) capacity to generate IgM. Chemical linkage of poly-saccharide to T-dependent antigens, such as diphtheria toxoid, or to *N. meningi-tidis* outer membrane protein, has improved the immunogenicity such that children under 2 years of age respond to polysaccharides.

At the other end of the age spectrum—in people older than 60 years of age—there also appears to be a reduced capability to mount a primary response to some antigens, such as influenza virus vaccine, but the elderly appear to retain the ability to mount a secondary response to antigens to which they have been previously exposed. The healthy elderly also respond well to bacterial polysaccharides, so that administration of pneumococcal polysaccharide vaccine can usually induce protective levels of antibody. Other groups, besides the elderly, who are especially susceptible to pneumococcal pneumonia (see section on active immunization selective application, following Table 22.2) should also be immunized. The same groups as those who have enhanced susceptibility to the encapsulated respiratory pathogen *Streptococcus pneumoniae* and to persons at high risk of exposure (e.g., residents of nursing homes and medical personnel) should receive influenza vaccines also.

USE OF MIXED, MULTIPLE ANTIGENS

Routine immunization against some infectious agents is simplified by their having a single antigenic type (e.g., the toxins of diphtheria and tetanus, polysaccharide of *Haemophilus influenzae* type b, and various viruses such as measles, mumps and rubella). However, immunization against other agents (e.g., poliovirus and pneumococci) must provide protection against several antigenic types. The host can be vaccinated simultaneously with several antigens and still generate adequate responses, although in some instances the generation of sufficient immunity requires repeated (booster) administration of antigen(s). The usual, initial immunization of children entails the injection of diphtheria and tetanus toxoids, whole killed cells of *Bordetella pertussis*, and the oral administration of attenuated polioviruses types 1, 2, and 3 (Sabin vaccine). The estimated 10^{12} lymphoid cells in the human body appear to be capable of responding to a huge array of antigens without significant competition. Although there is a possibility that a live viral vaccine may inhibit the immune response to a second live viral vaccine given a few days later, this interference does not appear to be of practical importance. Thus, it has been ascertained that simultaneous injection of **measles, mumps**, and **rubella** vaccines provides a protective response to all three of these viruses.

PRECAUTIONS

Site of Administration of Antigen

The usual site of *parenteral* (intradermal, subcutaneous, intramuscular) administration of vaccines is the arm, in particular the deltoid muscle. Studies have shown a suboptimal response to hepatitis B vaccine when given by intragluteal injection, as compared with injection in the arm. The parenteral administration of inactivated polio vaccine may induce a higher antibody response in the serum than the attenuated oral polio vaccine, but the response to the latter, which includes secretory IgA, affords adequate protection.

Some vaccines may provide a greater antibody response when given by the *respiratory* route than when given by injection (e.g., attenuated measles vaccine), but administration via the respiratory route has not yet supplanted parenteral administration.

Hazards

There are potential hazards associated with the use of some vaccines. Vaccines made from *attenuated* agents (e.g., measles, mumps, rubella, oral polio, bacille Calmette-Guérin) have the potential for causing *progressive disease* in the *immunocompromised* patient or in the patient on *steroid therapy*. In rare cases, reversion of attenuated poliovirus type III to virulence in the intestine of the vaccinated individual has caused paralytic polio; for this reason, some workers favor the *inactivated* polio vaccine, which is used exclusively in some countries.

The attenuated organisms should ordinarily not be given to pregnant women because of potential damage to the fetus. (The virions in rubella vaccine have been transmitted to the fetus, although without any recognized injurious effect.) Vaccination against smallpox is no longer carried out (except in some military personnel) since the disease has been eradicated; however, if vaccinia should be utilized in the future as a carrier for other antigens (discussed in a subsequent section), care must be taken because this virus can cause serious problems, not only in immunocompromised individuals but also in individuals with certain cutaneous lesions. Contact between vaccinated and vulnerable individuals must be avoided until the vaccinia lesions have healed.

Arthritis and arthralgia are common but transient complications following vaccination with attenuated rubella virus, particularly in adult women. Of the *inactivated* vaccines, the whole killed *Bordetella pertussis* bacterial vaccine in DTP has questionably been associated with serious side effects, such as encephalopathy in the infant. However, this has not been confirmed by recent evidence. The pertussis vaccine is recommended, since the complications of whooping cough outweigh any alleged risks of immunization. Obviously, pertussis vaccine should not be given to infants with a history of neurologic problems, such as convulsions. Tetanus and diphtheria toxoids may provoke local hypersensitivity reactions. Because an adequate initial series of immunizations in childhood appears to give immunity that lasts some 10 years, the use of "booster" injections of tetanus toxoid should be guided by the nature of an injury and the history of immunization. The increased hypersensitivity to diphtheria toxoid of adolescents and adults necessitates use of a smaller dose of diphtheria toxoid than is used for children. [Usually the diphtheria toxoid (D) is given with tetanus toxoid (T), the lower dose of diphtheria toxoid being indicated by a lowercase d, as in Td.] Increased incidence of neurologic complications (***Guillain–Barré syndrome***) followed use of the 1976 swine influenza vaccine, but they are not a significant problem with the influenza vaccines currently in use. Because the virus is cultivated in chick embryos, allergy to egg protein is a contraindication to vaccination against influenza. Whole influenza virus vaccine is used in adults but gives side effects in children, so a split-virus component vaccine is recommended for persons under 13 years of age. Some vaccines contain ***preservatives***, such as the organomercurial compound thimerosal (Merthiolate), or antibiotics, such as neomycin or streptomycin, to which the vaccinated individual may be allergic.

RECENT APPROACHES TO PRODUCTION OF VACCINES

Advances in ***recombinant DNA*** technology and in the technology of rapid, automated ***synthesis of peptides*** and other areas of bioengineering (e.g., monoclonal antibodies) hold promise for improvements in available vaccines and new approaches to the production of vaccines.

Vaccines Produced by Recombinant DNA

Production of vaccines against hepatitis B from yeast by recombinant DNA technology simplifies the production of greater quantities of a safer vaccine than the vaccine prepared from blood plasma of humans, although even the latter has not been associated with significant side effects. Indeed, hepatitis B vaccine produced by recombinant DNA is currently used for immunization of humans. Other vaccines produced by recombinant DNA technology are in various stages of clinical testing.

Conjugated Polysaccharides

Allusion has already been made to the poor response of young children to polysaccharide antigens. Conjugation of such (bacterial) polysaccharides or oligosaccharides (e.g., of *Haemophilus influenzae*), to protein such as diphtheria toxoid has provided vaccines that are effective in this age group.

Synthetic Peptide Vaccines

Because of their greater purity, synthetic peptide vaccines may afford protection that is associated with fewer side effects. The design of the synthetic peptide vaccine is based on knowledge of the amino acid sequence of the protein antigen. Analyses of potential epitopes are performed using various algorithms and a series of peptides is synthesized and tested for immunologic activity either conjugated to carriers or if unconjugated, depending on peptide size. (Conjugates usually consist of <15–20 amino acid residues.) In general small synthetic peptides require effective and safe carrier molecules. Several synthetic peptide vaccines are currently in clinical testing. A word of caution: if the vaccine consists of a peptide comprising an epitope recognized by B cells and a carrier recognized by T cells, no anamnestic (memory) response should be expected when the immunized individual encounters the B-cell epitope on a different carrier such as, for example, on the natural antigen from which the B-cell epitope has been taken (the carrier effect, described in Chapter 11).

Blocking of Specific Receptors

Specific receptors on host cells serve as the sites of attachment of some pathogens. Several vaccines that can block access to the receptors, such as by molecular mimicry of the ligand on the pathogen, are currently in clinical testing.

Anti-idiotype Vaccines

An antibody (idiotype) induced to a specific epitope of an antigen has a combining site that structurally fits the epitope. If that antibody, in turn, is used as an immunogen to induce an antibody (an anti-idiotype) that reacts with the antigen-combining site of the idiotype, the anti-idiotype may structurally mimic the epitope. This structural mimicry is referred to as an "internal image." Because of the resemblance of the anti-idiotype and the original antigen epitope, its internal image (anti-idiotypic antibody) can be used as an immunogen to induce antibodies against the original epitope (Fig. 22.3).

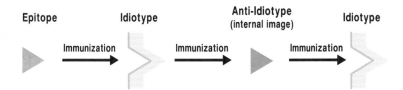

Figure 22.3.
A representation of an anti-idiotype (internal image) immunogen.

An example is an immunogen consisting of antibodies made in mice against a monoclonal mouse antibody to hepatitis B surface antigen. Immunization with these anti-idiotypic antibodies that contain the "internal image" of an epitope on the hepatitis B surface antigen induces antibodies to that epitope. When the toxic effects of certain biological toxins preclude their use as antigens, anti-idiotypic antibodies can be used to elicit an antitoxic response.

Virus-Carrier Vaccine

It has been possible to introduce into a live virus, such as vaccinia, adenovirus, or poliovirus by means of a vector, a gene from another organism that codes for a desired antigen. The vaccinia virus construct replicating in the host serves as a vaccine to that particular antigen. This approach is useful only provided that the vaccinia virus is not hazardous to the host (as it may be to an immunocompromised individual). This virus-carrier vaccine has the additional advantage in that it induces cell-mediated as well as antibody-mediated immunity to the incorporated antigen. Additional vaccines involving baculovirus, a virus that infects insect cells, has been used to produce components of the HIV virus in attempting to produce an experimental vaccine against HIV.

Bacterium-Carrier Vaccine

Analogous to virus carriers are attenuated bacteria such as strains of *Salmonella typhimurium, Escherichia coli*, and BCG into which foreign genes can be introduced. Introduction of these recombinant bacteria in a host can lead to their generating antigens, coded by the foreign genes, to which the host would become immunized. *S. typhimurium*, an intestinal pathogen, could be used to induce mucosal immunity to the foreign antigens.

It is also possible that introduction by transduction of DNA of the suspect infectious agent into cells of the mammalian host could permit synthesis of immunogenic antigens by the host cells.

Some of these molecular approaches may provide practical, safer and more effective means of immunization than are currently available. Indeed, dozens of vaccines produced by the approaches described above are being developed, some are already used in clinical trials on humans, and others are already used for immunization of humans (against hepatitis B) and of domestic animals.

PASSIVE IMMUNIZATION

Passive immunization results from the transfer of antibody or immune cells to one individual from another individual who has already responded to direct stimulation by antigen. It can be divided into ***natural*** and ***artificial*** passive immunity.

Natural Passive Immunity

MATERNAL IMMUNITY VIA THE PLACENTA. The presence of maternal antibody confers passive protection to the fetus, which is effective in those circumstances when ***IgG*** suffices, for example, as an antitoxic and antiviral antibody or as an antibacterial antibody, such as against *Haemophilus influenzae* (type b) or *Streptococcus agalactiae* (group B). Adequate active immunization of the mother constitutes a simple and effective means of providing passive protection to the fetus and infant in the first few months of life. (However, some premature infants may not acquire the maternal antibodies to the extent that full-term infants do.)

MATERNAL IMMUNITY VIA COLOSTRUM. Human milk contains a variety of factors that may influence the response of the nursing infant to infectious agents. Some of these factors are natural selective factors that can affect the intestinal microflora, namely, by enhancement of growth of desirable bacteria and by nonspecific inhibitors of some microbes, by the action of ***lysozyme, lactoferrin, interferon***, and ***leukocytes*** (macrophages, T cells, B cells, and granulocytes). ***Antibodies*** (IgA) are found in breast milk, the concentration being higher in the ***colostrum*** (first milk) immediately postpartum (Table 22.5). The production of

TABLE 22.5   Levels of Immunoglobulin in Colostrum[a]

	Day postpartum				Approximate normal adult level (mg/dl)
	1	2	3	4	
IgA[b]	600	260	200	80	200
IgG[c]	80	45	30	16	1,000
IgM	125	65	58	30	120

[a]After Michael JR, Ringenback R, Hottenstein S (1971): J Infect Dis 124:445.
[b]80% of this is secretory sIgA.
[c]IgG$_4$ represents 15% of colostral IgG and 3.5% of serum IgG.

antibody in the mammary gland is related to antigens that enter the maternal intestine and the migration of antigen-stimulated B cells from intestinal lamina propria to the breast (the "enteromammary system"), part of the mucosa-associated lymphoid tissue (MALT) system. Thus, organisms colonizing or infecting the alimentary tract of the mother may lead to production of colostral antibody, which affords mucosal protection to the nursing infant against pathogens that enter via the intestinal tract. Antibody to the enteropathogens *Escherichia coli, Salmonella typhi, Shigella* species, poliomyelitis virus, and coxsackie and echoviruses have been demonstrated. Feeding a mixture of IgA (73%) and IgG (26%) derived from human serum to low-birth-weight infants who could not have access to mothers' breast milk protected them against necrotizing enterocolitis. (Antibodies to nonalimentary pathogens have also been demonstrated in colostrum—e.g., tetanus and diphtheria antitoxins, and antistreptococcal hemolysin.)

Tuberculin-sensitive T lymphocytes are also transmitted to the infant through the colostrum, but the role of such cells in passive transfer of cell-mediated immunity is uncertain.

Artificial Passive Immunity

HETEROLOGOUS VERSUS HOMOLOGOUS ANTIBODY. World War I afforded unusually suitable, if regrettable, circumstances for testing the value of passive immunization with tetanus antitoxin. In 1915, antitoxin produced in the horse was used to treat the wounded British troops and resulted in prompt reduction in cases of tetanus. This experience allowed the determination of the minimum concentration of antitoxin needed to provide protection and also showed that the period of protection in the human was brief. The basis for the latter is

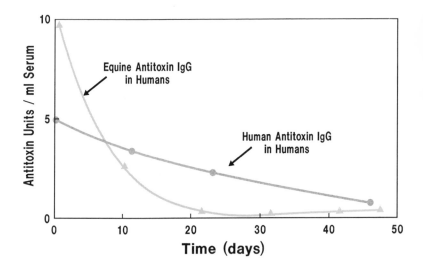

Figure 22.4.

Serum concentrations of human and equine IgG antitoxin following administration into humans.

shown schematically in Figures 22.4 and 22.5. The heterologous equine antibody in the human undergoes dilution, catabolism, immune complex formation, and immune elimination. In contrast, the homologous human antibody, which reaches a peak level in the serum about 2 days after subcutaneous injection, undergoes dilution and catabolism with a reduction to half the maximal concentration in about 23 days (the half-life of human IgG_1, IgG_2, and IgG_4 is 23 days; that of IgG_3 is 7

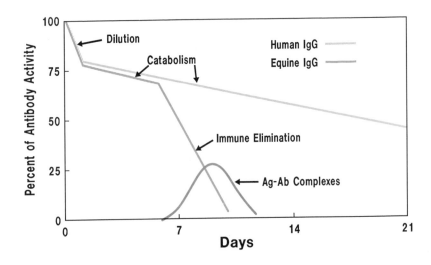

Figure 22.5.

The fate of human and equine IgG following administration into humans.

days). The protective level of the human antibody is thus sustained considerably longer than that of the equine antibody. *Heterologous antibody*, such as that from the horse, can cause at least two kinds of hypersensitivity reaction: *type I* (immediate, anaphylaxis) or *type III* (serum sickness from immune complexes). If no other treatment is available, it is possible to use the heterologous antiserum in an individual with type I sensitivity by administration of gradually increasing but minute amounts of the foreign serum, given repeatedly over several hours. Some preparations of heterologous antibody [e.g., equine diphtheria antitoxin and anti-lymphocyte serum (ALS)] are still used in humans.

USE OF HUMAN IMMUNE SERUM GLOBULIN. The use of globulin from human serum apparently began in the early 1900s, when serum of patients convalescing from measles was given to children who had been exposed to measles but had not yet developed symptoms. Additional attempts in 1916, and later, showed that early administration of measles convalescent serum could protect against emergence of clinically apparent measles. In 1933 human placentae were also recognized as a source of measles antibody.

In the early 1940s Cohn and colleagues devised a method for separation of the "gammaglobulin" (γ-globulin) fraction from human serum by precipitation with cold ethanol. This *"Cohn fractionation"* represented a practical and safe method for production of homologous human antibody for clinical use.

It is likely that specific monoclonal antibodies of human origin will become available for certain uses from the application of hybridoma technology.

PREPARATION AND PROPERTIES OF HOMOLOGOUS IMMUNE SERUM GLOBULIN. Plasma is collected from healthy donors or placentae. The plasma or serum from several donors is pooled and the preparation is termed *immune serum globulin (ISG)* or *human normal immunoglobulin (HNI)*. If the plasma or serum is from donors who are specially selected after an immunizing or booster dose of antigen, or after convalescence from a specific infection, the specific immune globulin preparation is designated accordingly [e.g., tetanus immune globulin (TIG), hepatitis B (HBIG), varicella-zoster (VZIG), or rabies (RIG)]. Large quantities can be obtained by *plasmapheresis*—removal of the plasma while returning the blood cells to the donor. The fraction containing antibody globulin(s) is precipitated by cold ethanol. The resultant preparation (1) is free of hepatitis virus and the HIV of AIDS, (2) concentrates many of the IgG antibodies about 25-fold, (3) is stable for years, and (4) can provide peak levels in blood approximately 2 days after intramuscular injection. Preparations that are safe when administered intravenously (called IVIG or IVGG) involve cold alcohol precipitation followed by various other treatments, including fractionation using polyethylene glycol or ion exchangers; acidification to pH 4–4.5; exposure to pepsin or trypsin; and stabilization with maltose, sucrose, glucose, or glycine. Such stabilization reduces aggregation of the globulins that can trigger anaphylactoid reactions (see Precautions section, below). In these newer intravenous preparations, IgG is present in about one-third to one-fourth its concentration in the intramuscular immune globulin preparations and there is only a "trace" of IgA and IgM (see Table 22.6).

TABLE 22.6   Composition of Human Immune Serum Globulin

Source	Immunoglobulin (mg/100 ml)		
	IgG	IgA	IgM
Whole serum	1,200	180	200
Immune serum globulin	16,500[a]	100–500[a]	25–200[a]
Placental immune serum globulin	16,500	200–700[a]	150–400[a]

[a]Intravenous preparations contain 3,000 or 5,000 mg IgG per 100 ml and only trace amounts of IgA and IgM.

The commercially available immune globulin contains higher concentrations of IgG (of all subclasses) than those in whole serum (see Table 22.6), but there is a relative deficiency of IgA and IgM. Deficiency of the latter could be significant if protection is required against lipopolysaccharide endotoxin or whole gram-negative bacteria, which are adversely affected by IgM plus complement.

INDICATIONS FOR USE OF IMMUNE GLOBULINS

Specific Immune Globulin. Antibody (Rhogam) to RhD antigen is given to Rh⁻ mothers within a 72-hour perinatal period to protect against their immunization by fetal Rh⁺ erythrocytes. As discussed in Chapter 15, the role of Rhogam in this protection is attributed to its removal of Rh⁺ fetal cells to which the mother is exposed during parturition, and thus avoids sensitization of the Rh⁻ mother by Rh⁺ antigens. *Tetanus immune globulin (TIG)* (antitoxin) is used to provide passive protection after certain wounds and in the absence of adequate active immunization with tetanus toxoid.

Varicella-zoster immune globulin (VZIG) is given to leukemics who are highly vulnerable to the varicella-zoster (chickenpox) virus and to pregnant women and their infants exposed to or infected with varicella virus.

Cytomegalovirus human immune globulin (CMV-IGIV) is used prophylactically for recipients of bone marrow or renal transplants.

Rabies immune globulin (RIG) is given together with active immunization with human diploid cell rabies vaccine to individuals bitten by potentially rabid animals (human RIG is not universally available so equine antibody may be necessary in some areas).

Hepatitis B immune globulin (HBIG) may be given to a newborn child of a mother with evidence of hepatitis B infection, to medical personnel after accidental stick with a hypodermic needle, or after sexual contact with an individual with hepatitis B. (ISG may also be used against hepatitis B; see below.)

Vaccinia immune globulin is given to eczematous or immunocompromised individuals with intimate exposure to others who have been vaccinated against smallpox by live attenuated vaccinia vaccine. Such compromised individuals can develop destructive progressive disease from the attenuated vaccine.

Immune Serum Globulin (ISG or IVIG). ISG or IVIG has been used in certain circumstances: hepatitis A—ISG can be used for both pre- and postexposure protection; hepatitis B—ISG preparations in recent years have been regarded as sufficiently potent to substitute for HBIG in some circumstances; hepatitis C—ISG *may* offer protection against this blood-associated disease; and measles—ISG is used for the protection of infants exposed to measles prior to vaccination with attenuated measles virus. IVIG has ameliorated the effects of cytomegalovirus in bone marrow transplant patients and of echovirus-induced chronic meningoencephalitis. ISG or IVIG has been useful in children with immunosuppressive conditions and in premature infants; in hypogammaglobulinemia and primary immune deficiency disease repeated injections of ISG are required. In immune idiopathic thrombocytopenic purpura (ITP) the higher dose of IgG in the ISG presumably blocks the Fc receptors on phagocytic cells and prevents them from phagocytosing and destroying platelets coated with autoantibodies. IVIG has also been used with varying success in other immune cytopenias. It has had significant success against group B streptococcal infections in premature neonates and against Kawasaki's disease, a condition of unknown etiology. It has been useful in reducing bacterial infections in patients with hematopoietic malignancies, such as chronic B cell lymphocytic leukemia or multiple myeloma.

PRECAUTIONS. The preparations of globulin other than IVIG have been given by the *intramuscular route*, since *intravenous* administration is contraindicated because of possible *anaphylactoid* reactions. These are probably due to aggregates of Ig formed during the fractionation by ethanol precipitation. These aggregates activate complement to yield anaphylatoxins (IgG_1, IgG_2, IgG_3, and IgM by the classical pathway; IgG_4 and IgA, by the alternative pathway). The IVIG safe for intravenous administration has been increasingly used, particularly when repeated administration is required as in agammaglobulinemia.

One unique contraindication to the use of the usual immune globulin preparations is in cases of congenital deficiency of IgA. Since these patients lack IgA, they recognize it as a foreign protein and respond by making antibodies against it, including IgE antibodies which can lead to a subsequent anaphylactic reaction. The IVIG preparations with only a trace of IgA may pose less of a problem. Table 22.7 presents a compilation of available vaccines and antisera.

IMMUNOTHERAPY

Immunotherapy (treating an existing disease) has been attempted but has *limited applicability*. Thus, except for the postexposure immunization described above, there is little applicability of immunotherapy to the treatment of infectious diseases. Some efforts were made to treat bacterial meningitis in humans by administration of heterologous antibody via intrathecal and other parenteral routes. The success of this approach was questionable, and the advent of antimicrobial agents (sulfonamides and antibiotics) lessened the zeal for studying immunotherapy in cases of bacterial meningitis and other infections. Restoration of immune capability, such as in treatment of burn patients who incur serious infections, is receiving attention, and prospects for combined use with chemotherapy are generating renewed interest in immunotherapy.

Antibody directed against cytokines that may produce undesirable effects in certain clinical situations may provide a useful immunotherapeutic modality. Thus, passively administered antibody specific for TNF-α may be beneficial in reducing mortality associated with "septic shock" of infectious origin. Septic shock is a physiological response of the host to substances produced by infective agents. This response leads to the release of cytokines, arachidonic acid derivatives, kinins, and other substances. These substances affect endothelial, myocardial, and other cells, with resultant organ dysfunction, such as oliguria, hypotension, and altered mental status.

Monoclonal antibody directed against the receptor for IL-2 on T lymphocytes has been effective in preventing acute rejection of renal transplants in humans.

TABLE 22.7   Immunizing Preparations (Vaccines and Antisera) Useful in Humans

Vaccine	Type of vaccine
Bacterial	
Anthrax	Killed bacteria; alum-precipitated antigen from culture filtrate
Botulism	Toxoid, limited use in research workers
Brucellosis	Attenuated live *Brucella abortus* strain 19 (limited use in humans only outside the United States)
Cholera	Killed *Vibrio cholerae*
Diphtheria	Toxoid
Haemophilus influenzae	Type b polysaccharide, alone or conjugated to protein
Meningococcal meningitis	Polysaccharide, group A,C,Y,W135 of *Neisseria meningitidis*
Pertussis	Killed *Bordetella pertussis,* subunit
Plague	Killed *Yersinia pestis*
Pneumococcal infection	Polysaccharide (capsule) of 23 serotypes of *Streptoccocus pneumoniae*
Tetanus	Toxoid
Tuberculosis	Attenuated live bacille Calmette-Guérin (BCG)
Typhoid	Killed; or attenuated *Salmonella typhi* Ty21$_a$;Vi antigen
Rickettsial	
Typhus fever	Formalin-inactivated *Rickettsia prowazekii,* restricted applicability
Viral	
Hepatitis A	Inactivated or attenuated HA
Hepatitis B	Inactivated HB surface antigen or recombinant (yeast)
Influenza	Inactivated whole or "split" (subunit) virus
Japanese B encephalitis	Inactivated
Measles	Attenuated
Mumps	Attenuated
Polio	Attenuated or inactivated
Rabies	Inactivated
Rubella	Attenuated
Varicella	Attenuated
Antisera	
Black widow spider	Equine antivenin
Botulism	Human immune globulin, equine immune globulin
Coral snake bite	Equine antivenin
Crotalid snake bite	Polyvalent equine antiserum
Cytomegalovirus	Human immune globulin
Digoxin	Ovine
Diphtheria	Equine immune serum

(*continued*)

TABLE 22.7   Immunizing Preparations (Vaccines and Antisera) Useful in Humans (Continued)

Vaccine	Type of vaccine
Hepatitis A	Pooled human serum globulin (ISG)
Hepatitis B	Specific anti-HB (HBIG) or ISG
Hypogammaglobulinemia	Pooled human ISG
Measles	Pooled human ISG
Rabies	Human immune globulin (RIG), equine immune serum
Rh_0 (D)	Immune (human) globulin vs. Rh_0 (D) factor
Tetanus	Human immune globulin (TIG)
Vaccinia	Vaccinia immune globulin
Varicella-zoster	Zoster immune globulin (VZIG)
Antilymphocyte serum	Equine
Antithymocyte globulin	Rabbit

Nonspecific Immunostimulation

Attempts to arrest growth of tumors have involved nonspecific immunostimulation with various microbial or mammalian cell products. Induction of local contact hypersensitivity with dinitrochlorobenzene (DNCB) at the site of a tumor occasionally, on subsequent topical application of DNCB, leads to diminution in the size of some cutaneous malignancies.

Specific Immunostimulation

TRANSFER FACTOR. Transfer factor (TF), a dialyzable extract of peripheral blood leukocytes (lymphocytes), was originally reported to transfer delayed-type hypersensitivity to antigens to which the leukocyte donor reacts. However, no unequivocal usefulness has been demonstrated for TF, and it is mentioned here for historic interest only.

SPECIFIC IMMUNOTARGETING. The use of "immunotoxins," i.e., specific antibodies with attached toxins, e.g., ricin, or radioactive isotopes to attack tumor cells, was discussed in Chapter 21. Such immunotoxins may also be useful in preparing a recipient for a bone marrow or organ transplant by damaging certain T lymphocytes that could react against the transplanted tissue. Such immunotoxins directed against receptors in macrophages with intracellular parasites (e.g., *Leishmania*) may lead to damage of the cell and to the intracellular organism. Fibrin-specific antibody with conjugated fibrinolytic enzymes has shown clot-specific lysis, a means of treating thrombi in blood vessels.

Plasmapheresis

While *plasmapheresis* (the separation of blood cells from plasma) is used for collection of specific, antibody-rich plasma for use as ISG or other globulin preparations, it has also been used to remove detrimental antibody to afford clinical improvement in some patients. For example:

1. In *myasthenia gravis*, an antibody to the acetylcholine receptor protein leads to muscle weakness.
2. In *Goodpasture's syndrome*, there is autoimmune antibody to renal glomerular basement membrane.
3. In one type of *autoimmune hemolytic anemia*, antibody is destructive to erythrocytes.

It is evident that the cellular production of autoantibodies would continue in all cases and that plasmapheresis can provide only transient benefits. However, transient benefits may provide time for development of more durable therapeutic interventions.

Leukapheresis

Selective removal of leukocytes from patients' blood has also been used therapeutically, such as in some otherwise unresponsive cases of rheumatoid arthritis.

SUMMARY

1. Protection against diseases may be achieved by active as well as passive immunization.

2. Active immunization may result from previous infection or from vaccination, while passive immunization may occur by natural means, such as the transfer of antibodies from mother to fetus via the placenta, or to an infant via the colostrum; or by artificial means such as by the administration of immune globulins.

3. Active immunization may be achieved by administration of one immunogen or a combination of immunogens.

4. The incubation period of a disease and the rapidity with which protective antibody titers develop influence both the efficacy of vaccination and the anamnestic effect of a booster injection.

5. The site of administration of a vaccine may be of great importance; many routes of immunization lead to the synthesis predominantly of serum IgM and IgG; oral administration of some vaccines leads to the induction of secretory IgA in the digestive tract.

6. Immunoprophylaxis has had striking success against subsequent infection; immunotherapy has had limited success in infectious and noninfectious diseases.

REFERENCES

Buckley RH, Schiff RI (1991): The use of intravenous immune globulin in immunodeficiency diseases: New Engl J Med 325:110.

Doller PC (1993): Vaccination of adults against travel-related infectious diseases, and new developments in vaccines. Infection 21:1.

Donnelly JJ, Ulmer, JB, Lui MA (1994): Immunization with polynucleotides. A novel approach to vaccination: The Immunologist 2:20.

Gardner P, Schaffner W (1993): Immunization of adults: New Engl J Med 328:1252.

Peter G, Halsey NA, Marcuse EK, Pickering LK (eds) (1994): Report of the Committee on Infectious Diseases, 23d ed. Elk Grove Village, IL: American Academy of Pediatrics.

Rabinovich NR, McInnes P, Klein DL, Hall BF (1994): Vaccine technologies: view to the future. Science 265:1401.

U.S. Department of Health and Human Services (1994): General recommendations on immunization. Recommendations of the Immunization Practices Advisory Committee (ACIP). MMWR (January 28) 43 No. RR-1.

World Health Organization (1986): Expanded Programme on Immunization. 86/7, Rev 1. Geneva, Switzerland.

REVIEW QUESTIONS

For each question, choose the ONE BEST answer or completion.

1. The best way to provide immunologic protection against tetanus neonatorum (of the newborn) is to
   A) inject the infant with human tetanus antitoxin
   B) inject the newborn with tetanus toxoid
   C) inject the mother with toxoid within 72 hours of the birth of her child
   D) immunize the mother with tetanus toxoid before or early in pregnancy
   E) give the child antitoxin and toxoid for both passive and active immunization

2. Active, durable immunization against poliomyelitis can be accomplished by oral administration of attenuated vaccine (Sabin) or by parenteral injection of inactivated (Salk) vaccine. These vaccines are equally effective in preventing disease because
   A) both induce adequate IgA at the intestinal mucosa, the site of entry of the virus
   B) antibody in the serum protects against the viremia that leads to disease
   C) viral antigen attaches to the anterior horn cells in the spinal cord, preventing attachment of virulent virus
   D) both vaccines induce formation of interferon
   E) both vaccines establish a mild infection that can lead to formation of antibody

3. The administration of vaccines is not without hazard. Of the following, which is least likely to affect adversely an immunocompromised host?
   A) measles vaccine
   B) pneumococcal vaccine
   C) bacille Calmette-Guérin
   D) mumps vaccine
   E) Sabin poliomyelitis vaccine

4. The administration of foreign (e.g., equine) antitoxin for passive protection in humans can lead to serum sickness, which is characterized by all of the following *except*:
   A) production by host of antibody to foreign antibody
   B) onset in 24–48 hours
   C) use of homologous antitoxin
   D) deposition of antigen–antibody complexes at various sites in the host
   E) although delayed, the reaction is not a cell-mediated, delayed, type IV immune response

5. The pneumococcal polysaccharide vaccine should be administered to all *except*:
   A) individuals with chronic cardiorespiratory disease
   B) elderly (over 60 years of age) persons
   C) children (under 2 years of age)
   D) persons with chronic renal failure
   E) individuals with sickle-cell disease

6. The following statements about human immune serum globulin (ISG) are true *except*:

A) the source is human placenta
B) the globulins are obtained by precipitation with cold ethanol
C) the concentration of IgG is more than 10-fold greater than in plasma

D) IgA and IgM are present in concentrations slightly lower than in plasma
E) the ethanol precipitation does not render preparation of globulin free of hepatitis virus

ANSWERS TO REVIEW QUESTIONS

1. **D** The simplest and most effective way to protect the newborn infant against exotoxic disease, such as tetanus and diphtheria, is to induce antibody in the mother. The antitoxic IgG passing through the placenta will provide the necessary protection. While tetanus antitoxin could be used to provide short-term passive protection, it would be more costly and require an otherwise unnecessary and painful injection. Injection of toxoid in the mother within 72 hours of delivery of the child would not allow time for induction of antibody. While antitoxin and toxoid could provide immediate passive and future active protection, the latter would have to be accompanied by future injections of toxoid and the former is expensive; both would require undesirable injections.

2. **B** Both attenuated and inactivated vaccines lead to formation of circulating antibody, which would provide protection by intercepting the infecting virus before it reaches the target tissue in the central nervous system. While the Sabin vaccine induces mucosal gut IgA that may intercept virus at the portal of entry, the parenterally injected Salk vaccine is not effective in inducing mucosal IgA. Viral antigen in the vaccine might attach to the anterior horn cells in the nervous system, but it probably would not provide durable immunity. Induction of interferon would represent potentially only brief protection. Only the Sabin vaccine, being attenuated and "live," would induce a mild infection.

3. **B** The pneumococcal vaccine consists of capsular polysaccharides from *Streptococcus pneumoniae* and represents a nonviable vaccine, which cannot lead to infection. Measles, mumps, and Sabin polio vaccines contain attenuated viruses, and BCG is an attenuated bacterium. These attenuated organisms are capable of proliferating in the human host. The normal host limits their replication, but the immunocompromised host may not be able to do so, and progressive infection may occur.

4. **B** The reactions that constitute serum sick-

ness follow administration of the foreign substance within 6–12 days. During this time, the host produces antibody that reacts with the foreign substance(s), which persists in the host and leads to antigen–antibody complexes that can be deposited in joints, lymph nodes, skin, and elsewhere. The manifestation of the immune reaction, although appearing later, nevertheless are classified as type III rather than cell-mediated, delayed (type IV) hypersensitivity because they involve antibodies rather than T cells.

5. *C* Children under 2 years of age do not respond adequately to immunization with pure bacterial capsule polysaccharide vaccine. Therefore, vaccinating them may be useless. The various other individuals listed are particularly vulnerable to infection with *Streptococcus pneumoniae.* While some of them may mount a suboptimal response to the vaccine, they should nevertheless be vaccinated.

6. *E* The potential hazard of hepatitis viruses in human plasma is overcome by the separation of ethanol-precipitated globulins. The concentration of IgG is about 16,500 mg/dl, compared with 1200 mg/dl in plasma. Whereas the IgG thus becomes highly concentrated in ISG, IgA and IgM are relatively depleted, and their concentration in the ethanol-precipitated ISG is close to their original concentration in the plasma.

PARTIAL LIST OF CD MOLECULES

CD no.	Other name	Function	Ligand
CD2	LFA-2	T-cell adhesion molecule	CD58
CD3		TcR signal transduction	
CD4		TcR coreceptor, signal transduction	MHC class II, HIV
CD8		TcR coreceptor, signal transduction	MHC class I
CD11a, CD18	LFA-1	Adhesion molecule	ICAM 1, 2, 3
CD19		B-cell signal transduction	
CD20		Ca^{2+} channel in B-cell activation	
CD21		Involved in B-cell activation	EBV and complement
CD28		T-cell costimulator molecule	B7 (CD80 and CD86)
CD32	FcγR II	Low-affinity receptor for IgG	Aggregated IgG and antigen–antibody complexes
CD34		Marker for early stem cells	
CD44	PgP-1, H-CAM	Lymphocyte adhesion to HEV	Hyaluronic acid
CD50	ICAM-3	Adhesion molecule	LFA-1
CD54	ICAM-1	Adhesion molecule	CD11a, CD18; rhinovirus
CD58	LFA-3	Adhesion molecule	CD2
CD62L	L-Selectin, MEL-14	T-cell adhesion to HEV	
CD74	Invariant chain	Associated with MHC class II	
CD79a	Igα	Signal transduction molecules	
CD79b	Igβ	associated with Ig	
CD80	B7.1	Costimulatory molecule on APC	CD28, CTLA-4
CD86	B7.2	Costimulatory molecule on APC	CD28, CTLA-4

453

GLOSSARY

Accessory cell: Cell required to initiate immune response. Often used to describe *antigen-presenting cell* (*APC;* see below).

Adjuvant: A substance, given with antigen, that enhances the response to the injected antigen.

Adoptive transfer: The transfer of the capacity to make an immune response by transplantation of immunocompetent cells.

Affinity: A measure of the binding constant of a single antigen combining site with a monovalent antigenic determinant.

Agglutination: The aggregation of particulate antigen by antibodies. Agglutination applies to red blood cells as well as to bacteria and inert particles covered with antigen.

Allelles: Two or more alternate forms of a gene that occupy the same position or locus on a specific chromosome.

Allelic exclusion: The ability of heterozygous lymphoid cells to produce only one allelic form of antigen-specific receptor (Ig or TcR) when they have the genetic endowment to produce both. Genes other than those for the antigen-specific receptors are usually expressed codominantly.

Allergen: An antigen responsible for producing allergic reactions by inducing IgE synthesis.

Allergy: A term covering immune reactions to nonpathogenic antigens, which lead to inflammation and deleterious effects in the host.

Allogeneic: Genetically dissimilar within the same species.

Allograft: A tissue transplant (graft) between two genetically nonidentical members of a species.

Allotypes: Antigenic determinants that are present in allelic (alternate) forms. When used in association with immunoglobulin, allotypes describe allelic variants of immunoglobulins detected by antibodies raised between members of the same species.

Alternate complement pathway: The mechanism of complement activation that does not involve activation of the C1–C4–C2 pathway by antigen–antibody complexes, and begins with the activation of C3.

Anamnestic: Literally, means "does not forget"; it is used to describe *immunologic memory*, which leads to a rapid increase in response after reexposure to antigen.

Anaphylatoxin: Substance capable of releasing histamine from mast cells.

Anaphylaxis: Immediate hypersensitivity response to antigenic challenge, mediated by IgE and mast cells. It is a life-threatening allergic reaction, caused by the release of pharmacologically active agents.

Antibody: Serum protein formed in response to immunization; antibodies are generally defined in terms of their specific binding to the immunizing antigen.

Antibody-dependent, cell-mediated cytotoxicity (ADCC): A phenomenon in which target cells, coated with antibody, are destroyed by specialized killer cells (NK cells and macrophages), which bear receptors for the Fc portion of the coating antibody (Fc receptors). These receptors allow the killer cells to bind to the antibody-coated target.

Antigen: Any foreign material that is specifically bound by specific antibody or specific lymphocytes; also used loosely to describe materials used for immunization. Compare to *immunogen.*

Antigen-binding site: The part of an immunoglobulin molecule that binds antigen specifically.

Antigen-presenting cell (APC): A specialized type of cell, bearing cell-surface class II MHC (major histocompatibility complex) molecules, involved in processing and presentation of antigen to inducer *T cells.*

Antigen receptor: The specific antigen-binding receptor on T or B lymphocytes; these receptors are transcribed and translated from rearrangements and translocation of V, D, and J genes.

Antigenic determinant: A single antigenic site or *epitope* on a complex antigenic molecule or particle.

Apoptosis: A form of programmed cell death caused by activation of endogenous molecules leading to the fragmentation of DNA.

Arthus reaction: A hypersensitivity reaction produced by local formation of antigen–antibody aggregates that activate the complement cascade and cause thrombosis, hemorrhage, and acute inflammation.

Atopy: A term used by allergists to describe IgE-mediated anaphylactic responses in humans, usually showing a genetic predisposition.

Autochthonous: Pertaining to "self."

Autograft: A tissue transplant from one area to another on a single individual.

Autoimmunity (autoallergy): An immune response to "self" tissues or components. Such an immune response may have pathological consequences leading to autoimmune diseases.

Autologous: Derived from the same individual, "self."

Avidity: The summation of multiple affinities—for example, when a polyvalent antibody binds to a polyvalent antigen.

B lymphocyte (B cell): The precursors of antibody-forming plasma cell; this cell expresses immunoglobulin on its surface.

Bence–Jones protein: Dimers of immunoglobulin light chains in the urine of patients with multiple myeloma.

Blocking antibody: A functional term for an antibody molecule capable of blocking the interaction of antigen with other antibodies or with cells.

Bursa of Fabricius: Site of development of B cells in birds; an outpouching of the cloaca.

Carcinoembryonic antigen (CEA): Antigen present during embryonic development that normally is not expressed in the adult but reappears in the malignant cells.

Carrier: A large immunogenic molecule or particle to which a hapten or other nonimmunogenic, epitope-bearing molecules are attached, allowing them to become *immunogenic.*

Cell-mediated cytotoxicity (CMC): Killing (lysis) of a target cell by an effector lymphocyte.

Cell-mediated immunity (CMI): Immune reaction mediated by T cells; in contrast to humoral immunity, which is antibody-mediated. Also referred to as *delayed-type hypersensitivity.*

Chemokines: Cytokines of relatively low molecular weight released by a variety of cells, which have effects on other cells.

Chemotaxis: Migration of cells along a concentration gradient of an attractant.

Chimera: A mythical animal possessing the head of a lion, the body of a goat, and the tail of a snake. Refers to an individual containing cellular components derived from another genetically distinct individual.

Class I, II, and III MHC molecules: See *Major histocompatibility complex (MHC).*

Class switch: See *Isotype switch.*

Classical complement pathway: The mechanism of complement activation initiated by antigen–antibody aggregates and proceeding by way of C1 to C9.

Clonal deletion: The loss of lymphocytes of a particular specificity due to contact with either "self" or foreign introduced antigen.

Clonal selection theory: The prevalent concept that specificity and diversity of an immune response are the result of selection by antigen of specifically reactive clones from a large repertoire of preformed lymphocytes, each with individual specificities.

Cluster determinant (CD): Cluster of antigens with which antibodies react that characterize cell-surface molecules.

Combinatorial joining: The joining of segments of DNA to generate essentially new genetic information, as occurs with Ig and TcR genes during the development of B and T cells. Combinatorial joining allows multiple opportunities for two sets of genes to combine in different ways.

Complement: A series of serum proteins involved in the mediation of immune reactions. The complement cascade is triggered classically by the interaction of antibody with specific antigen.

Complete Freund's adjuvant (CFA): See *Freund's complete adjuvant.*

Congenic (also co-isogenic): Describes two individuals who differ only in the genes at a particular locus and are identical at all other loci.

Constant region (C region): The invariant carboxyl-terminal portion of an immunoglobulin or TcR molecule, as distinct from the variable region at the amino terminal of the chain.

Coombs' test: A test named for its originator, R.R.A. Coombs, used to detect antibodies by addition of an anti-immunoglobulin antibody.

Cross-reactivity: The ability of an antibody, specific for one antigen, to react with a second antigen; a measure of relatedness between two different antigenic substances.

Cytokines: Soluble substances secreted by cells, which have a variety of effects on other cells.

D gene: A small segment of immunoglobulin heavy-chain and T-cell receptor DNA, coding for the third hypervariable region of most receptors.

Delayed-type hypersensitivity (DTH): A T cell-mediated reaction to antigen, which takes 24–48 hours to develop fully and that involves release of lymphokines and recruitment of monocytes and macrophages. Also called *cell-mediated immunity.*

Determinant: Part of the antigen molecule that binds to an antibody-combining site or to a receptor on T cells; also termed epitope (see *Hapten* and *Epitope*).

Differentiation antigen: A cell-surface antigenic determinant found only on cells of a certain lineage and at a particular developmental stage; used as an immunologic market.

Domain: A compact segment of an immunoglobulin or TcR chain, made up of amino acids around an S–S bond.

DP, DQ, and DR molecules: MHC class II molecules of humans found on B cells and antigen-presenting cells.

Enhancing antibodies: Antibodies that enhance the survival of a graft or of a tumor.

Enzyme-linked immunosorbent assay (ELISA): An assay in which an enzyme is linked to an antibody and a colored substrate is used to measure the activity of bound enzyme and, hence, the amount of bound antibody.

Eosinophil chemotactic factor of anaphylaxis (ECF-A): A substrate released from mast cells during anaphylaxis that attracts eosinophils.

Epitope: An alternative term for *antigenic determinant.*

Equivalence zone: In a precipitin reaction, the region in which the concentration of antigen and antibody leads to maximal precipitation.

Exon: The region of DNA coding for a protein or a segment of a protein.

Fab: Fragment of antibody containing one antigen-binding site; generated by cleavage of the antibody with the enzyme papain, which cuts at the hinge region N-terminally to the inter-heavy-chain disulfide bond and generates two Fab fragments from one antibody molecule.

F(ab')₂: A fragment of an antibody containing two antigen-binding sites; generated by cleavage of the antibody molecule with the enzyme pepsin which cuts at the hinge region C-terminally to the inter-heavy-chain disulfide bond.

Fc: Fragment of antibody without antigen-binding sites, generated by cleavage with papain; the Fc fragment contains the C-terminal domains of the immunoglobulin heavy chains.

Fc receptor (FcR): A receptor on a cell surface with specific binding affinity for the Fc portion of an antibody molecule. Fc receptors are found on many types of cells.

Fluorescent antibody: An antibody coupled with a fluorescent dye, used to detect antigen on cells, tissues, or microorganisms.

Freund's complete adjuvant: An oil containing killed mycobacteria and an emulsifier which, when emulsified with an immunogen in aqueous solution, enhances the immune response to that immunogen following injection. Termed "incomplete" Freund's adjuvant if mycobacteria are not included.

Genotype: All the genes possessed by an individual; in practice it refers to the particular alleles present at the loci in question.

Germ line: Refers to genes in germ cells as opposed to somatic cells. In immunology, it refers to genes in their unrearranged state rather than those rearranged for production of immunoglobulin or TcR molecules.

Graft-versus-host reaction (GVH): The pathologic consequences of a response initiated by transplanted immunocompetent T lymphocytes into an allogeneic, immunologically incompetent host. The host is unable to reject the grafted T cells and becomes their target.

Granuloma: An organized structure in the form of a mass of mononuclear cells at the site of a persisting inflammation; the cells are mostly macrophages with some T lymphocytes at the periphery. It is a typical delayed hypersensitivity reaction which is persistent due to the continuous presence of a foreign body or infection.

H-2 complex: The major histocompatibility complex situated on chromosome 17 of the mouse; contains subregions K, I, D, and L.

Haplotype: A particular combination of closely linked genes on a chromosome inherited from one parent.

Hapten: A compound, usually of low molecular weight, that is not itself immunogenic but that, after conjugation to a carrier protein or cells, becomes immunogenic and induces antibody, which can bind the hapten alone in the absence of carrier.

Heavy chain (H chain): The larger of the two types of chains that comprise a normal immunoglobulin or antibody molecule.

Helper T cells: A class of T cells that help trigger B cells to make antibody against thymus-dependent antigens. Helper T cells also help in the differentiation of other T cells such as cytotoxic T cells.

Heterophile antigen: A cross-reacting antigen that appears in widely ranging species such as humans and bacteria.

Hinge region: A flexible, open segment of an antibody molecule that allows bending of the molecule. The hinge region is located between Fab and Fc and is susceptible to enzymatic cleavage.

Histocompatibility: Literally, the ability of tissues to get along; in immunology, it means identity in all transplantation antigens. These antigens, in turn, are collectively referred to as histocompatibility antigens.

HLA complex: The human major histocompatibility complex situated on chromosome 6; stands for "human leukocyte antigens." It contains several subregions.

Humoral immunity: Any immune reaction that can be transferred with immune serum (as opposed to *cell-mediated immunity*). In general, this term refers to resistance that results from the presence of specific antibody in the serum.

Hybridoma: A hybrid cell that results from the fusion of an antibody-secreting cell with a malignant B cell; the progeny secrete antibody without stimulation and proliferate continuously both in vivo and in vitro. Also applies to a hybrid T cell resulting from the fusion of T lymphocytes with malignant T lymphocytes; the hybrid proliferates continously and secretes cytokines upon activation by antigen and APC.

Hypersensitivity: State of reactivity to antigen that is greater than normal for the antigenic challenge; hypersensitivity is the same as *allergy* and denotes a deleterious outcome rather than a protective one.

Hypervariable regions: Portions of the light and heavy immunoglobulin chains that are highly variable in amino acid sequence from one immunoglobulin molecule to another, and that, together, constitute the antigen-binding site of an antibody molecule. Also, portions of the T-cell receptor that constitute the antigen-binding site.

Ia: "Immune response-associated" proteins; an old term now replaced with *MHC (major histocompatibility complex)* class II molecules.

Idiotype: The combined antigenic determinants *(idiotopes)* found on antibodies of an individual that are directed at a particular antigen; such antigenic determinants are found only in the variable region.

Immediate-type hypersensitivity: Hypersensitivity tissue reaction occurring within minutes after the interaction of antigen and antibody.

Immune adherence: The adherence of particulate antigen coated with C3b to tissue having cells with C3b receptors.

Immune modulators: Substances that control the expression of the immune response.

Immunogen: A substance capable of inducing an immune response (as well as reacting with the products of an immune response). Compare with *antigen*.

Immunoglobulin (Ig): A general term for all antibody molecules. Each Ig unit is made up of two heavy chains and two light chains and has two antigen-binding sites.

Immunoglobulin superfamily: Proteins involved in cellular recognition and interaction that are structurally and genetically related to immunoglobulins.

Interferon: A group of proteins having antiviral activity and capable of enhancing and modifying the immune response.

Interleukins: Glycoproteins secreted by a variety of leukocytes that have effects on other leukocytes.

Internal image: A spatial configuration of the combining site of an anti-idiotype antibody that resembles the epitope to which the idiotype is directed.

Intron: A segment of DNA that does not code for protein: the intervening sequence of nucleotides between coding sequences or *exons*.

Isograft: Tissue transplanted between two genetically identical individuals.

Isohemagglutinins: Antibodies to major red blood cell antigens present normally as a result of inapparent immunization by cross-reactive antigens in bacteria, food, and other substances.

Isotypes: Antibodies that differ in the constant regions of their heavy chain (Fc portion); distinguishable also on the basis of reaction with antisera raised in another species. These differences also result in different biological activities of the antibodies. Also known as antibody *classes.*

Isotype switch: The switch which occurs when a B cell stops secreting antibody of one isotype or class and starts producing antibody with a different isotype but with the same antigenic specificity. It involves joining V-region genes to a different heavy-chain constant region gene.

J chain (joining chain): A polypeptide involved in the polymerization of immunoglobulin molecules IgM and IgA.

J gene: A gene segment coding for the J or joining segment in immunoglobulin DNA; V genes translocate to J segments in L chains, and to D and J segments in H chains. Also, codes for a portion of the T-cell receptor.

K cell: An effector lymphocyte with *Fc receptors* that allow it to bind to and kill antibody-coated target cells.

Killer T cell: A T cell capable of specifically killing a target cell expressing foreign antigen bound to MHC molecules on the surface of the target cell. Also called *cytotoxic T cell.*

Light chain (L chain): The light chain of the immunoglobulin molecule; occurs in two forms: κ and λ.

Linkage disequilibrium: The frequency, in a population of linked genes, which is governed by factors other than change.

Lymphocyte: Small cell with virtually no cytoplasm, found in blood, in all tissue, and in lymphoid organs, such as lymph nodes, spleen, and Peyer's patches, and bears antigen-specific receptors.

Lymphokines: Soluble substances secreted by lymphocytes, which have a variety of effects on lymphocytes and other cell types. Cytokines secreted by lymphocytes.

Macrophage: A large phagocytic cell of the mononuclear series.

Macrophage-activating factor (MAF): Comprises several lymphokines, including interferon, released by activated T cells, which together induce activation of macrophages, making them more efficient in phagocytosis and cytotoxicity.

Major histocompatibility complex (MHC): A cluster of genes encoding polymorphic cell-surface molecules (MHC class I and class II) that are involved in interactions with T cells. These molecules also play a major role in transplantation rejection. Several other proteins are encoded in this region.

Memory: In the immune system, memory denotes an active state of immunity to a specific antigen, such that a second encounter with that antigen leads to a larger and more rapid response.

MHC class I molecule: A molecule encoded by genes of the MHC that participates in antigen presentation to $CD8^+$ (cytotoxic) T cells.

MHC class II molecule: A molecule encoded by genes of the MHC that participates in antigen presentation to $CD4^+$ T cells.

MHC restriction: The ability of T lymphocytes to respond only when they are presented with the appropriate antigen in association with either "self" MHC class I or class II molecules.

Minor histocompatibility antigens: Multiple antigens encoded outside the MHC which stimulate graft rejection, but not as rapidly as MHC molecules. In contrast to MHC molecules, minors do not stimulate primary responses of T cells in vitro, nor do they serve as restricting elements in cell interactions.

Mitogen: A substance that stimulates the proliferation of many different clones of lymphocytes.

Mixed lymphocyte reaction (MLR): When lymphocytes from two individuals are cultured together, a proliferative response is generally observed, as the result of reactions of T cells of one individual to MHC antigens on the other individual's cells.

Monoclonal: Literally, coming from a single clone. A clone is the progeny of a single cell. In immunology, monoclonal generally describes a preparation of antibody or T cells that are homogenous; derived from a clone of cells with the same specificity toward an epitope.

Monokines: Soluble substances secreted by monocytes, which have a variety of effects on other cells.

Myeloma: A tumor of plasma cells, generally secreting a single monoclonal immunoglobulin of unknown specificity.

NK cell: Naturally occurring, large, granular, lymphocyte-like killer cells that kill various tumor cells; they may play a role in resistance to tumors. Also, they participate in ADCC. They do not exhibit antigenic specificity, and their number does not increase by immunization.

Opsonin: A substance, usually antibody or complement component, which coats a particle such as a bacterium and enhances phagocytosis by phagocytic cells.

Opsonization: Literally means "preparation for eating." The coating of a bacterium with antibody and/or complement that leads to enhanced *phagocytosis* of the bacterium by phagocytic cells.

Paratope: An antibody combining site that is complementary to an epitope.

Passive cutaneous anaphylaxis (PCA): The passive transfer of anaphylactic sensitivity by intradermal injection of serum from a sensitive donor.

Passive immunization: Immunization by the administration of preformed antibody into a nonimmune individual.

Phagocytosis: The engulfment of a particle or a microorganism by leukocytes.

Phenotype: The physical expression of an individual's genotype.

Pinocytosis: Ingestion of liquid or very small particles by vesicle formation in a cell.

Plasma cell: The antibody-producing end-stage of B-cell differentiation.

Polyclonal activator: A substance that induces activation of many individual clones of either T or B cells. See *Mitogen*.

Polymorphism: Literally, "having many shapes"; in genetics, polymorphism means occurring in more than one form within a species; the existence of multiple alleles at a particular genetic locus.

Primary lymphoid organs: Organs in which the maturation of T and B lymphocytes takes place and antigen-specific receptors are first acquired.

Primary response: The immune response as a consequence of the first encounter with antigen. The primary response is generally small, has a long induction phase or lag period, and generates immunologic memory. In the primary B-cell response, mainly IgM antibodies are made.

Prophylaxis: Protection.

Prozone: A region of diminished agglutination or precipitation of antigen–antibody complexes in titration curve due to excess antibody.

PSA: Prostate-specific antigen.

Radioallergosorbent test (RAST): A solid-phase radioimmunoassay for detecting IgE antibody specific for a particular allergen.

Radioimmunoassay (RIA): A widely used technique for measurement of primary antigen–antibody interactions, and for the determination of the level of important biological substances in mixed samples. It takes advantage of the specificity of the antigen–antibody interaction and the sensitivity that derives from measurement of radioactively labeled materials.

Reagin: Allergist's term for IgE antibodies.

Reticuloendothelial system: A network of phagocytic cells.

Rheumatoid factor: An autoantibody (usually IgM) that reacts with the individual's own IgG. Present in rheumatoid arthritis.

Second set rejection: Accelerated rejection of an allograft in a primed recipient.

Secondary lymphoid organs: Organs in which antigen-driven proliferation and differentiation of mature B and T lymphocytes take place following antigen recognition.

Secretory component: A surface receptor on epithelial cells lining mucosal surfaces that binds dimeric IgA and transports it through the cell into mucosal secretions.

Serum sickness: A hypersensitivity reaction consisting of fever, rashes, joint pain, and glomerulonephritis, resulting from localization of circulating, soluble, antigen–antibody complexes, which induce inflammatory reactions. Serum sickness was originally induced following therapy with large doses of antibody from a foreign source, such as horse serum.

Slow-reacting substance of anaphylaxis (SRS-A): A group of leukotrienes such as released by mast cells during anaphylaxis that induces a prolonged contraction of smooth muscle. This prolonged contraction is not reversible by treatment with antihistamines.

Suppression: A mechanism for producing a specific state of immunologic unresponsiveness by which one cell or its products act on another cell.

Syngeneic: Literally, genetically identical.

Syngraft: Same as *isograft;* grafting tissue from one area to another area on the same individual.

T cell: A lymphocyte that differentiates in the thymus.

T-dependent antigen: An immunogen that requires T helper cells to interact with B cells in order to induce antibody synthesis.

T-independent antigen: An immunogen that induces antibody synthesis in the absence of T cells or their products; antibodies synthesized are generally only of the IgM isotype.

Titer: The reciprocal of the last dilution of a titration giving a measurable effect; e.g., if the last dilution giving significant agglutination is 1:128, the titer is 128.

Tolerance: Antigen-specific turn off or unresponsiveness of B or T cells; usually produced as a result of contact with that antigen under nonimmunizing conditions.

Toxoid: A nontoxic derivative of a toxin used as an immunogen for the induction of antibodies capable of cross-reacting with the toxin.

Transport piece: Same as ***secretory component.***

Unresponsiveness: Inability to respond to antigenic stimulus. Unresponsiveness may be specific for a particular antigen (see ***Tolerance***), or broadly nonspecific as a result of damage to the entire immune system, for example, after whole-body irradiation.

Vaccination: Any protective immunization against a pathogen. Originally referred to immunization against smallpox with the less virulent cowpox (vaccinia) virus.

Xenogeneic: Originating from a foreign species.

Xenograft: A tissue transplantation between individuals belonging to two different species.

INDEX